Ariadne's Thread

Case Studies in the
Therapeutic Relationship

Eric W. Cowan

James Madison University

LAHASKA PRESS
HOUGHTON MIFFLIN COMPANY
Boston   New York

Publisher, Lahaska Press: Barry Fetterolf
Senior Editor, Lahaska Press: Mary Falcon
Editorial Assistant: Lisa Littlewood
Senior Project Editor: Tracy Patruno
Senior Manufacturing Coordinator: Marie Barnes
Marketing Manager: Brenda L. Bravener-Greville

Cover image: Woman with a Candle (oil on canvas), Schalken, Godfried (1643–1706), Palazzo Pitti, Florence, Italy. Reprinted courtesy of the Bridgeman Art Library.

Credits appear on page xii, which constitutes a continuation of the copyright page.

Lahaska Press, a unique collaboration between the Houghton Mifflin College Division and Lawrence Erlbaum Associates, is dedicated to publishing books and offering services for the academic and professional counseling communities. The partnership of Lahaska Press was formed in late 1999. The name "Lahaska" is a Native American Lenape word meaning "source of many writings." The small eastern Pennsylvania town of Lahaska, named by the Lenape, is the home of the Lahaska Press editorial offices.

Printed in the U.S.A.

Library of Congress Control Number: 2002116642

ISBN: 0-618-37028-5

23456789-QUF-08 07 06 05 04

✕ ✕

Contents

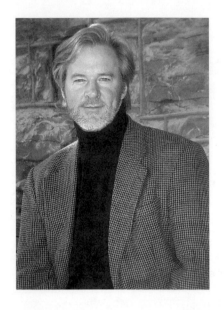

About the Author

Eric Cowan holds a doctorate in Clinical Psychology from Alliant University in San Diego, California. As an associate professor in the Department of Graduate Psychology in Counseling at James Madison University, he teaches individual therapy, group therapy, theories and techniques of intervention, process of counseling, practicum supervision, and psychopathology.

Eric served a two-year term as Director of Counseling and Psychological Services (CAPS) at James Madison University's outpatient clinic. The clinic provides a training setting for JMU graduate students in the counseling and clinical psychology programs. For the past nine years he has practiced as a licensed clinical psychologist in Harrisonburg, Virginia.

Eric lives in the woods of Rawley Springs at the foot of the Allegheny Mountains. When he is not sailing on the Chesapeake Bay, he and his wife enjoy hiking in the national forest adjacent to their home.

‍❧ ❧

Prologue

The king of the island of Crete, who dwelt in the palace of Minos, decreed that the Athenians must send across the sea to him an annual tribute. King Minos demanded that this tribute be a score of Athens' most beautiful virgin youth, for he intended to sacrifice the helpless victims to the Minotaur. Now the Minotaur was a monster— half man, half beast—a scourge and terror to men, a devourer of beauty. The Gods created the monster in wrath and retribution for the hubris and impiety of King Minos. Persecuted and fearful before this terror of the Gods, Minos created a kind of prison for the monster, desperate that his annual sacrifice to the beast might appease the Gods' anger toward him. King Minos commanded the renowned scientist Daidalos to construct a great labyrinth, a maze of corridors and passages that went deep into the earth. Upon entering the labyrinth, no person could find a way back out, and all passages seemed to lead further into the depths. Deep in the heart of the labyrinth, in its dark central chamber, lurked the Minotaur.

Aegeus, the Athenian king, had a son, Theseus, who was full of spirit and courage. Theseus deplored the injustice and tyranny of this sacrifice. He proposed to sail to Minos, enter the labyrinth, and slay the Minotaur. His father begged him not to venture to his certain destruction. But Theseus would not be dissuaded and set out in a ship for the island. As soon as he set foot on shore, however, he was captured by the king's soldiers and thrown into prison.

But King Minos had a daughter, and as she looked out of her white hall of alabaster, she saw Theseus step ashore. Knowing the meaning of his quest and seeing his beauty and courage, the king's daughter could not bear to see him devoured at the dark center. Her name was Ariadne. She was beautiful and wise, and she, too, deplored the sacrifice of so much youth, promise, and beauty. When darkness fell, Ariadne secretly entered the prison, stole the keys from the sleeping guards, and gave to Theseus the key to his cell. She armed him with a broad sword with which to do battle with the monster. She revealed to Theseus what she knew of the secrets and dangers of the labyrinth, and this served to steel Theseus's resolve, for he meant to slay the monster or be killed in the attempt.

Ariadne longed to go with Theseus but understood that he could only succeed in his quest by the strength of his own arm. So Ariadne spun a thread of silver for Theseus. The silver thread was thin but strong and as long as all the passages in the labyrinth. "Unwind the thread as you go deep into the labyrinth, and if by the grace of the Gods you slay the Minotaur deep at the center, follow the silver thread back through the maze, and it will guide you to the daylight."

So Theseus entered the labyrinth, his broadsword in one hand, his silver thread in the other. As he went through the maze, ever deeper toward the Minotaur's chamber, he unwound Ariadne's silver thread to mark the way. Deep in the central chamber he met the monster in the dark and, after a great battle lasting many days, slew him. Alone, wounded, and lost in the darkness, he remembered Ariadne's thread and followed its silver gleam back out of the winding and twisting corridors of the labyrinth to the surface. He was scarred from his battle, and Ariadne helped tend his wounds until he recovered his strength.

The myth of Theseus and Ariadne is a descriptive metaphor for the therapeutic journey. As in the myth, an exploration of the inner regions of human experience sometimes begins as a journey into the personal labyrinth. It often involves facing darkness, hardships, and trials, and sometimes the traveler can only prevail by some inner strength discovered along the way.

The silver thread that enables the client to journey into the heart of the labyrinth is the relationship between client and therapist. The thread is as long as the therapist's sustained empathy for the client. The therapist's attitude of empathic inquiry makes it possible for therapist and client to travel far into the client's inner world while still keeping a secure connection to familiar reference points. Like Ariadne, the therapist cannot take the journey for the client, cannot even know the way. But the therapist's relationship with the client can provide ways to drug the guards, unlock the cell, forge a new weapon or essential tool, and finally to grapple with core conflicts that devour the person's vitality and joy. The therapist's relationship with the client may spin a thread long enough to cover a great distance, but the client is the one wearing out his shoes.

The client knows there are no guarantees in such an enterprise. Individuals who come into therapy often fear revealing to the therapist, and to themselves, aspects of their lives that have long remained sequestered and hidden from view. They also learn that they must confront and battle old fears and overcome the ways in which they have chosen to live a diminished existence. Clients coming into therapy are tired of sacrificing virgins.

Pondering the entrance to the cave, however, the client often struggles with fear and doubt. The client wonders whether the thread will be long and strong enough. Both therapist and client may feel the trepidation inherent in the risk of real participation. Therapists, unlike Ariadne, cannot spin a perfect thread that infallibly follows the contours of the client's inner world. Will Ariadne's thread really be able to reach between the hidden chambers of the heart and the world of connection, participation, and relationship?

This is a book of stories about becoming a psychotherapist or counselor, two terms that, in this book, mean the same thing. It appears to be a book of stories about clients in therapy, and it is that too. However, contrary to popular belief, becoming a therapist is not something one learns only in graduate school, though that often helps. Psychotherapy is something one also learns from clients. As a therapist-in-training, my clients, each in a different way, shook up my closely held theories, beliefs, and methods, evicted me from comfortable and familiar surroundings, and tried to teach me how to create a therapy just for them.

During my postdoctoral residency, I gained my first experience teaching and training students in clinical skills. While we watched our students' videotaped sessions together, an esteemed senior colleague remarked, "Seeing these tapes reminds me that it takes 10 years to become a master therapist." He must have seen the dismay on my face because he laughed and said, "not that you can't be a very effective therapist before then. It takes five years to get your professors out of your head, and another five for your clients to teach you what your professors meant to, to begin with." So this is a book of stories from *my* first 10 years of learning to be a therapist.

As I recalled these stories, looked over process notes, and thought back on the many sessions, especially those with my earliest clients, I felt nostalgia, even a sense of loss. Mostly, this was due to my recollection of those unique people and personalities who let me into their lives, honored me by making me important to their struggle and growth, and finally left my life, not realizing that I was also changed by our encounter. But I also realized that some of my feelings of loss were due to missing the same intensity of professional growth that attended the earliest years of revelatory, dynamic, and discovery-filled encounters wherein my own transformation as a therapist evolved out of my engagement with my clients. I would not have believed at the time that I would miss even my "mistakes." Though I would not choose now to re-create them (I'm too busy making new ones), I also know that what I thought of as error sometimes propelled the sessions forward with energy and vitality. Collecting these case studies reminded me, once again, of the Zen adage that only in the role of a student, not as an expert, can one learn anything new.

For each case study I have included a discussion of a clinical concept that seemed to me to best represent or illustrate some aspect of the unfolding therapy for that person. I probably could have used any of the cases to illustrate any of the ideas, but I looked for the best fit between case and concept. The therapeutic concepts themselves are chosen with a view to training therapists in a few of the essential ideas that inform clinical work. They are concepts that I struggled with as a therapist-in-training when I wished that I had some concrete illustration to flesh out the theory. The criterion for inclusion is simply that each concept represents an important element of the therapeutic *relationship*. I have, therefore, included ideas from different theoretical orientations that converge when emphasizing the interpersonal process and relational aspects of the client–therapist encounter. The therapist-in-training struggles mightily to construct an integrated and theoretically consistent approach compatible with his or her personality. My aim is to help provoke and stimulate ideas in this struggle rather than to provide pat solutions.

Sometimes the case narrative or following discussion centers on my own feelings, thoughts, fantasies, or struggles as I attempt to accommodate what is happening in the therapy. This exposure of my own personality in the therapeutic process seems to be at odds with most literature intended to help train clinicians. Many case studies, even those that purport to centralize the interpersonal process, seem to pretend that the therapist is merely a functionary and witness to the therapy. It is as if the therapist's half of the "personal" in *interpersonal* is missing. Perhaps this sanitization of case studies is an effort to represent a generic model for a responsible and effective therapeutic "stance" or demeanor, an important consideration. However, I find it useful and enlightening to learn what other therapists experience as they work with their clients. I want to understand how the therapist's own personality interacts with his or her client's as the process unfolds. Therapists-in-training also seem to long for this inside view, not only of the consulting room of their mentors but of the inside view of their internal process. I encourage these students not only to understand the effect of their personality on their clients but to understand and draw on their own unique qualities to give efficacy to their therapeutic relationships and the interventions they make within them. I do not intend that anyone should seek to emulate my particular style, but I hope to offer some examples of therapy in which the human encounter is central.

For me, part of the early discovery of working with clients involves something so fundamental and yet so elusive that one can never be said to have completed exploring its dimensions. Therapy that addresses itself to the deepest levels of human existence always occurs in the context of a healing relationship. It is self-evident, even cliché, that we do not exist as persons in isolation but become human as our lives intersect with others. But it is also in human relationships that we have the capacity to grow ill, and it is, therefore, in relationship that we also must heal. As Martin Buber (1958) observed, when two persons come together at the deepest levels of human meeting, the reality of that meeting exists not in one or the other of them but between them, almost as a third unique entity. Buber defines the qualities necessary for such an "I–Thou" encounter: mutuality, authenticity, openness and availability, inclusion, immediacy, and a sense of being fully present in the moment with another. It is often the lack of these fundamental qualities in human relationships that evoke in persons the protective and constricting maneuvers that lead to isolation, fear, rigidity, and existential sickness—in shorthand, to symptoms.

Existentially oriented therapists and thinkers created therapies that centralized the therapeutic relationship and embodied Buber's relational qualities, and these powerfully influenced my own development as a therapist. I am still puzzled when I meet practitioners for whom therapy is really a glorified form of car mechanics. This is not to say that some "repair work" cannot be accomplished without incorporating this ontological dimension of human meeting into one's clinical work. Many therapists address themselves to the work at this level and seem content. But for the "atrophied center" of the soul to be touched, I believe the cultivation of this relational possibility is essential. As many have said, it is the relationship itself that heals in psychotherapy.

The rich heritage of analytic theorizing also contributed to my formation as a therapist. This influence occurred mostly through the more recent derivations that move past the reductionism and determinism of drive theory and centralize the importance of development in relation. Harry Stack Sullivan's interpersonal model and Heinz Kohut's "self" psychology explore relational themes in personality development that have been useful to me. Kohut especially broke with the traditional schools by emphasizing the importance of affective life over drives, promulgating empathy as the central investigative stance from which to explore the construction and experience of the self. This was, at least with respect to empathy, catching up to Carl Rogers's focus on the "heart" of the matter.

Postmodern "intersubjectivity" theory further broke with the analytic past, eschewing depth psychology's "myth of the isolated mind" (Stolorow & Atwood, 1992). Intersubjectivity theory articulates the relational and affective foundations of psychological life and addresses dimensions of the therapeutic relationship that I found myself experiencing with my clients. Writers in intersubjectivity theory tap into the rich heritage of analytic thinking but with greater awareness than other analytic schools of the ontological dimension of human encounter. These modern variants of analytic therapy redefine the meaning and expression of many traditional analytic concepts, such as resistance and transference, in a way I find useful in my work with clients.

But enough of that. The influences I have mentioned were important in that they pointed a finger in the right direction, gave me a language to name the landmarks along the way, and described the experiences of those who had traveled the road. However, the wonderful and infinite variations of human experience, as life is inflected through each person, ensure that for any two travelers the way is never completely the same. The therapist must also make it up as he or she goes along.

This book is dedicated to all of those who spin the silver thread and to those with courage enough to unwind it as they journey into the labyrinth.

Acknowledgments

I would like to thank the following for their contributions to this book: Susan Facknitz for being a great writing mentor and a wonderfully perceptive and sensitive editor; Lennie Echterling and Ed McKee for being great colleagues, for reading parts of the manuscript, and for much more; Jack Presbury, another great colleague, for his significant contribution to the discussion section of Chapter four; all the Thursday afternoon choirboys for discussing ideas and cheerfully tolerating, as friends must, my constant musings on the progress of the book. Mike Nichols for his careful reading of parts of the early manuscript and whose suggestions helped to structure the other chapters; Mary Falcon, Barry Fetterolf, Merrill Peterson, and the folks at Lahaska Press for their vision and support; the reviewers for Lahaska—Clifford Brooks, Shippensburg University; Susan Gray, Barry University; Teri McCartney, Adams State

College; Tracy Stinchfield, Idaho State University; and Geoffrey Yager, University of Cincinnati—who all offered many helpful observations and criticisms. Kay Mikel for copy editing the manuscript; Karen Hanam for typing the references; and my students and supervisees for their various readings, feedback, and contributions.

I would also like to thank the clients whose experiences went into writing these cases. Of course their identities, circumstances, and predicaments have all been significantly altered to protect confidentiality as well as to convey a concept. In a couple of cases I have even fused the therapies of two different clients to illustrate different clinical ideas while remaining faithful to the spirit of therapeutic experience. Although I made reference to audio or video recordings for some of the sessions, most of the conversations recounted in the cases are based on recollection of the encounters and the course of the sessions over time. In this sense the clinical data presented in the cases must be viewed as apocryphal. Any imagined recognition of the persons in these pages will certainly be an error.

Most of all I would like to thank my wife, Johnna, who not only made significant editorial contributions but whose love, support, and companionship are the living embodiment of all the best ideas in the book about what it means to be in relationship with others.

Credits

ᔓ ᖾ

Once, My Lovely . . .

Those with whom we are truly intimate
sometimes with hands and organs,
sometimes with the paste of words alone,
the creatures for whom the hollow
places of our solitude are open wide
to shimmer with the lighted lamps of love,
we shape ourselves to hold them.

—Marge Piercy

All tho new thinking is about loss,
In this way it resembles all the old thinking.

—Robert Hass

I'll bet you slept with her! And in our very own bed too!"
"No, and I resent you saying that. Anyway, I'd be embarrassed to.
You haven't washed the sheets in weeks. Look, we had dinner and
talked, that's all. She's married too, you know."

"I don't believe you, you bastard. You think just because you say
things in here that it's okay? You think because you're being 'open' that
that makes it any better? I can't believe you, or her."

As I listened to this exchange, I had the sense that the past three
months of sitting once a week with this smart, beautiful couple had
never happened. Where had all that coaching gone about using "I" messages and speaking from one's own experience? We had been making good
progress. But when Samantha and Jeffrey got heated up, it all went out
the window. And at this moment Sam was mad. She had gone out of
town, and Jeffrey had visited with a former girlfriend. Because they
were both very intelligent, their battles were often as elegant as a

swordfight or a dance. I knew they would be all right. I decided to let them go on for a little longer.

"I can't believe she would do this to us! She was at our wedding for Christsake!"

"Do what to us? You're freaking out. You're the one that's all about 'openness,' and here I am being open right now and you're bashing me for it."

"Open! *Found out* more like."

"How do you figure that; I'm the one who told *you*. Though you do have a way of lying in wait and then pouncing when what I have to say is not to your liking."

"Oh. Right! You only said it after I asked you how your 'meeting' went."

"Entrapment! I decided to tell you because I knew that my 'meeting' was something you'd want to know about when you got past your PMS-ing insanity."

"Don't even go there! What a weasel, blaming your dishonesty on my hormones. How far ahead did you know she was coming here?"

"Just a few days."

"'Just.' And you knew I was going out of town when you made plans?"

"Yes, I did know. And I thought of telling you, but I knew that because things were all screwed up, and we had just had that big row, that you would make a big deal out of it."

"You're right. I would have made a big deal out of it. So you lied."

"No, I just didn't say everything I knew. I didn't want *this* to happen. I knew you were sensitive about it, and I just didn't want to deal with your crap about it. And now that I have told you, it appears I was right. Look, I'm not going to give up my women friends just because we're married."

"She's a little different, don't you think? You dated her."

"That was over 10 years ago!"

"And you know she's cheating on Robert."

"She wanted to talk about her relationship, and *I* told you about her infidelity with Robert."

"And you know she's always been jealous of you marrying me. It's an accident waiting to happen. And then she sends a letter saying, 'Oh, what a wonderful visit!'"

"Oh, so now you've been reading my mail! You knew about this before you set me up, questioning me about the 'meeting.' And it wasn't a letter; it was a postcard. Why would she send a postcard instead of a letter? She obviously didn't care if you read it or not."

"I'm not reading your mail. You just said it was just a postcard, right? If she didn't care, then why should you care if I read it? Apparently, it's the only way I'm going to get any straight information."

"I told you about it for Christsakes!"

"Yeah, but I had to find it out from a postcard first, didn't I?"

"I didn't know you were reading my mail, so my confession still counts."

"I wasn't reading your mail, remember? You said it was a postcard, which makes it different. So you didn't tell her that you were keeping your meeting from me?"

"Are you kidding me? That would be humiliating. I'm not going to ask you for permission to have friends."

Yes, Sam and Jeffrey were great fighters. Arguing for them had a quality of the sweet science. They were both articulate, perceptive, ruthless combatants—great debaters with a good sense for any weakness. I admired the choreography of their conflicts, and I think that secretly they did too. They were also very much attached to one another and at times capable of such obviously deep love, empathy, and affection that in the presence of it I sometimes had to narrow my eyes and attempt to look wise to avoid the expression of my own upwelling grief, a sense of my own losses that their sudden tenderness evoked and set in relief. I liked these two a lot.

"Okay, time out," I finally intervened. "Sam, I'd like you to tell Jeffrey what you would like to have happen here from your perspective. Jeffrey, please don't speak."

"Gladly . . . what's the point?" he said, slumping back on the sofa on which they sat side by side across from me. I tilted my head toward him in a "don't make me come over there" kind of warning. I could see him mask a wry grin.

She looked at me, "What I want is for him to . . ." I interrupted her by casually pointing my finger toward Jeffrey. She turned her body and face toward him.

"What I want from you is to be totally up-front," she said heatedly. "You say you didn't tell me because we fought and you didn't want to deal with my reaction, but I can't deal with that. I feel taken out of the conversation when that happens, and it feels like you're trying to pull something over on me. It feels not only like you're just not mentioning something I might object to, which is bad enough, but that you are lying to me. If I'm going to trust you, you have to be straight with me," she appealed. "And if I find out that you've been screwing Amanda, I'm going to murder you while you sleep."

"Good, Sam. You were really able to stay grounded in your own experience of it. Jeffrey, can you tell Sam what she just expressed to you? Sam, please don't speak." She nodded obediently.

"God," he said, "we're back to this? I feel like we've been demoted back to session three." She looked at him skeptically. "Okay, *What I hear you saying,*" he said, straightening his back formally and assuming a condescending tone.

"Forget it," she reacted immediately, "if you're going to patronize me."

"Okay, okay. Seriously," he said, turning toward her and assuming an attentive expression. She crossed her arms and tilted her head skeptically in an expression that said, *"Well, I'm listening . . . you'd better get it right."*

"What I hear you saying," he began, and provided an accurate reflection of her concerns, ending with, "and Amanda was always uptight and frigid, so though I still love her very much, I have absolutely no desire to sleep with her, or anyone else but you, so keep your homicidal fantasies under control."

"Sam, did Jeffrey get it right? Do you think he heard you?"

"Yeah, but is he going to act on it?"

"Ask him."

"Are you going to act on it or not? Do you respect me enough to tell me stuff so that we can have some trust here?"

"Yeah, I'll do it better next time," he said resignedly. "It was only because we had just argued that I didn't mention it at all."

She paused, deliberating whether she was going to accept this or not. Then, "Is Amanda really frigid?" she asked, scrunching her face, the sudden change in tone causing Jeffrey and I to laugh.

"She really is . . . at least she was until last Tuesday," he taunted.

"Don't start, Jeffrey, we're out of time here," I warned.

Sam and Jeffrey came to therapy, like most married couples, at the female partner's insistence. But Jeffrey quickly warmed up to the process, especially when he realized that Sam would not just have a forum for complaining about his shortcomings, a vehicle for "fixing" him. Though he continued to maintain an indifferent and slightly patronizing disposition toward therapy, Jeffrey obviously valued the sessions. It turned out that Jeffrey had plenty to say to Sam that he was not voicing in their day-to-day conversations. They were both in their early 30s, college educated, articulate, and engaging. She worked for a publishing house doing editorial work as well as art direction. He was a writer. Jeffrey's short stories had appeared in magazines, and he had just published a first novel. They were approaching their 10th anniversary.

At first their reasons for coming to therapy were less apparent to me than the random conflicts in which they engaged with such energy, conflicts that seemed to stand in for some less tangible reality between them that neither of them could say. They just wanted, Sam explained, "to work on our marriage" and "improve our communication." They were still "grinding the edges off of one another," learning how to make their personalities compatible.

So we started on what was apparent. Jeffrey had married a woman he valued for her "steadiness and level headedness," a nature loving woman who had "both feet on the ground." She knew "how to negotiate the ordinary with grace" and was "wonderful with people." But now he wished she were less controlling, more spontaneous and fun loving, less conventional. And what had happened to her reverence for his talent that she had shown in those early years?

Samantha had married Jeffrey because he was romantic, charismatic, and fun loving. Yes, he was moody, but there was a beauty and energy in his temperament that lent a sense of vitality and directness to life. But now she wished that he was a little more mature, less impulsive, and followed through on things better. And couldn't he pull his weight around the house a little more? She still admired his talent, but she wished his life were more structured, like people's lives who have to go to work every day; the hours he kept were random and unpredictable.

Like most married couples, some of the unique qualities that had attracted them to each other became the very attributes that didn't wear so well over time. We each marry our shadow. We gain access to qualities that we do not possess, but which our personalities can tolerate only in measure. But the more they talked, the more I felt as if we were addressing the mundane misunderstandings and problematic communication patterns that were the outward expression of something nameless.

They had quickly come to understand the technical aspects of "active listening," of speaking from one's own subjective experience of an event, and of taking responsibility for their individual reactions and feelings about shared experiences. It was good; the basic stuff of couples therapy. And we three had a good connection. In the language of systems work, they had let me "join" with them. We were even having fun. Still, it felt like there was something more there that our work was not touching, something that none of us could name, laying like a fault line under the ground, storing up energy over time, and calling into question all the building going on above.

At some point, all couples therapy comes to a central question: What holds these two people together, sustains their connection, keeps them in one another's orbit, like binary stars circling one another in the gravity of attachment? For some the gravity is almost entirely the pull of complementary neuroses. For Sam and Jeffrey this did not appear to be true. They were both fairly integrated, self-aware individuals with great interpersonal skills. It seemed apparent that they loved one another deeply. They were romantically attracted, often sexually fulfilled, affectionate, concerned for one another, self-sacrificing, mostly sincere, and respectful.

But over time I began to notice a pattern that I suspected was central to their relationship and yet invisible to each of them. It was difficult for them to find an acceptable way to back away from their intense periods of connection and affiliation. It was as if they were afraid of what they did so well, and that conflict, far from being expressive of their remoteness from one another, was the dance by which they loosened their hold and pushed away. Who would first need to close their eyes while making love, loose the grip when parting, turn the head elsewhere into the world? How was it possible to get away? Was what I was sensing a kind of nausea in feeding on so much richness, I wondered.

Unlike most couples I had seen who struggled with the fearfulness of love's fulfillment, there seemed to be no pattern for it, neither one seemed to be less capable of sustaining their wonderful and fearful oneness. They seemed to take turns in departure. As they talked about themselves, I could see that whichever one turned away first, the other would slowly pursue, feeling both the sudden relief as well as the loss of intimacy and connection. It was an elegant dance, for each of them was capable of sometimes pausing in the center, where they briefly met, circling in oneness and communion. Then they went spinning away into the loneliness and safety of their individual existences. It's the best that anyone can do, though some wise couples find a way to understand and welcome that parting with one another, knowing that otherwise love can get greedy and feed on what sustains it, and like the snake that eats its own tail, consume itself entirely.

Sam and Jeffrey didn't understand or accept their partings with one another, and they had not discovered a way to incorporate this experience. It was the paradox of love and marriage revealing itself to them: that one can never really possess another, and that in marriage there is the potential to lose most what one loves best. Someone once said, "Love is an ideal thing. Marriage is a real thing. A confusion of the ideal with the real never goes unpunished." In the high terrain of their oneness they breathed the pure air together, but down in the town where the world spins, they were flung away from one another and injured themselves, and each other, in the tumbling of it. It was as if Romeo and Juliet hadn't died but had gone on to get married, have a mortgage, take the subway to their jobs in the city, and split the house chores. It manifested in a hundred small ways.

———

"So, we're lying there together having just made love," Jeffrey says heatedly in a later session, "and it's great, you know, there's this nice afterglow, and she starts talking about something so trivial and mundane that it's mind numbing . . . like we have to solve this stupid problem right away or some calamity is going to happen. And I'm thinking, what the hell is that? Here we are, having just had this great experience, and she wants to talk about a new system that Ted from work recommended for handling the mail. I mean, a little sensitivity for Christsake."

"As you say it, Jeffrey, you seem upset by it even now. It seems like you feel that Sam discounted the great lovemaking experience by chitchatting about something trivial, and you feel hurt, almost offended, by the look of it."

"Well it is kind of offending. I mean, what's the message to me? Okay, let's move on to something else now that we've taken care of that. I mean, I'm lying naked with my wife and all of a sudden I've got Ted in my bed with his plan for the damn mail."

"Yet you say that you felt very connected to Sam, like it was a time that was special as you were making love. 'Not just a nice bonking,' you said."

"Yeah, that's why it's so annoying."

"Do you want to speculate on what was happening for Sam, or should we just ask her?"

"My guess is that she just did her normal 'Okay, time to move on to the next thing; let's get something done,' to hell with honoring the feelings about it."

"That's how you experience her? That she is not sensitive to the feeling dimension of your relationship? Last week you were saying that perhaps she was oversensitive to monitoring your moods. That it was hard for you to be in a funk because she has a tendency to resonate with your moods, and you didn't want to bring her down."

"Yeah, I don't know. It changes. Maybe it's just when it's around sex or something."

"Why don't we ask her?"

Sam had been patiently listening, occasionally shaking her head as if wondering, "What world are you coming from?"

"Well, you attribute all these motives to me," she said defensively. "I don't know what you're talking about. I was feeling very close to you, and I didn't think that making small talk was a big deal, you know, just kind of touching base with the little things in our lives. The time before, after we had sex, you started talking about planting the garden while we cuddled, and that was okay with me. So why is it not okay to talk about something that was on my mind?"

"There's a big difference talking about planting the garden. That was something we had planned to do together that very day. Not like some unnecessary project from Ted, some obnoxious detail."

"Jeffrey likes to sit after a movie and watch *all* the credits, you know. He doesn't leave until the lights go up."

"You equate lying together after making love with sitting in a movie theater?" protested Jeffrey.

"I'm just saying that talking about my project didn't diminish the pleasure of being with you after making love. It didn't ruin the mood."

"Oh yeah, it's really great for me too. The fact is, you must not have been into it or you would have had a little more sensitivity afterward."

Ah, I thought, there it is again, the worm of doubt, boring into the core of their *being* together. Each of them found ways to say it: I am connected with you in this brief moment, but somehow we know that we can't stay here, and I can't keep you from receding from me, and all the rest that is not this brief immortality floods in, and I am alone again.

"I think maybe you've got it backwards," I said. There was a long pause as they tried to work it out in reverse.

"What do you mean?" Jeffrey said finally.

"I don't know, this is just an impression I have, maybe it's right and maybe it's not, but I think Sam wanted to chitchat with you after making love precisely *because* it was a powerful experience for her. I have the sense that each of you has a hard time finding a way back from this consuming flame of intimacy that you stand in for a while. You haven't quite worked out how to do that gracefully yet, but perhaps it's because you are each such a powerful presence for the other that you can only stand the heat of that for a bit. In which case, Sam's seeming insensitivity to the mood of the moment is really a testament to the profundity of what preceded it—your mutual powerful lovemaking experience.

Maybe each of you needs to get away a little when that happens. Maybe that intimacy scares you a little. How does that sound to you?"

They both sat silently. I was proud of myself, and I felt like the timing of my reframing and interpretation was perfect . . . emerging out of an experience that they had offered, not to mention articulate and well delivered. How could they fail to have the sudden flash of insight I anticipated?

They didn't like it. I nodded and made nonspecific therapeutic noises as they both refuted it. They countered that their squabbles had nothing to do with fearing their intimacy. It was conflict, they argued, that kept them from being intimate. It was personality and the ways in which they were incompatible and rubbed each other wrong that was the problem. That's what they needed to work on they said. All the active listening in the world was not going to change who they were, noted Jeffrey. They just needed to learn to accept each other's differences, and be more sensitive, he added, slipping in his peeve for the day.

What, about my interpretation, I wondered, had sparked their strong negative reaction? They had circled the wagons together against it, which made me wonder if that was even more evidence that it was credible. Confronted with the idea that they might have to consciously acknowledge the need to deliberately give each other space, they seemed threatened. Was I messing with their mythology of themselves?

In the next session we stuck to the task of helping them work through conflict by communicating better. I suddenly felt like I was shooting spitballs at the sun. There was no way that tinkering with communication structure was going to resolve any conflicts here. They *needed* their conflicts. In the next two sessions they had nothing to resolve or discuss. Things were going along perfectly, and they were so in love. As I observed them, I realized that they were bilingual in the language of love. Conflict was the other tongue they spoke to stay connected and engaged when they could no longer tolerate the fuzziness of their own boundaries when they were feeling intimate. There seemed to be little tolerance for a middle ground, a ground where each of them might stand alone. Conflict was a paradox: it reestablished their sense of separateness while still keeping them locked together.

I began to see their relationship as more dependent than I had realized, and I thought my interpretation about the function of their conflicts was right. Neither one could tolerate the sense of being alone, and conflict kept them from that sense of isolation. Over the next few sessions I became more convinced that this was the invisible but dominating theme of their relationship. I also wondered whether their conflict didn't also scare them. Was that why they needed me to witness and mediate it, so it wouldn't spin out of their control and really cause them separation? As sophisticated as these two were, I thought they both had the same developmental vulnerability: insecurity in attachment. They also shared the same existential condition that was an exaggeration of a normal anxiety: a dread of being alone in the world. Fortunately they were also well suited to one another, and their relationship mostly satisfied their anxieties. When it didn't, sparks flew.

"I'm wondering how these sessions are going for you?" I asked during one meeting.

"Well," answered Sam.

"A little boring," admitted Jeffrey.

"I have felt a little less energy in the sessions too, the last couple of times, and it seems like we're going over the same ground. I think you two know how to talk to one another deliberately using the stuff we've been doing in here. Yet it seems that when things are going well, they're going really well, and when things go wrong, that you are prone to wrestle and fight and debate with one another in the same old way."

"Yeah, it's as if we forget what we do in here when we're at home. I think that's why it's good to come in here," offered Sam.

"I'm wondering another thing," I offered. "I'm wondering how these conflicts really are important to you, and why you would be reluctant to give them up?"

"I don't think they work for us at all; they just create bad feelings between us."

"Yes, but they keep you feeling bad *together*," I pushed.

"I think there's something to that," said Jeffrey, surprising me.

"What do you mean," Sam turned to face him.

"C'mon, you know that sometimes we get off on fighting. At least I do. Sometimes I just want to let you have it, and I feel all this intense negative energy that I just have to vent toward you. It's almost as if I have a grudge against you for no reason. It's as if we go from being totally connected to needing to contend without losing each other. And it feels like I have to do that sometimes. And moreover, I think you set me up sometimes, and provoke me into it, even though it looks like I'm the aggressor."

"How do I do that?"

"By not responding, especially when you dump something on me that gets me going and then you are not available to talk about it. That pisses me off, and you know when you are doing it. It forces me to get in your face."

"Well, I don't think our fighting is a good thing, even though I think we know each other so well that we know just what buttons to push."

"I think it might keep you close and interacting," I said. "It does something for you, perhaps protects you from a feeling of being isolated or alone when you're not in one of your close periods."

"Maybe so," she said. Sam looked out the window turning her head. She looked pensive and a little sad.

"What is it Sam?" I asked.

"I don't know if I should go into it," she replied. "Give me a minute."

Jeffrey looked at her, suddenly attentive, a curious look on his face.

"Before Jeffrey and I were married," she began after a long silence, "I became pregnant by him . . . by you," she said, glancing up at his face. "I didn't tell you because at the time we weren't sure if we wanted to marry, and I didn't want the pregnancy to force you into something you didn't want. I was waiting for some commitment from you before I told you. You didn't seem sure about what you wanted then. I mean, I knew that you wanted to be with me, but I didn't know if you wanted marriage and a kid all at once. I mean, I wasn't sure either, about having a child then. So," she heaved a long sigh, "so, I had an abortion." Sam sat staring down at her lap, very still, and a heavy silence hung over them both. She began again: "It's the only time I've ever kept anything from you. I think that somehow I have blamed you for it; I don't know why . . . you didn't even know."

There was a long silence. I was absolutely still in my chair.

"I did know," Jeffrey said, finally breaking the silence.

"You knew what?" she said, startled, turning her face to his.

"I knew about you being pregnant, and I knew that you were going in for an abortion."

"Meg told you."

"Yeah."

They sat for a long time saying nothing. A tear glided down Sam's cheek.

"We've been trying to get pregnant for a long time," she said, not looking up from her lap, where her fingers were slowly tearing apart the tissue she held, "but so far it hasn't happened."

"Why didn't you tell me you knew?" she said, turning to Jeffrey.

"I was confused about it too."

"You haven't resented me not telling you all these years?"

"Sometimes I have resented you, other times I'm glad that you didn't ask me because it got me off the hook. You had to take all the responsibility for the decision. I told myself that since you didn't tell me I didn't have to decide. I was being a wimp about it."

"Are you glad I made the decision I did?"

"I don't know."

"I don't know either. Right now I'm wishing I hadn't done it." A long silence. "We got married a couple of years later," she said, looking up at me. I nodded.

"I'm sorry," she said, turning to him and taking his hand.

"I'm sorry too," he said clasping it.

They experienced a honeymoon-like period after these revelations to one another. Everything was perfect, and they said that they were entering a new phase of their relationship that was more honest and open than ever before. They spent all their free time together. They bought a small house out in the woods. Jeffrey wanted to keep bees. Sam made an effort to do more fun things, and Jeffrey adjusted his work to a more normal schedule. The sex was great. They lingered after and felt no need to create any distance between them. They were not afraid, they assured me, of the closeness continuing. They had been trying to get pregnant. They reduced our meetings to one a month. They thought that they might be ready to end our sessions altogether, that they had found a new balance.

Then Jeffrey got sick. It wasn't a serious illness, but it was no common cold either. Viral pneumonia laid him out for weeks. They had to cancel their vacation to visit her parents in Florida. It had been a couple of months since I had seen them by the time he was fully recovered.

We had scheduled a final session to wrap things up. Halfway through this session, Sam remarked, "I was thinking about what you said a while back, about how we may use conflict to find a way to reestablish our separate space, you know, and something happened while Jeffrey was sick, I mean in my reaction that made me wonder about that."

Jeffrey looked at her questioningly.

"You mean you had a response to Jeffrey being ill that called that separateness–relatedness theme back to mind?"

"Yeah, though I don't know if it's the same thing or not, but it just surprised me. When he was ill . . . when you were ill," she said, "I found myself feeling angry toward you about it. At first I thought it was just because I knew you didn't want to go visit my parents, and I thought, 'Well, now you have a legitimate excuse, so you're probably glad about that.' But when you got sicker and bedridden, I started to get a little scared, and I found that my feelings were totally irrational. I mean, I was still a little angry with you for being incapacitated. I couldn't account for it."

"You even spent one night at your sister's when I was pretty bad off."

"I know, I think I didn't want to acknowledge that you were as sick as you were. I feel bad about it now. I feel like I should have been with you the whole time."

"You took good care of me for most of it."

"Yeah, but I sometimes felt mad at you, even though I didn't say it, and even though I said to myself that I was just frustrated for both of us. The truth is that I was mad at you for being . . . it sounds so stupid, for being ill."

"Sam, I heard you saying that you were angry about Jeffrey getting ill, but I also heard you mention in passing that you were a little scared about seeing him bedridden."

"Yeah, I mean, I knew that he was going to be all right, so it's totally irrational, but I did feel a little nervous about it."

"Why didn't you tell me what you were feeling?" Jeffrey asked.

"I didn't want to dump it on you while you were feeling bad, and I also felt guilty for feeling it in the first place. I was just going to forget it, but something made me think of it in here. Maybe because it bothered me that it made no sense."

"But let's take it a little further," I offered, "because usually people have the feelings that they do for good reasons, even though they may not make logical sense. As you sit here right now, check in with yourself and see if anything comes to mind about Jeffrey, other things that perhaps you are angry or upset about."

She sat for a few moments. "You know, I can't think of anything. I wondered that before, am I just mad at him for some other reason that I'm putting into this situation? But it didn't fit."

"Okay, let's try this. I'm struck that your being scared preceded your being angry. Imagine that Jeffrey got even sicker. That he was in serious trouble."

"I would feel awful, not mad. I wouldn't have the luxury of being irrational."

"And while you were feeling awful, what might you be thinking, what if he were going to possibly die?"

"I'm not sure I like where this conversation is going," Jeffrey quipped.

"I'd think I wouldn't know what to do with myself. I wouldn't want to go on without him. I'd think, hell, get up, *you're not allowed to die on me, that's not part of the bargain.* I'd be lost. I'd probably have to . . ."

I interrupted her. "You're not allowed to die on me," I repeated carefully and deliberately, "that's not part of the bargain." We sat in silence for a moment.

"Yeah, I mean, I know that you can't really make that kind of bargain."

"I'm not sure that you do know," I said quietly. More silence.

"Before I got sick," Jeffrey broke the stillness, "and we were doing so well and were so happy, I had the fantasy that something was happening between us that was like a shield around us. You know, like nothing bad could touch us. I was actually a little surprised to get sick, you know, as if my immune system was so strong because of my state of mind that no bugs could get me."

"Yeah, exactly. I wonder if you two might not have a contract with one another to provide something that you can't possibly fulfill." They sat with this for a moment.

"I think in our best times we do fulfill it," Sam said. "When we're in that zone, it seems like the world is our puppy . . . but that we expect that nothing else is good enough. I guess that's a problem. When Jeffrey was sick, I felt alone because he was out of it, and I didn't like it. Not that I can't spend time alone, I can, but alone in a much bigger sense knowing he was sick. I mean, I did think what would happen if he were not there with me. I guess somehow I made it part of your job," she said turning to him, "to keep me from feeling that sense of *really* being alone. It's not an illusion," she said turning to me. "It's real."

"Oh, I know," I responded. "It's where real life happens. When I feel connected and loving with someone on all those levels, I feel most myself, and most fulfilled." Sam starts nodding.

"But it still can't keep us from the rest of life," Jeffrey interjected. "I think that at times each of us has resented the other for a promise that is not fulfilled. It wasn't stated, but it was implied by how we met. We met at a writer's retreat," Jeffrey explained, "and it was this incredibly creative and charged atmosphere, full of ideas and ideals. We fell in love in this kind of insulated, in some ways unreal, world, and it was so intense. It felt as if what happened between us could enable us to transcend other things more than is possible for anyone."

I was pleased that they responded to my directing the discussion into this area, but even more pleased that they were then able to get to the heart of the matter themselves. I knew that in this, as in most interventions aimed at insight and change, merely "telling them" what I thought was the problem, or how they might need to change, would have little effect. It is always much better to set up the conditions for change, to help, nudge, or perturb and hope that clients can come to it themselves.

I thought I understood now where the fault line ran through their union and the thing that kept them from being able to move easily between various levels of their relationship. Conflict may have been the method by which they both became separate while still connected, but their conflicts also expressed an underlying sense of betrayal: "You didn't protect me from parts of my own existence."

I glanced at Sam, and she had turned her head away and was gently but anxiously gnawing a knuckle on her closed hand.

"Sam, where are you right now? You just went off by yourself."

Without turning her head back to face either of us she said, "I was thinking of that . . . I was thinking, when Jeffrey said that we sometimes privately resent each other for a promise not fulfilled . . . I was thinking we could have had that baby." Tears began running down her cheeks. Jeffrey took her hand and we all sat for a while in silence.

"It's going to happen, it's just a matter of time," he offered.

She nodded silently. Then turning to him said, "I'm sorry I didn't take better care of you when you were sick."

"You took great care of me."

Our time was almost up. We spent the last part of the session saying our goodbyes and expressed to one another how much we had appreciated our time together. It was like many endings to a course of therapy; it felt, in a small way, like a metaphor for life and death itself— unfinished, ragged around the edges, with none of the loose ends tied up. I had been a fellow traveler for a brief time. With clients with whom I have felt especially close, there is always a sense of loss.

Time passed. I heard that Sam and Jeffrey had moved to Denver. When I assumed directorship of the university's outpatient clinic as part of my faculty duties, I decided to scale back my private practice. I could always see clients through the clinic. More time passed. One morning I listened to a new client, a woman in her early 30s, reflecting on the death of a friend. By her description of the circumstances, I suddenly realized that she was talking about Sam.

Without disclosing my connection with Sam and Jeffrey, I somewhat disingenuously managed to have my new client say most of what she knew about it. Sam had died of ovarian cancer that was fairly far advanced by the time it was discovered. She had finally consulted a physician about her inability to get pregnant, and they discovered the spreading malignancy. Jeffrey stayed on in Denver for five or six months, but he had recently returned to the house in the woods that he and Sam had bought before they left, and which my new client had recently vacated.

A couple more months went by, and I wondered if Jeffrey would contact me. He didn't. I thought of both of them often and decided that there was no reason for me not to call him. He appreciated the call and accepted my condolences with the conventional responses. To my remark that I was always "available to talk," he replied sardonically that he wouldn't know what to say if Sam were not there to bust him for it.

But a few months later, Jeffrey came to see me. He looked terrible. His face was thin and pale, except for the black of scruffy stubble. His hair was unkempt, and his clothes hung about him loosely, his jeans full of holes. He reeked of cigarettes.

"I'm not doing too good," he said sitting in the same spot on the couch as when he and Sam were there together.

"You don't look too good."

"Thanks," and there was the ghost of his wry smile. "I can't write. I can't think. I've been drinking a lot, and smoking a lot . . . both kinds. I'm so messed up. I'm not bouncing back from this. I mean, I did at first. It was as if after Sam died I had this sense of her still being with me, and I was heroic, you know. All through the funeral and the weeks after, I had this incredible sense of strength and courage. I felt almost caught up in something bigger than I was, as if there was some kind of cosmic significance to the drama being played out, as if she were helping me rise to the reality of it all. Maybe part of it was that she was so brave throughout the whole thing. I seemed to see my own life in all its dimensions, physically, spiritually. It was as if the partitions between this existence and the next where she was . . . none of those partitions existed."

"Then the door slammed in your face." He looked up at me curiously, as if he was surprised by my comment.

"Yeah, exactly. It was as if all of a sudden, bam, all that energy around me just stopped. I remember at the funeral I put my hand on Sam's casket, and I could feel this, I don't know, almost a hum of energy coming off of it. It was a physical sensation. I was surprised by it. It was as if her life was still vibrating with mine. Now I feel *nothing*. I'm already dead. I'm just passing time and waiting for the rest of me to catch up. I don't care about anything."

"Except that you're here. Some part of you knows you're not dead yet, that you still have to make an effort. I'm glad you came."

"It's a very small part that wants to make an effort."

"I know. Tell me about everything that happened."

Jeffrey described their finding out about the cancer, about their brief battle with it. Sam had decided against prolonged treatment in a lost cause, wanting her remaining days to be free of hospitals and nausea. They had both held each other and cried many times as she declined, but he had not wept a tear, he said, since the day she died. He described how she had turned her head and smiled at him before she eventually sank into a state where the world receded from her and all that was left was him, waiting for her body to cease.

The pathos of it all, he said, briefly connected him to something larger that included her, and he felt that he would live filled with a new and different sense of being. He saw her everywhere, and everything seemed to speak of her, as if he had not fully lost her. But then the world went suddenly gray and she was gone. He felt more alone than he had ever known was possible. He had no way back to her in anything. He was lost, he said, and he was having a hard time remembering her exact look as she gazed on him those last few lucid days. There was a pause, and then he recalled some of the meetings the three of us had shared together. We even smiled together remembering one incident when the two of us had laughed at Sam when she had, in a heated moment, misspoken and used the word *masturbate* in place of *exacerbate* when describing Jeffrey's tactics in their arguments. We sat together in silence. Had we, together, conjured up

Sam in that moment? Is that why he had come, to recapture something of what had happened in this room? I felt very close to him in that moment.

"It felt as if there was some purpose to it," he said finally. "It was more tolerable if Sam's death were part of something that God had in mind, you know?"

"Yeah, I know." I had the sense that he wanted me to say, "Yes, it was part of God's plan for you and Sam. Something greater will come from it."

His jaw looked firmly set, and his eyes were narrowed and intense; he hardly seemed to breathe. It looked to me as if unexpressed grief were simmering down into distilled anger.

"Jeffrey, I have the sense right now that if you took a deep breath and let it out all at once, that some of those missing emotions would be right there, as if they're just below the surface."

He took a deep breath, exhaled while keeping his eyes fixed on mine. "See, nothing in there," he said with a touch of the cynical voice he sometimes used in our former sessions.

"Maybe you're taking me a little too literally," I said with wry smile.

I almost had the sense that he was being defiant. He didn't want to talk about people in his life upon whom he could rely for support or companionship, and he didn't want to talk about alternatives to his substance use. He brushed off my expression of concern that he seemed to have shut himself off from his grief and was looking depressed instead.

He also didn't want to make any appointments for the future. He would, he said, be in touch if he needed to.

———

It was a month and a half before I saw Jeffrey again. He looked as tired and disheveled as before. He had been drinking and smoking pot, "way too much." He didn't care. He had gotten no work done and had been "keeping pretty much to myself." He seemed guarded and defensive, and he fended off with short replies any attempts on my part to engage him. Halfway through the session I was feeling at a loss as to how to proceed. I was just about to say this to him when he offered, "So Amanda came by last week."

"Amanda, is she a friend?"

"Yeah, remember Amanda. Sam was all freaked and jealous about my visit with her that time."

"Oh, yeah, yeah, Amanda, I remember. You've known her for a long time."

"Yeah. She came by. It was good to see her. She wanted to see how I was doing, and she's going through some rough times too in her marriage. It was good to see her."

I waited for him to say more. He didn't. "You were saying that you've been keeping to yourself, that you don't want to see anybody, but it was good seeing her."

"Yeah, we go a long way back, you know?"

"Yeah." Silence.

"I should go," he said suddenly.

"We still have lots of time. Why do you suddenly want to go?"

"I don't know, I don't know why I came. I mean, what's the point? I'm wasting both our time."

"So don't waste it. I'm having a rough time reading you today. You're here, but you don't seem to want to be, and I see that coming out in our conversation."

"Oh Christ. Now it's my fault."

"I didn't say it was your *fault*. I'm just noticing that you seem like you're having a hard time getting going. I really want to know what is happening for you right now."

"But it's all on me. I need to keep this going? What about you? Do you just get to sit there and wait for me to hold up both ends of the conversation?"

"I feel like I'm right here in the room with you holding up my end. Do you feel like I'm not responding to you or that I'm not getting something here?"

"Do you always answer a question with a question?"

"You seem angry now."

"Brilliant!"

"Sarcastic too!"

"Give the man the Nobel fucking prize."

I had to keep tabs on a sudden and rising annoyance. But what was happening was also uncharacteristic and I knew expressive of something I didn't yet grasp.

"You don't know everything, you know," he said. "You just saw a small piece of our lives. There were plenty of things you never saw about us. Our marriage was not like some book that you could edit by changing our communication. Sometimes we would leave here and say, 'What in hell are we going to that guy for? We don't need some divorced marriage coach changing the way *we* talk to one another.'"

That one stung, and I found myself saying, "So why did you continue then?" and knew that this was the wrong question to ask.

"Because Sam was more easily taken in than me."

"All right. Let's stop for a minute. Let's go back. We were talking about Amanda coming to visit you and something changed and you got angry. I'm wondering whether I missed something. What happened that made you feel like I didn't get what you were trying to say to me?"

"Nothing, there's nothing to get. Amanda came over. It was good to see her. She hung out and we got stoned together. We walked in the woods. We fucked. We listened to music and got stoned again. She went home to her rotten marriage. End of story."

"You said you made love with Amanda."

"No, I said I fucked Amanda."

"Okay, so that strikes me for a number of reasons."

"Why, because you guys think that sex is behind everything?" he said, baiting me.

"No, because as far as I know this is the first sexual experience with anyone since Sam died, and that seems important to wonder about in terms of how it felt to you."

"It felt great. How's it supposed to feel? You want the details?" he said, sarcastically. "Anyway, it was a mercy fuck; I think she just felt sorry for me."

"And second," I continued undaunted, "because it was Amanda that you had sex with, and Sam was jealous about your relationship with her in times past."

"Yeah, well in case you hadn't noticed, Sam is dead, so she doesn't get a say in it, does she?"

"You sound angry when you say that."

"So what, it's not going to kill you."

"No it's not, even though that's an interesting way to put it, and even if I thought that your anger was about me."

"What's that supposed to mean?"

"It means that I don't think this anger is really about me at all, even though I'm the target right now."

"You just have endless stores of this stuff, don't you? You think you see all kinds of stuff that isn't there."

"I'll tell you what I do see." In the back of my mind I was thinking, "impulse control, impulse control, impulse control," but what I said was, "I see you screwing up your life with drugs and alcohol because you can't manage to deal with Sam's death. You say you accept it, but you don't, and you keep avoiding it by getting depressed."

"She died, for Christsake. People get depressed."

"Yeah, but it's better if they have the courage to grieve instead. I see you being angry with me, and maybe there's something to that that I'm not getting, but I think you're really angry with Sam for dying on you. And that's why you had sex with Amanda," I said, as it came to me, "You got her back, didn't you: that'll teach her to die on you won't it? So does Sam know about it somewhere? Is she pissed at you? Does that connect Sam with you if she's mad at you?"

At the same moment I realized that this was why he was trying to fight with me, and perhaps why I was responding. He was doing with me what he used to do with Sam when he needed to feel apart, but connected with her. Was I standing in for her? Was he accessing her through me because of our shared experiences? Or did he want to feel close and to contend with me. It felt like all of these motivations could be true at once.

He sat there speechless. I half expected him to get up and walk out. But no, that's not how this fight was supposed to go. I was aware of my own emotional arousal and the charged feeling in the room. I wondered if it was too much too soon. Still, he sat there looking down at his lap. Was he taking this in? Maybe, I thought, he had elicited in me what he needed, in a way that he needed, through a process of conflict that was familiar to him. I was going on intuition. Though it always feels a little ambiguous, I thought, one can't always be deliberate. After a while he looked up and broke the silence.

"The hell with you," he said lamely. The energy had gone out of his anger. "Anyway," he continued, "I only felt anger toward Sam at first. I felt mostly guilty afterward, like I had let her down sleeping with Amanda."

"Ah." I said softly.

"It's also about needing some contact too, you know. I mean I've been alone in this for so long. What's wrong with feeling that? There's a lot more in it than just resenting Sam for leaving me."

"I know. There's nothing wrong with feeling the need for some solace. Sorting something like that out must be full of all kinds of emotions."

"All but the right ones."

"How so?"

"I have been staying stoned and drinking too much. I mean after Amanda left, I was feeling all this anger and guilt, and I didn't want to because . . . I'm not stupid . . . I know the grief and sadness is just behind . . . and I cried for the first time since all that wailing when Sam died. But the problem with that is that it means that she's *really* gone."

"If you're not crying and grieving and expressing it, then maybe she's not really gone. To grieve, and to come to the other side of that grief into some other life means to let her go. It's a life that doesn't include her."

"Yeah. It almost feels like I'm letting her down . . . I don't know."

"Like you would be disloyal for letting her go."

"Yeah." A long pause. "Listen, I'm sorry for giving you so much shit."

"I want you to be able to say what you want in here without editing, so don't worry about it. You're doing what you're supposed to be doing. I'm sorry for clobbering you over the head with all of that at once." I was suddenly aware that we sounded like Sam and Jeffrey making up after a fight.

"No, it's good. Sometimes I need to be clobbered." He sat still for a moment. "Sometimes I miss her so much I feel that if I let myself go, I'd never stop crying," he said, his eyes misting.

"Yeah, maybe. But even if you did stop crying someday, she'd still be with you. Sam owns big rooms in your heart. Don't worry. You'll never get over her."

"That's actually good to hear," he said, a tear finally rolling down his cheek. "Everyone's been saying things that imply the opposite."

I saw Jeffrey one more time in my office. It was about seven months later. I noticed that this time he sat in the middle of the couch. He had pulled himself together, he said, and quit numbing his sensibilities with so much alcohol and pot. He was still trying to face up to Sam's death but felt like he was being more honest with himself. His grief had come pouring out, and for a while he punished himself by obsessively recounting in his sleepless vigils all the ways in which he felt he had failed her. He regretted every unkind word, real or imagined. He wished he had forced her to seek medical treatment sooner. Most of all, he chastised himself for not having been more courageous in the years before he and Sam had married when she needed him most to help her make a decision about the pregnancy. He never imagined it would be their only chance, he said mournfully.

"You describe this as a period you went through. How did you do that . . . stop obsessing and forgive yourself for all of the kinds of things that people who are married manage to do to one another?"

"I don't know. I think it had something to do with a dream I had, though I can't say how. I just felt differently in the weeks following the dream. In the dream I was sitting by a stream whittling this branch with a pocketknife. It still had some dead leaves on it. Every time I would strip them off and trim off the bark and make some progress, I would look down and all the dead leaves and bark would be there again. I saw Sam across the stream, walking up the bank, and when she came parallel to me she waded in. When she got to the center of the stream, it was deeper than it looked; the water came up to her chin, and I was afraid she would be swept downstream, but she came up on my side. Strangely she was dry and smiling. She said, 'What are you doing?' I said, 'I'm whittling this branch, but every time I do it just goes back to the way it was.' She put out her hand, and I gave it to her. She examined it and then casually tossed it in the water, and it floated downstream. She said, 'Don't waste your time with that, you've got a deadline coming up. Let me know if you want some help with the editing.' That's all I remember about the dream.

"It was weird because two things happened after that. One was that after a while I stopped thinking about all the things I wish I had done differently. I mean, it didn't matter. In life, you know, we were great together. I think that somehow I wished I could have protected her from what happened, and I was pouring it all into wishing I had done all these little stupid things better."

"You didn't need to whittle that branch anymore."

"Yeah, but something else about that dream stuck with me when she said you've got a deadline coming up and she would help me with the editing. I mean she did that in real life, and it was great. I feel kind of lost without her help in my writing. She always knew what I was after."

"Okay, so that's what happened in real life. What were your feelings in the dream when she said that?"

"It was like, bam, forget that branch thing, it's unimportant. Like she knew what was important and was trying to tell me."

"As you recall it now, what new associations come up in response to her saying that? What comes to mind right now?" He paused and tilted his head reflectively.

"What comes to mind right now is that I was having some kind of sketchy periods where I was wondering if I was losing it. At first I thought it was coming off of all the shit I was drinking and smoking. But I was having some panic-like stuff, not bad, but upsetting. I was also having some apocalyptic dreams about terrorist stuff after Septem ber 11th. So my association now is that she was saying I have a deadline coming up . . . just like she had a deadline coming up and didn't know it. Pay attention to the important things because it's coming."

"Your own death will come; you don't know when."

"Yeah, because after that dream I didn't think so much about mortality stuff. It was like she said it so easily, and it stuck that way somehow."

"As if you had reached some kind of tolerance of the idea?"

"No, as if I might be more than okay about it. For a while before that I was really incredibly angry, at God, at people in general, at the nature of life. I decided it was all crap. Sam would have gotten mad at me for that; she had a lot of natural spirituality and a suspicion of all organized religion. I was exhausting that whole cliché about how could a merciful God do this or that. And then I thought this is just a bunch of mythological drama in my own head, but then I fell into despair. Not even about Sam, but about how all meaning had drained out of everything, and I thought I got to the bottom of it, which is that things just are, and there's nothing behind it, nothing to discover about it. I was sick with it and with myself. I kicked a God I didn't any longer believe in out of my own head, but I didn't have anything to replace it with. This was before that dream. It was the worst point, and I thought, man, this means that even if I put a gun in my mouth I won't see Sam again. That when she's gone, she's gone. I felt sick about that."

"But something happened about that too."

"Part of it was seeing Sam in that dream. That made me doubt my doubting, so I never really resolved that. But also, this really happened, I was walking down this path by our house. It was a walk through the woods that we used to take together all the time. I was sitting on a log, just sitting there for a long time all alone. I guess I had been there so long that the birds were getting used to me, because this incredible pileated woodpecker, you know, the kind with the big plume on its head, flew down to a dead log not 20 feet from where I sat. I was excited to see it again. This was the same bird that Sam and I had seen the previous spring. She always got excited when we would see it, but we never saw it up close. This beautiful bird lands on this stump, gets on the stump's side, and begins using its beak to methodically pry away the bark, eating bugs with each section that falls off. It was a wonderful thing to see it work around the stump until every bit of bark was gone, and all the bugs eaten. It lasted maybe half an hour. That's it. I mean, it was just a singular and beautiful thing that existed in the world in that moment, and I didn't give a damn about it meaning anything. But the beauty had a kind of eternity packed into it as well. So I thought, who cares about meaning? I'm alive, and for a while Sam was alive with me, and that was so fine."

"As you say it now, I can see that you've taken it into you in a new way. Your grief is present like a backdrop to your life, but you haven't lost her for not having it fill up the horizon."

"No, it seems that I remember stuff that was so much a part of our lives that I wouldn't have imagined I would recall it as something separate. She would always ask me to tell her a story. I always balked, and told her I didn't know any stories—that was part of the ritual—and she'd say, 'You're a writer, make one up.' Or she'd say, 'Tell me a story about us.' I'd always give in. We'd be lying naked in bed, and I'd always begin the story with the opening 'Once, my lovely . . .' Every time. That was what I'd call her," he said with a sweet, sad smile. "She loved that."

About a year later I saw Jeffrey again. He was standing on a low wooden bridge that spanned the South Fork of the Shenandoah River at Seneca Rock in West Virginia. The bridge was perhaps 10 feet above the water. The towering rock loomed high off to the right of the river. As I glided down in my kayak, I could see the climbers scaling the sheer face of the granite spire. They looked like insects, spiders hanging on silk threads, dangling in the air. As I approached the bridge, the water moving slowly, I recognized Jeffrey in the center of the span, leaning against the wooden rail. He was standing next to a woman who also leaned on the rail. They looked relaxed, and they were smiling. It was spring, and the water and air were clear, and the sun was high.

Without any change of posture or facial expression, Jeffrey saw me and said, "Hello Eric."

"Hello Jeffrey."

"It's a beautiful day."

"Yes, it's very fine."

I floated under the bridge, stroking gently, down the stream and away.

CASE ONE DISCUSSION
The Human Context of Therapy

PEOPLE USUALLY COME into therapy because they are suffering and looking for relief. They have often tried many different methods to alleviate their pain but found that all their efforts have failed. In distress, they seek help in a place that they formerly viewed, perhaps, as an unlikely possibility: the therapist's consulting room. I doubt that Sam and Jeffrey, as they were lovingly reciting their wedding vows, ever imagined that they might be sitting together in an office like mine.

The client in the waiting room anticipating the first appointment hopes that behind that door he or she can unshoulder this burden, perhaps leave it behind forever. Therapists-in-training, in particular, often resonant with the client's hope. They often behave under the misconception that it is the therapist's main task to eradicate the client's suffering and to quickly make the client feel better. Seasoned clinicians know that this is not only undesirable, but impossible.

Suffering is as much a part of growth, change, and life as are periods of happiness and fulfillment. Suffering is one of the "existential givens" of life, a part of the human condition. The most that any therapist can offer is to help the client suffer honestly and productively, not neurotically in a self-defeating fashion. The therapist's assumption must be that client self-exploration and understanding will likely lead to relief from nonproductive anxiety and discomfort. The therapist assumes that with new tools gained from the therapeutic process, the client can meet the future painful vicissitudes of life with a greater capacity to tap into his or her potentials. But for the client, it often gets worse before it gets better.

It certainly got worse for Jeffrey after Sam died. By the time he came to me, his grief had formed so deep a pool around the little patch of land on which he stood that he could not get to any other solid ground. The one thing occurred that he (and every person) most dreads: the loss of a dearly loved one. Sam and Jeffrey were so deep into one another, had places in their existence so mutual, that Jeffrey felt as if all meaning had drained from his life when she died. The portrait of a loved one is always painted against a background of inevitable loss.

Jeffrey had only partly grieved. He denied Sam's loss. Jeffrey's drug- and alcohol-induced numbness represented his attempt not to face the challenge that his own life called him to meet: life after Sam. He became committed to his self-destructive, drug-saturated response, and the story he told himself about it was that this was an expression of loyalty. It was perhaps even a little romantic for the writer to be lost in a stupor because he believed that to mourn outwardly, and to carry that grief forward into present life, was to deny the greatness of the love that Sam and he shared. He thought of his suffering as a memorial. In this, Jeffrey suffered no less than if he grieved honestly for Sam. But to grieve honestly, *aware of all the dimensions of his grief,* also brought up feelings that threatened him. These were the irrational and forbidden feelings of anger and resentment, the feelings of betrayal, that Sam had abandoned him. To become open to all the dimensions of his loss meant that he must also allow these unwelcome emotions to surface. A person cannot suppress one dimension of emotional life without losing other dimensions as well.

If, for the client, it often gets worse before it gets better, the real question then becomes, "In what ways are the client's difficulties an unproductive and repetitive form of suffering that prevents the person from responding fully to his or her existence?" This is not to say that all therapy must be like Jeffrey's, addressing itself directly to this dimension of the client's situation. Some client problems and issues are quite discrete, and their roots do not reach as deeply into the ground of the person's being. But without being aware of the contextual relevance of the larger human dimension of therapy, the therapist may only be tinkering with the client's real concerns. There is a very real danger in the current economic climate of mental health care delivery that the field of counseling and psychotherapy could increasingly become a marching ground for an army of therapy "technicians." To prevent this, those who value the healing power of the therapeutic relationship must be mindful of the larger human context in which it occurs.

A conception of the client's problems, therefore, needs to be multidimensional. At the psychological level the therapist takes interest in such things as the client's presenting complaints: What is bringing the person into therapy, and why at this particular time? The therapist may want to understand something of the client's developmental history, the formative and current relationships that shape the person's experiential world and self-concept. It is also useful to understand ways in which the client's behavior and efforts to actualize his or her potentialities have been successful or frustrated.

At a larger contextual level, the therapist may also wonder how these psychological aspects of the client's reality are embedded in the life concerns that affect all people. This is relevant to therapy because though these themes are universal they become inflected through the life of each person in a unique way. The therapist may want to understand how a client's natural tendency to create meaning from experience gives rise to the particular story or narrative that this person tells about the world and his or her place within it. The therapist may wonder how the client is oriented or reconciled to the uncertainties and ambiguities of existence. How do this person's relationships reflect the human aversion to alienation and need for love and deep connection with others? How does this person exercise the will and freedom to create his or her own life within the constraints and limitations of basic humanity? What has this person come to value in terms of work, ideas, or aspirations? How do all of these realities have their influence on the person's ability to accommodate inevitable losses, the finite nature of life, the finality of death?

The types of problems for which individuals seek therapy often express their anxiety in responding to these unavoidable, and often unarticulated, questions. But one cannot tolerate anxiety that is pervasive and amorphous. Anxiety wants to become fear (May, 1983). That is, formless "existential" anxiety seeks a container or object that can be identified (and potentially avoided): a *specific* fear, or "psychological" symptom, that is discrete and identifiable. In Jeffrey's case, anxiety wants to become Amanda. His sexual relationship with Amanda externalized and discharged many ambivalent and oppressive feelings that he found difficult to hold within himself: his anger at Sam, his sense of loss, his guilty conflict over longing for contact with someone new, his fear of isolation.

In other words, the psychological becomes embedded in the freedoms and limitations that form the context of the person's being. The client's unique needs alert the therapist to what degree these contextual and existential considerations connect to the particular work to be done. Psychological inquiry tends to become trivial unless it connects on some level to these larger themes of life.

In the marital part of my work with Sam and Jeffrey, I found this to be especially true. It was not that their problematic communication patterns, for example, were not important and relevant; they were. But these communication problems outwardly manifested a much more profound and universal struggle, one that reached deep into the very nature of their human connection: love and finitude. Part of our work together involved exploring the previously unspoken pact between them that each of them would protect the other from the uncertainties and vagaries of life. Of course, each person hopes to derive from his or her closest relationships an antidote to isolation and some measure of strength to face the inevitable losses in life to sickness, injury, and death. But Sam and Jeffrey, more than most couples, placed an added burden on their relationship by expecting the other to *shield* them from the anxieties and realities of these experiences. They each looked to their love to provide more than it could possibly give and were alternately delighted and disappointed in their relationship's strengths and limitations.

This is, perhaps, the most common and appealing of all illusions: that love can finally transcend and conquer the defining limitations inherent in life and death. Sam and Jeffrey drew tightly together and held onto one another closely, reassuring one another that their union was present, immediate, and secure. But in this blending they began to lose touch with the outline of their own identities and felt the need to blow apart to prevent the fusion in which they each lost themselves. At either end, fusion or isolation, they seemed to encounter a sense of annihilation. They occasionally found a graceful dance of communion at the center of these oscillations. But often their conflicts kept them separate but reassuringly engaged and bound together. Addressing the structure and style of Sam and Jeffrey's methods of conflict helped them to civilize their fights, and to prevent more misunderstanding than was useful to their objectives.

Ultimately, however, the therapy evoked and made visible themes with much more pathos: the hidden fears, frailties, and longings, the secret expectations expressive of the reasons for their conflicts. In revealing themselves to one another more completely, Sam and Jeffrey needed to rely less on their old repetitive ways to secure their union. The special interpersonal climate of trust that therapy provides enabled them to disclose secrets to one another that they had been unable to reveal on their own. These secrets attenuated their capacity to be fully available to the other and formed an unspoken barrier between them for many years.

Spinning the Thread

Repeated throughout these pages is this maxim: It is the *relationship itself* that heals in psychotherapy. The therapy relationship is a type of human connection that is, in structure, unlike any other available in ordinary life. The therapist brings his or her presence into relation with the client solely in service of the client's growth and healing. In this sense the relationship is not reciprocal. The client does not, as in all other relationships, need to take care of the "other side," worrying about how his or her words, feelings, or fantasies affect the other person. Unlike marriages, friendships, and family connections, the client can be fully self-expressed in therapy, saying and revealing anything without endangering the relationship. In fact, the successful therapy relationship *actively excludes* many of the ordinary rules and conventions that characterize most social intercourse. This goes for the therapist as well as the client. In therapy the relational economy is different because the relationship itself exists solely for actualizing the potentialities of the client.

The therapy relationship is collaborative and active. Many clinicians-in-training seem to assume (perhaps misunderstanding Rogers) that merely listening compassionately to the client constitutes effective therapy. Joining with the client is certainly essential, but therapy involves a working alliance between client and therapist whose common goals are exploration, change, struggle, and hard-won gains in self-awareness. The therapist must contend for (and sometimes with) the client, as both join in a battle to overcome what stands in the way of actualizing these goals (Friedman, 1989). The therapist must sometimes "throw a wrench in the gears" to help the client disrupt old patterns and ways of being that frustrate the freedom to make productive changes. This is not an attitude of "me against you" but rather "you and me against your demons," so to speak.

The therapy relationship is healing not merely because of the "functions" the therapist provides or the techniques he or she employs. It is a real *human* relationship that rests on a foundation of trust, empathy, and unconditional positive regard. The therapist cannot hide behind a role or method and expect these potentials to be realized. The worlds of therapist and client come into contact with one another in a real encounter, elemental and palpable, which can be very powerful for *both* participants. Therapists-in-training are sometimes intimidated by these relational aspects of therapy. They would often rather "do something to" rather than "be someone with" the client. Strong emotions, disturbing revelations, sexual attractions, and confusing transferences are all potential parts of the therapy relationship. The therapist must be able to maintain his or her reference points while deeply engaging and participating in the inner world of the client. A strong and secure sense of self is necessary for the therapist to remain unthreatened by this level of participation. The therapist must learn to use (not neutralize) his or her unique personality to stay grounded in the relationship and to facilitate the interventions and goals of therapy. There is no generic or one size fits all method or style of intervention.

The therapist must strive to create, by his or her presence and encouragement, a *holding environment* or container for all of the client's emerging feelings, thoughts, and self-expressions (Winnicott, 1945). The client sometimes needs to "borrow" the therapist's ego to strengthen the client's own ability to contain all the powerful impulses, fantasies, and emotions elicited by the unique therapy environment. Sam and Jeffrey relied on me to help them modulate, control, and share feelings that might have been too dangerous, disruptive, or overwhelming for them to express individually or with each other. It was no accident that in the safe climate of therapy they were able to talk about the abortion that neither one of them had been willing to acknowledge on their own. After Sam's death, Jeffrey was able to express his continuing grief in therapy in spite of the fact that it felt like a "quicksand" that might suck him completely under. The therapist's reliable and consistent presence enables the client to borrow the therapist's strength to unwind the silver thread, allowing the emergence of self-states that the client might otherwise perceive to be too dangerous or overwhelming.

When this collaboration is established, the therapeutic relationship gains in healing potential. Sensing the therapist's sustained empathy, the client's deepest areas of injury begin to become accessible. The client begins to use the relationship to address old wounds experienced with others in an effort to remediate them in the here-and-now. The immediacy of the therapy relationship "stands in" for other important relationships in the client's life as a kind of prototype for the authentic human connection for which he or she longs. Areas in which the client has become developmentally "stuck" become apparent. Defenses and resistances often appear precisely because the new opportunity to get archaic needs met in the relationship with the therapist also elicits old fears that the therapist is unreliable, or will respond in the same hurtful ways as others in the client's life. The client secretly fears retraumatization by the therapist. This is especially true if the client reveals what he or she imagines are the disgusting, forbidden, or shameful things that will destroy the therapist's regard or drive the therapist away. However, when the therapist does not respond in the injurious ways the client expects, but rather maintains an attuned and validating presence, this provides the client with a new and healing relational event. Franz Alexander called this a "corrective emotional experience" (Alexander & French, 1946).

Another way in which "it is the relationship that heals" is that real encounter with another person happens in the here-and-now. The past is already gone, the future is always a breath away; it is the present moment in which life happens. When therapists attempt to make explicit a client's behaviors, thoughts, and emotions that emerge in response to the immediate events unfolding between them, they refer to this as working in the "process." When therapists are working in the process, they are "tracking" the flow of the events, making "process comments" about what is taking shape at the intersection between the client's and therapist's subjective worlds. Tracking the process illuminates dimensions of the current relational exchange, promoting greater awareness. This enables the client not only to pay special attention to emerging self-states but to have an opportunity to understand how he or she is being perceived and experienced by another. This sort of "illumination of the obvious" is often prevented by normal social manners and customs that aim to obscure precisely what the therapist would like to reveal. Working in the process gives therapy energy and dynamism and provokes emotional arousal. Emotional arousal is important because significant life events are rarely merely intellectual or cognitive; they are infused with a sense of "happening." Therapists, who want what the clients gain in therapy to stick, are attentive to working in the process.

By the end of my work with Sam and Jeffrey, we had a profound appreciation and fondness for one another. I made no attempt to hide my affection for them and for their marriage together. I think that seeing this spontaneous expression on my part helped them to appreciate themselves and their marriage more fully. With Sam's tragic death, Jeffrey felt the oppression of others' hopes that he would "pull back together" and "get over it." When it came time for him to do the "soul work" he needed to do, he remembered a place, a human relationship with me, where he could reveal and "contain" the forces pressing for expression. He knew that I would accept him where he was, that he wouldn't have to "feel better." He sensed that I would honor his suffering and stand with him in it, not just as a therapist but as a fellow human being. But he also understood that I would not leave it at that; I would challenge him in our relationship to rise to his full potential.

Martin Buber (1958) argued that the essence of what he termed the "I–Thou" encounter resides not in either person but in the third reality that exists between them as they come together at the deepest levels of engagement. If one drew two overlapping circles, like a Venn diagram, the place that belongs to both but that outlines a middle separate area in itself would be a metaphorical representation of this meeting. In the "between," as Buber termed this level of meeting, persons encounter each other fully oriented to the possibilities in themselves and the other. They participate with one another openly, authentically, and spontaneously and are sensitive to the nuances of their unique encounter as their individual subjective worlds come into contact. The principles of human encounter apply to the therapeutic dialogue. It is a real human meeting that includes the subjectivity of both participants. However, the therapeutic process places an added demand on the therapist. The therapist must be fully present and yet concurrently be able to reflect on what is experientially occurring at any given moment. The process demands that the therapist balance subjective participation with the client while cultivating a reflective and observant "objectivity" so as to be able to make sense of the unfolding process (Hycner, 1991). This blending of processes is no easy task. Some therapists excel in the empathic dimensions of encounter but lose the opportunity to elicit change through overidentification with the client's subjective reality. Other therapists possess a keen eye for the client's issues and conflicts and can produce the interpretations to prove their technical analysis, but they lack the empathic engagement that make these interventions effective. The skilled therapist walks the "narrow ridge" between these two dimensions of participation.

The I–Thou involves inclusion, which Buber describes as a "bold swinging" into the life of the other (as cited in Friedman, 1989, p. 179). Far more than mere emotional resonance, inclusion means to enter into and participate in the world of another, experiencing it the way that person does, understanding it on its own terms and principles. Inclusion is the fullest form of empathy. To enter the world of another fully is a difficult task, for to do so risks temporarily losing sight of one's own bearings, values, and reference points. But inclusion implies also comprehending and recognizing the other person in their *potential* as well as their current existence.

Beginning therapists often struggle with Rogers's exhortation to exercise unconditional positive regard for the client because they believe this means accepting and endorsing all of the client's actions and behaviors. To unconditionally accept another in his or her essential humanity and potential, however, speaks to this deeper level of inclusion. At this level I see and accept you in your current state of development, but I also see that you have unrealized potentialities. You are a *being in the process of becoming.* Again, Buber argues that the therapist sensitive to this level of engagement may have to contend *for* the client and *with* the client to help the other realize his or her potential. This contention is not based in mere persuasion or rational argument; it emerges from the new opportunities and realizations that such levels of participation with another create.

Buber's "dialogical" perspective on human relationships is not some mystical state or idea. The I–Thou experience is present in all human relationships where there is mature, deep, and authentic participation with another. Sometimes the I–Thou exists for a brief instant, even with someone we have just met. Sometimes, as with Sam and Jeffrey, and between them and me, it manifests at different levels in the context of sustained relationships. Buber (1988) argued that each of us needs the I–Thou in our lives, from the time we are cradled as infants to that final parting with others through death. He argued that it is in the I–Thou relation to others that we constitute ourselves as fully human. If it is nowhere in our lives, then we live a diminished and shrunken existence.

Of course, we cannot live with such a high degree of participation all the time. In some ways, this is what Sam and Jeffrey wanted and feared in their union: that they might continually bask in the fullness of one another's presence. Perhaps this was another function of the secrets they kept from each other. The I–Thou meeting is a reference point for those experiences that emerge spontaneously when two people create the interpersonal conditions. When therapists seek to foster better communication skills through couples therapy, the ultimate goal is often to make possible these moments of full participation that transcend the mechanics of the communications.

The I–Thou represents one pole on the continuum of interpersonal participation; the other pole of this continuum is described as the "I–it" way of relating to others (Buber, 1958). Here others become objectified and are seen merely as a representation of the functions they play in the person's experience. The I–it way of being causes one to see only the exterior of other people. When I am stuck in the DMV line and the clerk hands back my problematic papers and sends me to the end of another line, I am inclined to see her entirely in the I–it modality. My hostility dehumanizes her and reduces her to merely a barrier to my desires, a source of my frustration. If the I–it modality becomes pervasive and characterizes a person's attitude toward waiters, gas attendants, teachers, students, lovers, or people in general, then that person robs his or her interpersonal world of all richness. In the extreme I–it mode, we see others only as furniture with arms and legs moving around in the living room of our life.

In the Oscar-winning film *Monster's Ball,* Billy Bob Thornton plays a prison guard entrenched wholly in the I–it mode of relating to others. He is devoid of the ability to resonate with the life of anyone around him. When his son, who is also a prison guard, botches the electric chair execution of a prisoner, Thornton's rage is not due to the prisoner's increased suffering or his son's remorse but because the procedure was not carried out properly. We are not surprised when the son, raised in such an interpersonal wasteland, points a gun at himself and pulls the trigger. For most of us, when we oscillate into the I–it mode of relating to others, it is not so extreme, but merely utilitarian. Buber argues, however, that modern culture is becoming increasingly dehumanized and impersonal as persons become interpersonally divorced from others, from nature (also an I–Thou type communion), and ultimately from themselves.

The interhuman meeting is at once both the starting and end point of the therapy process (Trüb, 1964a). Psychopathology, by definition, hinders the client from participating fully with others. As therapist and client attempt to establish a dialogue, the barriers to such an I–Thou meeting will manifest and be explored in the unfolding relationship. As new experiences with the therapist increasingly demand the interhuman dimension of engagement, the client is "called out" to fuller participation, not only with the therapist but with the larger community. This is what Hans Trüb (1964b) meant by the phrase "healing through meeting." The therapist, keeping an eye on this level of interpersonal process and on how the client's problems manifest in relation to the larger themes of life, creates a context for therapy in which such healing can occur.

✗ ☡

Daddy Dearest

You do not do, you do not do
Any more, black shoe
In which I have lived like a foot
For thirty years, poor and white,
Barely daring to breath or Achoo

—"Daddy," by Sylvia Plath

Theresa, can you tell something about what's bringing you here to meet with me today?"

The woman in front of me tilted her head slowly but curiously, as if trying to make sense of my question, as if I were speaking a foreign language. Silence.

"I know you just came from a week at an inpatient center," I offered. "How did you come to be there?" A pause.

"I checked myself into a crisis house."

"Ah, and why did you do that?"

"Because I was in crisis."

"Okay. Perhaps you'd like to say a little more about that?" She closed her eyes for a moment, as if she were considering whether this might be too much effort. Her face seemed flat and still, and the gray baggy sweats she was wearing made the rest of her appear like an inert lump of laundry piled in the chair. The languid lids opened, and she stared at me with her large brown panther-like eyes, their tops still partly veiled. She looked to me like some kind of stunned animal that has just been hit by a car and suddenly finds itself among surrounding alien humans with no capacity to run away.

"I had the feeling that my skin was going to blow off," she said slowly. "I was going to explode." Her monotonous and lifeless delivery conveyed no such energy now.

36

I nodded, but she sat still. "It felt as if your skin was going to blow off," I said after a moment.

"I went in to buy some groceries and the price wouldn't come up on an item, and the guy behind the counter was clueless. As I stood there waiting, I just wanted to strangle him. After I left there I went to the bank, and the machine wouldn't accept my card. The man was just closing the doors. I had seen someone else enter a few moments before, but it was right on the hour. I had the urge to just punch him and break down the door." She paused, and then, "So I knew I was losing it, and I wanted to just fall," she said, lifting her thin hand, palm outward, and opening it slowly, as if to convey some delicate idea, "to let go . . . not care anymore, or be responsible for anybody. I didn't want to take anybody else into account. I just wanted to crawl under a rock and be left alone . . . before I killed somebody," she said, turning up the palm of the suspended hand as if at a loss to understand. The expressive gesture, contrasting as it did with her gray stillness, seemed strange in its grace, almost theatrical.

"So you were feeling like you couldn't hang on any longer, and you were having all these violent impulses and fantasies. I get the impression, as you say that, that those violent feelings were new or surprising."

Again, a long pause and a Buddha-like stare. "I'm a peaceful person. I don't know where that was coming from."

"You're a peaceful person, so when all these incredibly strong feelings of anger and rage came out, it felt like you were losing it, and you went to the clinic." I hoped with these simple reflective remarks to confirm her experience but also to draw her into a deeper engagement around the issues that had engendered her crisis.

She took a deep breath and exhaled. I had the sense that she had resolved to engage in our conversation, to try to reach into herself, and with effort, to share with me what she drew up. "I was really losing it. So I knew about that place, I don't know how, and I just went there, and they had a spot, and I stayed there. I had to let myself fall into this hole," she said, as if talking more to herself than me, "and I thought that I would never stop falling, that it was endless. But something happened because I stopped caring if I would land. The falling itself became not so bad. I knew that even if I never landed I would be falling into a part of me. It was still me, not some hell of someone else's imagination. There was something reassuring about that. At least it was my despair, and I wrapped it around me like a blanket and rocked myself to sleep. I was utterly alone in it, and that had never been allowed to happen before, and I thought, hell is not so bad." She paused, as if what she

had just said had cost her the rest of her energy reserve. "They gave me
the name of this place when I left, so when I left there yesterday, I came
here today."

"I'm glad you came. It seems like something happened when you
were able to have some time all to yourself. You were able to let go and
allow yourself to take in all the feelings you were keeping pushed away
because you feared they would completely disrupt your life. It seems
like there was no way you could both 'let go' and keep your regular life
going at the same time. That your own hell was better than living in
someone else's idea of heaven."

At this last statement, a ghost of a smile played across her mouth,
and a hint of human presence seemed to siphon up from some protected
inner well and back into her eyes.

"There's more in that than you can know," she said. After a pause she
observed, "Letting my life shut down like that . . . it's not something
anyone can understand . . . or that I would let people see. It surprised
even me, more so because it helped. I'm not sure I was even looking for
that, to be helped by it, it just seemed imperative. It was good to have
all the grunt stuff taken care of . . . meals and stuff. I wasn't alone all of
the time. I went to the therapy groups and met with the shrink. He put
me on an antidepressant. I'm not sure what effect that is having. I don't
know if I was ready to leave. But at least I'm walking around."

"Yeah, and you were able to get yourself in here."

"I don't know what I'm going to do in here though," she said with a
tired sigh, "I feel numb."

"I get that. It looks to me like everything is an effort for you right
now. Your voice is very quiet, you sound very tired."

"Exhausted, and I feel like I've been drugged or something. I can't
believe I'm in this kind of shape; so depressed. I was always someone
who's on top of it, the one who's got it under control. Another part of
me feels embarrassed realizing that I'm so screwed up I had to check
into a place like that. My normal consciousness is reasserting itself, I
guess. My kids seemed to understand. My father just thinks I'm being a
whiner. He refused to acknowledge it by not coming to see me."

"Ouch."

"Yeah. 'No time for a drama.'"

"You mean he thinks you're faking?"

"No, not quite faking; just being a whiner. You know, too
weak willed."

"Just pull yourself up by your bootstraps and get on with it."

"Yeah, 'the fight is 12 rounds.'"

"You take your shots."

"Yeah, there's nothing to contemplate about it. You just fight, and if you get banged up, well, that's life. You go your 12 rounds. Why make it harder than it is?"

"Between rounds you get a breather."

"That's not something he would understand. I'm not sure I do myself, that I would wind up there."

"It's not the kind of place you imagined you would ever need to go to?"

"No. I never thought I would feel that out of control and be ready to assault someone. I was ready to really whack that woman; I was seeing red."

Her head drooped and she was quiet, as if she were suddenly elsewhere, and I again felt alone in the room. I asked her for some basic information to keep her engaged.

Theresa related that she is 47 years old and has sons ages 16 and 18, and a daughter age 23. Her daughter left home a few years before, but her sons live with her. She has been divorced for seven years and works part time doing office work. She seemed to recollect herself a little, so I segued back to her presenting concerns.

"Theresa, I'm curious about what led up to your checking in to that crisis house. From what you've said, it seems like you normally are able to get on with life pretty well, but that to do that you've been ignoring big parts of how you think and feel. Then there was a pretty sudden experience of being out of control. Did something happen that was upsetting or traumatic for you that made you feel fragile or sent you off into a rage?" She shook her head.

"Nothing out of the ordinary, really. Well, I did stop drinking a few months ago. Even though I started drinking when I was 15, it wasn't that hard. But I think when I quit that things just kind of built up . . . not like a single event. If it was a single event I could say, wow, that was bad . . . but it's just not that easy to get at. It's everything combined, and that's the feeling that my skin is going to blow off, like I can't even live in my own skin, because I just want to get out."

"You seem to imply that stopping drinking after so long made you more aware of parts of yourself that you might have been able to ignore before." She nodded. "So there might be a lot to explore that your drinking has kept on hold, things that have built up over time. What's the first thing that comes to mind about what's going on in your life before you checked into the crisis house? Perhaps even a little thing that stands out?"

Theresa paused for a moment, then sighed. "It's a picture of my sons sitting at the kitchen table joking around, just teasing each other and putting one another down in a friendly sort of way. And my father comes over to the house. You know, he kind of knocks, but it's really more of a knock like, 'I'm coming in, like it or not.' Like he knocks and opens the door at the same time. He goes into the kitchen and sits there with the boys, and they're kidding around and it's good. But pretty soon he's lecturing them, you know. He's on his continuing mission to indoctrinate them into the Catholic Church, to make sure that they're good Catholic boys. And all that kidding and good feeling is just going out the window because my father is laying all this heavy morality on them: lecturing them about being virtuous, about God and drugs and sex and marriage. Trying to get it all in at once."

"The way you describe it, it seems like you felt intruded upon."

"Big time."

"So you saw this scene at the kitchen table, and you had some response to it."

"I wanted to just smash him over the head with a frying pan. I wanted to say, 'No.' I wanted to scream, 'Don't you do this to them!'" Her voice, for the first time, seemed connected to some emotion. "There was this heavy atmosphere, and the boys were sullen but obediently listening. And that's what got me, the obedience, this sense that they felt powerless to fend him off. They just had to endure it."

"Just like you had to endure it. I can hear in your voice the anger that you feel about it. You say they were obediently listening. What about you, did you have any impulse to intervene for them, to alter the dynamic of what was happening?"

I could see that with this question I had overreached. It was a "what did you do" instead of a "how did you experience it" kind of question, and I was going too fast. I should have let her volunteer her own reaction. Theresa heard it as if I was punitively saying, "So why didn't you intervene?"

The lids closed again over her suddenly inscrutable eyes, and again I was alone in the room. I tried to recover, offering lamely, "I imagine that is pretty complicated." She nodded. Our time was up. We agreed to meet twice a week to start.

"You asked me what happened before I blew up," Theresa began in our next session. She seemed to have recovered some energy and appeared more able to engage in a dialogue. "I thought of another thing after I left. I had to go over to Georgetown University to do something for work. And I saw all these young women riding their bikes around, and wearing backpacks. They looked as if they could just go anywhere. Just like all the world was open for them."

"It seemed as if they were free to go where they liked, to do what they wanted."

"Yeah, they were young and free, and everything was before them. I was so wishing I could be there, and not be trapped."

"That feeling of trapped seems important."

"Yeah, trapped, and worse, that it's too late even if I weren't stuck, you know, that it's too late to do anything about it. I'm a 47-year-old divorced woman with three kids and not nearly enough money. What could I do even if I did have an idea of something?"

"You are trapped by your vitae?"

"What?"

"You are a 47-year-old divorced woman, and so on. It sounds carved in stone, like nothing new could happen. Life is over for you." Theresa looked at me as if I didn't know her; that I couldn't begin to comprehend the circumstances of her life that kept her from envisioning new possibilities. "You look skeptical as I say that. So what keeps you trapped?"

"An ill mother for one. Three kids. A crazy family for another. That's probably something I'd like to avoid going into for as long as possible."

"Never say that to a therapist. It's like a big flashing sign that says 'look here.'" She smiled, and I was struck to see an emotion pass over her blank face. "In what way is your family crazy?"

"Everybody is into everybody else's business," she said, her face again showing some signs of animation. "After my divorce seven years ago, I moved outside of Washington D.C., and my father wanted to be close by, so they moved too. It was hard financially, and my ex wasn't paying child support, so I had to rely on my father to help out. Somehow it just got out of control, and now I feel like I never left home in the first place."

Over the course of the following few sessions, Theresa expanded on this single theme. She explained that of her father's three daughters she had always been his favorite. She recalled that when she was a child, her father confided in her, and liked to take her with him, especially in all his activities related to the Catholic Church. She enjoyed being his helper, anticipating his needs, feeling special. As she grew older, however, she became increasingly aware of being "caught in the middle" between her parents. She became the "keeper of secrets," as each parent confided in her, especially during times of frequent marital stress. Once, she recalled, her parents had fought and her father had left the house for days. She remembered her mother's admonition that they must all be "extra nice" and never upset her father, or he might get angry and leave for good. She told herself that she would never upset him, never get angry and disrupt the "family mood." She prayed that God would help her to take good enough care of him so that he would always be with the family. And because her attention to him seemed to work, and was important to him, she seemed to have a "special place" in the life of the family.

But as Theresa grew, her special relationship with her father felt more and more uncomfortable. He increasingly turned to her for support and companionship. She was his "go-to" girl, he said, and the sports metaphors seemed to somehow make it seem innocuous. Especially in her teen years Theresa sensed that there was an emotionally incestuous quality to their connection. She could no longer be equally "between" her parents, and she felt the emergence of resentment from her mother as she regularly stood in for her at social and church events. As her mixed feelings of specialness and repugnance increased, she began to long for greater independence and freedom and began to contemplate going to college. Every attempt on her part to widen the distance between her and her father, however, was met with disapproval. He possessed a powerful personality and formidable demeanor. He insisted that she attend a Washington area college and live at home for, he said, financial reasons. In her sophomore year she discovered a new way to increase her independence from her family: she married.

Theresa soon found, to her regret, that she had not actually gotten away from her father, merely replaced him with a substitute. Many long years of unhappy marriage followed, finally ending in divorce. Her father had been there to help her financially after the divorce. He also found her a job at the church. As her mother became more incapacitated by illness, Theresa took over her mother's duties, including cooking and cleaning, for which her father paid her. But now, even in her 40s, she found herself playing a wifely role to her father, presenting a "good family front" to the church community, conforming to her father's demands. She felt powerfully the "obligation" to take care of her ailing mother and experienced a crushing guilt whenever her feelings of resentment got the upper hand. Theresa had developed her own interests in Catholic women's issues and "spiritual feminism," but her father ridiculed these as irrelevant and teased her about her "new age" attitudes. Her confusion resulted in what Theresa called her "dysfunctional Catholicism," as she could neither abandon nor reform for herself the faith that was so much a part of her family identity.

As Theresa unfolded her narrative over these beginning sessions, she seemed to slowly reinhabit her body. Her face became more expressive, she used language fluently to capture the pith of her experience, and the long pauses quickly gave way to flurries of associations that she wanted to capture and to tell all at once. She had waited long years to find someplace where she could vent her thoughts and feelings freely. The more she spoke, the more her anger surfaced, as if she were only now beginning to realize what a vast underground reservoir of rage was stored in her history.

A sense of rapport and trust began to emerge between us. At the same time, I could see important transference issues emerging that were expressive of Theresa's interpersonal relationships and the conflicts she felt within those important ties.

———

The first obvious transference enactment concerned a seemingly trivial "housekeeping" issue regarding our appointment. I had wanted to reschedule our meeting for a more convenient time for me, and she had readily agreed. When she later made a passing reference to the switch, I thought I heard an undertone of resentment that at first she denied.

"Really, it's fine. The time is no big deal," she dissembled.

"I don't know. What you are saying, and what I am feeling as I recall how you said it, feel like two different things."

"What did I say?"

"I don't remember the exact words, just that it felt to me like you had some feelings about the switch in time that you weren't openly acknowledging."

"Does the time work for you?" she persisted.

"Yes, but that's not the point. The point is, I would like to know how you really feel about it. I suspect that you resent the change of time."

"Well, I wouldn't say resent." A pause. "I would just say that it's not as good as the last time we had."

"I wonder why you didn't say that when we discussed it?"

"It seemed important to you, so I just kind of let it slide. I'll get over it."

"There's something to get over?"

"Yeah, I guess I was a little put out about it."

"Put out," I said dubiously.

"All right, pissed off. I guess I was just deferring. The fact that you're the 'Doctor'; you have the reins in your hands. I may have been angry, but, you know," she shrugged. "Also," she suddenly seemed to remember, "You were 10 minutes late that day! Why is every man I've ever met late? Is it genetic? It made me wonder if you were too busy to take me as a client. You know, if I really get into this, are you just going to not show up one day? That would be just like a man."

"So, you are mad about the change in time, and my lateness, but you hide those feelings from me because you think I have more authority here."

"Yeah."

"And you defer, or ignore your wishes, to placate me."

"Yeah. And then I feel resentful about it."

"Okay, I can see how this relates to what happened between us. Does this sound familiar to you, though?"

She sat looking at me, and a smile began to play on her mouth. "Yeah, I'm doing with you what I do with my father . . . putting my own needs aside to service him."

"And it pisses you off. Even though you try to hide it, it kind of leaks out."

"That's a good way to put it. It leaks out somewhere else, you know, and it might be somewhere that is far enough away from where it's really located that it can't be traced, you know. Like I am covering my tracks so nobody can point the finger and say, 'that's her.'"

"I'm guessing you do it as well with people other than your father. But you found a way to bring it back to me, though not directly."

"Yeah, I would kind of do the same thing with my father, that indirectness, but it would just go phissssh," she made a gesture of her hand passing over her head. "You know, he just wouldn't pick up on it. He's not what you might call a subtle person."

"So, even though this time I picked up on it, I wonder if you could do something different in here with me?" I asked.

"About this?"

"Why not?"

"Okay. You mean like redoing that same conversation?" I nodded. "So do you want to change the time of our meeting back to what it was?" she said tentatively.

"Not really," I said. She looked confused for a moment. I smiled. A mischievous look slowly spread across her face.

"Well, I do!" she said definitively.

"You're sure about that?"

"Yeah!"

"Then I guess we have to talk about what works for both of us, huh?"

Another small constellation of transference incidents emerged that we successfully addressed, and this seemed to deepen the bond between us.

———

As our twice a week sessions fell into a rhythm, Theresa expressed a growing feeling that therapy was merely a self-indulgence, a selfish activity that exaggerated the importance of her self-experience, which was really not worth such attention. "After all," she said, "everybody has problems. Everyone's mother dies." She related a dream in which an autobiographical paper she had written for a class came back to her with a grade of "A." As she watched, however, the grade kept changing on the paper to a lower grade, and finally to a zero. The paper also bore a note from the teacher that read, "This was supposed to be a biography." Later in our session together I noticed a change in the level of her immediacy and openness.

"Something has happened in the last few minutes in our conversation," I observed. "You were talking about this feeling of wanting to break free of all these rules you have in your head that keep you trapped and about how you can't live your life; you were very much here in the room with me, and then something shifted. You got more reserved or withdrawn or something."

"I guess I was just finished."

"It felt to me more like you felt interrupted or stopped."

"It's nothing."

"Okay, if you say so." A long silence.

"Well, actually . . . there is something, but it seems petty. I remembered that last session, you stifled a yawn, and then you shifted in your chair. As I was talking just now, I thought, maybe I'm just whining."

Though not remembering a need to yawn (I did not challenge her assertion), I encouraged her to tell me what my stifling a yawn had evoked in her. She explained that she thought that I must be bored with her, that her self-disclosures were not important, and that I must have clients who were much more interesting than she. Her subjective impression that I must be bored with her conjured up fears that maybe she was not important to me, not "special" and valued in the way that she found herself wanting to be. Theresa explained that I was the first person she had met to whom she could really talk openly and that she saw me as completely capable . . . that I must be "one of the talented ones." She worried that she might not be worthy of my "special abilities."

How much could be read into a stifled yawn! Theresa's frustrated but remerging developmental need for emotional resonance and to be accurately mirrored had slowly revived in the empathic connection between us. Her legitimate but frustrated needs to be "special" to another person had come out of hiding and began to move into the foreground in our relationship. Theresa's need to feel special and prized, however, had always been a devil's bargain for her: as long as she was willing to give up her own ground to conform to another's desires, she might win the approval she sought. With me she felt the possibility that she could be both valued and real, but she had little faith in this perception; she did not fully trust my reliability. Theresa's fear that I might punish her now alternated with her fear that I might withdraw from her if she really revealed herself. On one hand, her idealization of me as her therapist helped her to feel that I would always know what to do, that I would divine her needs, and that I was possessed of wisdom. This helped her to feel safe enough to tentatively bring out her private longings and fears. On the other hand, her idealization evoked in her feelings that she wouldn't be good enough, and that when I really understood her I would lose interest in her and abandon her.

I shared these impressions with Theresa and observed to her that the conflict she was feeling seemed to also be mirrored in the message of the dream she had earlier related: Not only should her autobiography receive a "0" instead of the prized "A+," but it should not be about her at all . . . it should be a *biography,* a narrative about some other, more interesting person! She took this all in.

"Yeah," she said after a while. "And in here, I'm suddenly afraid to turn the paper over and see what's on it, you know. It's like, I don't know, like I can't figure out how it started to matter to me."

"How it started to matter to you what I might think of your autobiography?"

"Yeah, before, when we started, you were like, 'any therapist USA.' You were like that tape recorder (I was recording our sessions), just a listener as I was spewing out all this junk and all these feelings. But somehow, over time, you became more of a real person. I'm not sure how that happened."

"You're not so sure how you feel about that, that somehow I became not just 'some body' in the room that seemed to nod and from whose face sounds sometimes emitted, but 'somebody,' a real person."

"Yeah, because if you're a real person, it's a little disappointing that now I have to take you into account." I cocked my head and raised my eyebrows in a "say more about that" expression.

"Yeah . . . like I have to worry about what you will think. Can I really say, 'What if you matter to me?' I mean what the hell did I care before what you thought? I only see you in here, and I can leave any time I want and would probably never see you again."

"If I matter to you, you might think, 'I had better edit what I'm willing to disclose, because I don't want Eric to have a negative opinion of me, or judge me, or punish me.'"

"Not so much punish me, but not, you know." She stopped.

"You were going to say something."

"It's embarrassing. You might not think I'm, you know, special . . . extraordinary," she said shyly. There was a pause, and I felt the pull to gratify her need for reassurance, to soothe her longing, to tell her she was special and exceptional. At the same time, I knew my praise would bounce right off of her, and it would be making a bargain with her that recapitulated her conflict. I would be in the position of evaluating or approving her. I told her I was thinking this, and said, "All I can say to that is that I find that the most extraordinary people I've known have somehow managed to go deeply into their own lives, to share their lives with others in a real and direct coming together, and that we have a good start with that. I'm very interested in your *auto*biography and imagine that the deeper you are able to tell it in here, the more we will both want to see what is on the next page. I don't remember if I needed to yawn or not, but I'm certainly not bored in here with you, and I like you very much. You said that I was becoming more important and real for you, and I feel that way with you too: you are becoming more important and real to me."

There was a long silence.

"How are you feeling right now?" I asked after a while.

"Strangely relieved. I somehow trust you a lot more now that we don't have to get into this approval thing. But then I think, it's not real, is it? I mean, I give money to come here, and you have to listen to me. It's your job to somehow make me feel better. You're smiling."

"Yeah, I'm smiling. So, you think you're going to feel better in here, huh? You said last week that your emerging impulse to become more independent was like 'killing off the family,' and that talking about your immediate life is conjuring up all these feelings of rage and despair that make you want to go back to numbing yourself with drinking. This has been a real picnic for you."

She laughed. "Yeah, maybe I look to some time in the future where I might have some hope of a picnic."

"I don't mean to make light of your bringing up the issue of money . . . the structure of therapy does seem a little artificial, doesn't it? The fact is that you are coming here for help from me in my professional capacity, but does it follow that the human elements that inform that are any less real?"

"I know; it's just so complicated. I can't tell you how it brings so much out. When I was coming here, I noticed my heart starting to beat, because I leave here, and it's like a tornado around me. I'm like, not in Kansas anymore Toto. I can't tell you all the conflicting thoughts and feelings that seem totally out of control."

"You have been telling me."

"Yeah, I guess I have. But I'm a little afraid at how fast it's all spilling out, and how I feel like, whoa, that's about as much as I can handle at one time."

"So we will need to be sensitive about how fast things are happening in here to make sure you can take this in and not be overwhelmed by it. Can you let me know how that's going for you?"

"Yeah. It's tough because things 'back up' during the week, and I come in here and I feel the floodgates open and feel relieved. But that opening conjures up all kinds of new stuff too."

———

Our sessions slowly changed after this. Over the following weeks Theresa seemed less hesitant, less interested in attenuating and monitoring her words and expression. Her face became increasingly expressive of the emotions and thoughts she related. It looked to me like her depression was beginning to lift and that she had more energy. Most of all, her eyes became less shielded and enigmatic. The stillness had given way to reflect the human presence behind them. They occasionally lit up with anger or excitement, or shone with appreciation and satisfaction when our meeting served to bring out what she described as the "pearls." These were sessions in which our talks enabled her to touch on parts of herself that she disallowed expression in all other contexts, even to herself. She had also thrown herself into her interests again. She began teaching her meditation classes and reengaging in her "women's studies" graduate curriculum at a local university. There, she was encouraged to explore other religious traditions, and she began helping to organize a series of lectures on comparative religion.

"I've been lying to you," she offered one session three months into our twice weekly sessions.

"How so?"

"Well, not exactly lying, but hiding from you parts that I still can't bring myself to talk about. No, that's not right either. I've been kind of showing you parts that are real but that keep you, and everyone else, from seeing the really ugly parts."

"The parts that you think I won't approve of."

"No, somehow I know now that you won't punish me, though everyone else would; it's more the parts that will, I don't know . . . that will *disillusion* you with who I am. It's that same thing, of wanting approval. But that's not right either. I thought that if I value all the things I want to be, all the things I'm working on in here, that this other part won't even *exist* . . . it will be gone. But last week I found out it's not gone."

"Something happened that let you know there are other parts of you seeking expression, and that surprised you."

"I don't know about surprised . . . just that have been dormant for a little while and have come back full force. Part of it is that I went barhopping last week. It's something I used to do quite a bit when I drank a lot. But I didn't drink; that wasn't a big deal. In my *past life,* before the crisis house, I did it a lot. I'd go over to a world, you know, that is this whole different world than the one I move in, with the nuns and all," she laughed. "I guess I've always gravitated to the wild guys, you know. I know where to find them. So I went out again. I don't know what it was. I thought I had gotten past it. It's too costly to the soul. Some bad things have happened in the past, but I somehow find myself driving down to Georgetown. I put on my sexiest dress, and it's like I'm this different person. I'm brash and 'out there,' and I get into my seduction process, and then things get kind of crazy."

"Your seduction process?"

"Yeah, I have a method," she said with a grin. She straightened up as if assuming a teaching stance to a group of students. First, you make eye contact to get him to come over to you. That's like turning the magnet on a guy. You can get him from across the room. He always comes over.

Then you engage in conversation and flirt just enough to keep him guessing, that's point two. Then, if you decide he's acceptable, you drop the remark."

"The remark?"

"Yeah, like guys say such stupid stuff when they're trying to seduce you. They might say, 'You sure look good in that red dress,' and I'd say the remark, like 'I look a helluva lot better out of it.'"

"Okay, that's point three; you make that one up as you go," I said, a little startled as I adjusted to this shift in Theresa's whole presentation.

"Yeah, I improvise. Then you go in for the kill: initiating physical contact . . . like putting your hand on his arm, or even leaning over and kissing him or something. After that, you don't really need a plan. Of course the whole process might take 30 minutes or a whole evening."

"Very scientific."

"Works every time."

A pause. "Theresa, as you describe your seduction process, you look—What's a good word?—almost *mischievous*. Your laugh comes back, and there's a tone of irony in your voice. I get the feeling that you look at yourself 'out there' from this vantage point in here, and you are amused and maybe a little baffled."

"Yeah, and 'out there' is kind of how I feel when I'm doing it. It's me and not me, and I look at it from in here, and I'm like, whoa!"

"You can hardly put the two together."

"Exactly."

"But you mentioned something else that doesn't fit with your sense of amused irony."

Theresa cocked her head and looked into my eyes. Had she ever looked at me so directly before? There was a suddenly reflective look on her face, the mischievous look left her eyes and they narrowed in an expression that made her face look suddenly serious and wise. The smile resolved to an almost imperceptible shadow of itself.

"Too costly to the soul," she said quietly. I let her remark hang in the air.

"Yeah," I said after a moment. "That seemed to contrast with the thrill of the hunt. I wonder how that fits in?"

"It doesn't fit in; that's the other side of it. You know, after, and you think, 'What in hell am I doing here?' There's another part of you that realizes that you're in some strange hotel room with some jerk with alcohol on his breath, and he doesn't even see you because he's done with you. And you think . . . I don't know, there's just a sense of nausea about it."

"Nausea."

"Yeah," she paused. "And one time I got myself into real trouble when I went with a guy out on his boat. It was late at night, and he brought his friend from the bar along, and it was all high hilarity, you know, racing around in his powerboat. But then he wanted me to have sex with both of them at once, and I refused," her gaze dropped to her lap. Then he said, okay, he would have to drop me off on shore then. I looked and all I could see was trees on the shore, just a house light here or there. I didn't know where in the hell I was, it was the middle of the night, and I was drunk. So I did it." She paused, raised her head from her lap, and looked up at me sadly. "Too costly to the soul," she said.

"So the seduction plan works well on one level, but when it comes down to it, it seems like it ends up costing you too much. It's a thrill at first, but you come away feeling unnourished, sometimes even coerced. It's as if you want to get close to a man, and that seems like it might be a way. But, Theresa, it also seems like there is a lot to do with power here. It's as if you feel that you can control a man with your prowess, with your sexuality."

"Damn it. Yeah, I guess it does. It's like I have to have control. I have to make sure I have the power. But sometimes that gets all blown to hell. I try to get some reins on this horse, but he keeps bucking," she said with a cynical laugh.

"I like your metaphor. Without thinking, tell me what horse you would most like to rein in . . . where you feel most dominated in your life."

"My father."

"You would like to get some reins on him?"

"Oh yeah . . . but then I would just tie him to a post and get out of town, and he couldn't follow me."

"As he did when you tried to move away and your parents moved to be near you."

"Yeah, and when you say that I had this thought, or impression, of something that happened yesterday. He had been drinking and was talking to someone on the phone about his daughters, and I was in the next room. He mentioned my name, and then said, 'Yeah, she's the good looking one.' And I just felt my stomach clench up real tight."

"Nausea."

"Not quite, but close."

"I mean there's a parallel process between what you just related and what you said before. You wind up in some strange place with a guy with alcohol on his breath; your seduction hasn't worked out by giving you power over the situation. Instead you end up with a feeling of help-lessness. It's as if you take this seemingly insoluble problem—you don't have any control in your relationship with your father, and there's some incestuous overtone to how he prefers your company to your mother, and you are his favorite daughter, and that makes you feel very uncom-fortable—and you try to work it out elsewhere, as if these other situa-tions are equivalent. Maybe all those other horses you are trying to get reins on aren't the one horse you want to subdue and tie up to a post."

"God, as you say that I kind of feel it right now."

"That tightening of the stomach."

"Yeah, it's strange because I think I would miss . . . this is hard to say . . . I think I would miss being my father's favorite because I want him to love me, and I know he does. But I can't stand the way it plays out, and I don't get what I need anyway. And Jesus Christ, I'm 47 years old; it's not as if I'm his adoring little girl anymore, so now it's all twisted. It's as if I bring it to all these other relationships, even ones that don't have anything to do with it."

"You are thinking of one now?"

"Yeah, even when I went to a meditation retreat to get away, I seduced my counselor. I mean, how far can I go with this? Even when I try to get away, I create the same thing."

"A counselor?"

"Well, he was more like an instructor; they're not real counselors."

"It's not something where you feel he crossed some kind of line."

"No, I knew what I was doing. That poor guy didn't know what hit him."

These conversations seemed to unleash, in the following sessions, a torrent of hostility: toward her father, toward her ex-husband, toward men in general. She gave vent to rage toward men as inconsistent, unre-liable, sex crazed, and self-absorbed. She railed against patriarchal reli-gion, sexual objectification of women, and the politics of power. She had had enough of the company of men. Theresa wanted to be with women who "run with the wolves," who celebrate their pagan sensibili-ties as givers of life with one another, who own their power.

The women in her graduate classes partly understood these things, but she longed for more. I could see clearly the split in her inner organi-zation between what she called the "spiritual" self and the woman of the methodical seduction process. She was not unaware of the discontinuity: "Studying women's issues, feminism and spirituality by day, and looking for the bad boys at night in the bars," she said ruefully. She hated men. I was the only man, she said, that she could bear to talk to right now.

I observed to her the split and told her I understood her reactivity, the sources of her rage as she struggled to recapture her own life from a family history of subtle and not so subtle bondage.

A few sessions later, however, Theresa's tone had changed. In addition to articulating how the "too close" relationship with her father had interfered with her becoming independent and able to form close ties with others, she also said that she had gotten a "reality check" to her negative view of men. She saw a television special in which imprisoned rapists were interviewed about how they thought about their victims. Theresa was appalled to realize that the objectification and depersonalization that they described resembled quite closely her own "use him and lose him" attitude toward her sexual partners. "It was like I could experience both the victim and the perpetrator's perspective," she said. She began to wonder, she said, what it might be like to revive an old wish of her younger years—to have a close relationship with a man that included real love and connection.

"You know, Theresa, as you talk about your feelings toward men, I wonder that you have chosen me, a male therapist, to do this work."

"Yeah, I thought about that too. It's like, why would I choose one of 'the enemy.' But you are the only man I feel I can talk to. Sometimes I feel myself wanting to fight with you, or contend, you know, like when you are putting something out there that's hard for me to hear. Sometimes I feel I'm standing on the edge of a precipice, but somehow it's okay. Somehow I trust you. I can't believe I can even say that."

"I'm glad you trust me. You know, in all these other areas of your life with men it seems like sex is a big part."

"Yeah," she smiled, "this is the one relationship I have with a man where sex is not a part of it."

"That's what I'm getting at. I wonder, do you think your four-point plan could work on me? That you might be able to seduce me as you have others?"

"I thought about that when we started, you know, but I didn't care. But after this started to become important to me, I thought of the danger of that and how that would just mess everything up when I'm trying to get out of this depression and get back on my feet. But, no, you're like a rock. I feel safe in here."

"I'm glad. We both know that part of why this relationship can be so powerful is that it has this boundary around it, and though sex had been a part of your other relationships, you have a sense that it would screw everything up, pardon the expression, if it intruded on this relationship."

"Yeah, I know it would. It's a relief to have that not be a possibility."

"How do you feel about me asking you about it?"

"Good, like it's just underscoring what is really here. It makes me trust you even more. You know, my mother's health is really failing now. I feel myself wanting to get away from it, and I feel all this guilt about it. I don't want to be stuck with my father. And there's this other piece: I wish she could have the experience I'm having now, that she could come to our sessions and get her own life to be more fulfilling. I even mentioned it to her, and she said, 'It's too late for me, honey.' That's really sad."

She revealed at this time that for a number of years she had been having an ongoing affair with a married man she liked. It was having a "man at a distance, there when I want him, gone when I don't," but that it felt like the only "respectful" relationship in her life that provided an outlet for her sexual desires that was "not so destructive" as her barhopping adventures.

"I wonder why you didn't mention this before?"

"I guess I was afraid that it might be taken away somehow . . . that talking about it might mean that I had to give it up."

"That I might say, 'This is no good for you, you'd better quit that.'"

"I suppose so. And maybe I'm just assigning that to you when it really belongs to me, because sometimes I want to. I mean, what the hell good is it to have a relationship that only comes out at night. Here I am, this nice little mistress, never making any waves, there when he wants and making few demands. And, of course, he's there when I want too . . . sometimes."

I could see that Theresa was still tentatively revealing herself to me. Each time she made some new disclosure, she feared I might disapprove, judge, or condemn her, and give her advice as her father would. She took new strength from our meetings when I did not behave as she expected but rather kept our conversations focused on illuminating her feelings, thoughts, choices, and motivations.

"There sure is a familiar pattern here."

"I knew you were going to say that," she said with an ironic laugh. "And yeah, I do that with my father . . . bend all my needs to his, clean his house for money, go with him to church and take his notes as he pretends to be a big shot with all of them in the running of the church . . . there when he needs me. It becomes more and more apparent to me how *all* my other relationships, especially with men, are expressing some part of this piece of never having really gotten away. Even my mother, you know. She calls at seven o'clock in the morning and says, 'Are you still in bed?' and the crazy thing is I feel guilty!"

"It's tough to be a 40-something-year-old woman who has to feel guilty about sleeping past seven."

"Yeah, and like how I'm so tuned in to my father's needs that all he has to do is make a motion with his hand when he's talking to his church constituents, and I know what he wants, like a pen or something, and I'm right there."

As her mother's health failed, something happened that proved a turning point in Theresa's willingness to maintain the status quo. Our therapeutic relationship continued to mature and deepen, and a fluidity, trust, openness, and immediacy charged the sessions with energy. A genuine feeling of affection had been growing up between us, and our sessions sometimes were lighthearted, sardonic, and full of banter as I challenged and confronted her or we uncovered some aspect of her life that was absurd or ironic. Just as often, our sessions were deeply felt, serious, difficult, and full of pathos. Theresa's mother was dying, and she felt her loss profoundly. At the same time, she feared further assuming her mother's role with her father. And now he wanted to draw her into a secret pact to keep from the other family members that he did not want the doctors to take any more measures to keep her alive. He wanted, he said, to let her die with dignity.

"So now, here I am, stuck with one more secret. What? You've got this look on your face . . . just say it."

"Horseshit."

"What?" she said with a laugh.

"You know *what;* you are setting me up to say it to you. I'm not buying it. You know you can change the rules anytime you want to."

Her face got suddenly serious. "There's something about this situation that *is* different. I mean, as I've been getting back on my feet, and my depression has faded so much, I have been shaking things up some, and he has resisted and complained and thrown his fits where he gets in a bad mood and drinks and even chides me for not drinking. I even yelled at him, 'How many people have to die in this family before we look at the role of alcohol in our problems,' and he said, 'Just one.' My heart practically stopped, and I said, 'Who me?' and he said, 'No, me.' It's like any change is impossible to contemplate, but something about this is different. I can't carry these secrets anymore . . . I'm so god-damned sick of it!" she said with uncharacteristic vehemence, and it was the first time I had heard her use anything other than mild profanity.

Some force had been slowly collecting in Theresa like a small stream filling a reservoir. I had not been aware as I observed her depression give way to a sense of increasing energy and vitality that some inner source of vital power had been slowly pooling, rising, and now was ready to be released. Then Theresa opened the floodgates.

She adamantly refused to keep her mother's medical treatment a secret from the rest of the family. She explained to her father that she no longer wanted to clean his house, and when he balked and put a guilt trip on her, she defiantly refused. She worked extra hours because she declined his financial "assistance" (more like indenture, she said). She quit going to his church, and instead revealed to him (and to me) that in addition to her women's studies she was pursuing a long-time interest in "alternative" religions that her father derided as "new age."

In the following months her clothes became more colorful, flowing, and draped about her in folds. I could see that a faith that seemed to her completely outside the realm of her father's experience was appealing to her, and that her religious interests seemed reactive as a means of differentiation. She challenged her father to seek help for his alcoholism. She presided over her mother's death in her own way, sharing with her all of the new things she was propelling herself into, and her mother was happy for her. When she died, Theresa broke with the somber funeral rites her father wanted and introduced poetry and music into the ceremony. When her father gave her all of her mother's clothes and pestered her to wear one of her dresses that he particularly liked, Theresa took every garment to a local charity, and despite her father's outrage, gave them away. He ridiculed her involvement in therapy and blamed the therapy for "filling her head with psychological crap."

Her long delayed rebellion culminated in a ferocious argument in which she articulated openly what she insisted were the destructive rules that secretly governed their lives. She wanted no more of it, she said, and was going to live life on her own terms, whether he liked it or not. He didn't like it. After this argument, Theresa struggled mightily with her guilt over "killing off the family." She felt as if she were betraying everyone who was close to her. She imagined as she drove away from the sessions that a lightning bolt would come down from the

sky and strike her dead. But she held her ground, and to her amazement, her father adjusted somewhat to the changes. He didn't disown
her or excommunicate her from his life. Though he refused to acknowledge any problem with alcohol, he did admit that he was prone to bullying her, dominating those who were closest to him, and said he had
been overbearing for too long to change now. They would all just have
to find a way to forgive him and get over it. But somehow in all of this
(Theresa thought the death of her mother had revealed a new vulnerability in him) he managed to find a way to express to her and her siblings that he loved them. For Theresa it was a victory, and to her own
surprise, she found herself tentatively loving him back.

Months went by, and Theresa hit her stride. She was making new
plans and became increasingly involved in her educational pursuits,
helping to bring in new speakers at her school and organizing meditation classes. I tracked her growing independence, efficacy, and ability to
be reflectively self-aware. I remembered the lump of clothes that had
once sat in the chair where now sat an articulate and animated person. I
realized that Theresa was one of the most engaged, interested, and capable clients I had ever seen. I certainly looked forward to our meetings.
Though I realized that her continuing idealization of me would eventually give way to disillusionment, I did wonder if this were not one way
in which I had allowed her to seduce me. She credited me with ushering
her into a new life.

"I felt like I had to walk into this great dark cave in me, and
you knew how to help me to do that. And I've come out the other side,"
she said.

Though I continually reminded her that it was her hard work
that had made our sessions valuable, I felt pride in our work and in
her progress.

Theresa's idealization of me took a hit, however, when she found her
vitality giving way, once again, to bouts of depression. Sometimes our
sessions no longer helped. Sometimes she left feeling like she did in
early sessions: confused, alienated, asking more questions than she had
answers for. She seemed fitful, frustrated, as if she wanted me to do
something for her that she could not do herself. She got angry with me

for "letting the genie out of the bottle and not knowing how to get the cork back on." She thought of quitting therapy.

"It's too much. I'm sick of struggling and fighting, walking into this darkness. At least before I could run away, but now I don't know how to get away from myself. I've destroyed everything I knew, and I'm walking blind."

But these periods alternated with her sense that she could make new choices. Over time she understood, she said, that not only were these depressive episodes no longer incapacitating, they had a certain utility. Her depressive dips let her know "where the work is" and served as a barometer of how well she was "paying attention."

"I know when I'm getting depressed that it means that something is looming and I don't feel ready to deal with it yet. Then, if I do, I get a breather."

She found herself being better able to tend to her inner states without my being there to help her. She noticed a decreasing sense of dependence on me, but felt a growing equality, partnership, and mutuality. Through our many sessions she had gotten to know me as a real person. It was reassuring, she observed, to know that I was a person who had to face my own growth struggles, who had feet of clay, and in that sense was just like her. I wasn't cut out of some other material.

In one session, about six months into therapy, Theresa began, "So I'm taking this class called Sexuality and Spirituality," she said, returning to the theme from our earlier conversations.

"I imagine that if you titled the class it would be called Sexuality *versus* Spirituality," I replied, thinking that since the subject had come up again it was time to more directly address this part of her inner world that was fragmented and conflicted.

"Wow . . . yeah, wow. God. I guess to put it like that kind of brings up all kinds of stuff. It's not easy to hear."

"You hadn't put it like that to yourself, and it shakes you up a bit to hear me say that."

"Yeah, but it's true. For me they are two different worlds. Tell me what you see in me about that."

"Just that. I have the impression that in the past sexuality and spirituality have been mutually exclusive. It's as if you have these two regions in your experience. You cultivate this meditative and artistic sensibility, you study women's issues and empowerment, but your erotic self seems disconnected from the things that are important to you there. I guess I've wondered what it would be like for you to be sexual and intimate with someone in a relationship. Maybe that's what I mean: How are sexuality and intimacy connected for you?"

"The first thing that I think is, shit, I hear what you're saying and it's right on."

"But . . ."

"But I want to be farther along, you know; this is an area that hasn't kept up with all this other growth, and, I mean, how could it? I haven't even been paying attention to 'man' issues because I'm too busy. I guess I thought I could take this class and clear it all up," she said with a laugh.

"Well, as you contemplate it now, are there places in your life where you can locate this conflict?"

"Well, of course in my barhopping exploits, though right now that seems like another life in the past; I have no desire for that. But I think about my relationship with my ex-husband. When we would have sex it was like I wasn't, or couldn't be, there. There was something just so oppressive about it. It was like 'sex on demand,' regardless of how I felt about it, and even though we were married, it's almost as if it was like rape, not intimacy. I guess I am just so reactive to any sense of intrusiveness you know. I learned to be detached, almost out of my body when it was happening, and I thought, 'How can I dislike and have sex with my husband at the same time?' We didn't last long after I realized that. I think it was probably a legacy of my push-pull relationship with Dad, how intimacy with him was what I most wanted, but was what felt most dangerous and disruptive. God, I hate that so much of this stuff feels connected to that."

"It seems as if there were things going on in your marriage that might make intimacy dangerous, even if you didn't have this sensitivity with your father. But what about intimacy? Has there ever been a time when your sexuality seemed expressive of intimacy with someone, where the two were connected?"

"I used to think that I used sex to get intimacy, but after all this," she spread her arms to indicate the room we sat in, "I think it's more that I have used sex to *prevent* intimacy. It's a way of being close without being close. But now, I want these parts of me to all be connected. But it's terrifying. I don't want it to be sexuality versus spirituality, and intimacy with someone does seem to be the connector between these two worlds that I flip-flop back and forth in," she waggled her head as if she were being bounced back and forth like a rag doll. "And I've only been able to discover that these days with women . . . and that's new, this sense of being close and intimate with *anyone,* and somehow that's happening with important women in my life now. It's so fantastic and new. I wished the other day that I could be a lesbian, you know; it would all be so much easier. I'd be done! I'd have intimacy and sex in one place. But I'm not attracted to women sexually . . . bummer huh . . . in fact, I haven't been sexually attracted to men for a few months now. It's as if something's just been turned off. I see a guy looking at me, and I just don't want to play anymore. It all seems so pointless."

It was now our seventh month of therapy. For the previous couple of months our work had focused on issues of independence, autonomy, her blossoming relationships at school, and her future plans and new possibilities. She was distressed to realize that her sister was now increasingly taking over her previous role with her father; doing his laundry, cleaning the house, and even contemplating moving in with him.

"It's as if she can't even see it. She doesn't know what she's walking into. It's as if I left this big void, and now she's going to step into it and get her life sucked away."

"I wonder if you feel any sense of remorse for having given up that role, or any sense of jealousy that she is now filling it," I challenged her.

"Ha! She can have it," she laughed. "The only remorse I feel is that if I had stayed in it she would be spared, and I care about her. But I want to say to her: 'Run for you life!'" she laughed. There is so much good stuff happening for me right now. I had this amazing meeting with this woman I've wanted to meet and get to know better. She has this kind of self-possession and sense of herself that she can speak her own truth, you know, and not worry about every little reaction that someone might have. She has what I've been slowly gaining in here, and I thought she is like a role model for me. I'd like to be more like her. Once she was talking about her husband, and there was such love in her voice, and I thought, wow, what must *that* be like, you know, to have that with a man. And I realized that I would have missed it before . . . that I never would have been open to that kind of spontaneous sharing that we had in that meeting with one another. I was kind of . . . I don't know . . . it was kind of bringing what happens in here out into the real world, and doing something different. I felt connected, like I do in here sometimes, you know?"

"Yes, I feel that too. We've come a long way together, haven't we, and I'm happy that this sense of connection is making it possible for you to go out into the 'real' world and feel this with others in your life. It's as if all kinds of new things are happening for you that you would never have expected . . . this sense of possibility."

"Yeah, we have come a long, long way." There was a long pause, and the silence seemed full of echoes of the words that we had just spoken. "So!" she suddenly exclaimed, "What's up with you?"

I laughed. "Well, that was quite a shift, what just happened there."

"Nothing, it's just that I haven't fully arrived with being able to sit in that kind of . . . what, I don't know. I guess it's that we're talking about it, not just experiencing it, and I like move in and out of this feeling when I stumble into this land that's more intimate, and not familiar. So, it's like I step into there, and I don't feel grounded yet."

"And you just said, sometimes we seem to connect with one another, and this makes possible these new things with others. And, just now, there seemed to be that shared experience between us, and then the desire . . ."

". . . to retreat," she filled in the rest.

"Okay, that's a descriptive word, to retreat."

"And I did that with this woman too."

"Ah. I think it's important what you are saying, that you recognize this need to retreat. But I also think it's important to understand what that retreat is about . . . to get at the feelings and thoughts involved with what that retreat means."

"So the retreat would be . . . God, this is hard . . . I guess an aborting of any feelings of closeness or caring or appreciation. It's like this picture (on the cover of her journal). There are four hearts, and each one is less obscure than the one before it. So up here is the part that is very protected, and here it is wide open. So these two obscure hearts feel safer, for whatever reason. And recently I've had glimpses of this unobscured heart. But I still feel some reluctance to have this open heart to you, or to anyone, although I've had glimpses of it, which is why the meeting with this woman was so great. But somehow to stay there. I don't know enough about it to stay there."

"And I don't know that anyone can stay there," I offered.

"Whew!" she said, her eyes widening.

"That's a relief to you?"

"I was just thinking that when you said it, but it was good to hear you say it. I just need to deal with this fear of going there at all; my stumbling on this sense of connection. Like moments of . . . I don't know."

"Grace?" I offered.

"Exactly! But there is something noticeable when you have a moment of grace. It sets up . . . it puts other things in motion. So the chances of having another one are much more possible. So, it's like there's no going back. And that's where this teetering comes in. It's like this limbo, and it's much more familiar to be back in the closed heart position. But that's not my desire anymore, because once you have a glimpse of the future, it's like you are propelled toward that. It's like the in-between of letting go of the comfort, and allowing for the stretch, but there's nothing to base it on."

"Nothing to base it on but the new experiences themselves, and deciding whether to trust them or not."

"Yeah, I've got no reference points, like from my family or past relationships, for any closeness that's not going to cost you."

Over the following sessions I noticed something different in our conversations. Theresa occasionally seemed to lose her train of thought, pause, and try to resume where she had left off. At other times, even when I thought our sessions were going very well because they were immediate and present focused, a distracted look would pass over her face, and I felt suddenly alone in the room. These bumps in the conversation, which looked like brief periods of dissociation to me, were very different from the earliest sessions when Theresa's depression seemed to draw her away from any external contact. Now these brief periods of blankness looked like an *interruption* from some other corollary process not accessible to her in the moment. Of course, I noted my impression to her. She observed that sometimes our sessions triggered so many thoughts and feelings that she was flooded with the deluge and had to take a second to choose which of them to give attention.

I accepted her explanation, and, as I had throughout our work, encouraged her to give voice to all of these associations, even if they were only half formed or didn't seem to make any sense. She agreed that she would try to remain in touch with her inner process during these moments.

A few sessions later, however, Theresa again became distracted in our session.

"I'm sorry, I'm just a little dizzy."

"Would you like a glass of water?"

"No, I'm okay, it's nothing, I'm just really tired."

I wasn't buying it. "I think maybe something else is going on," I said.

"What do you mean?"

"What was going on for you right before you began to feel dizzy?"

"Well, to tell you the truth, you were responding to something I had said, and I wasn't listening to you. Your mouth was moving, but I couldn't really pay attention to what you were saying."

"Yeah, I get that a lot." We both laughed. "Before that happened, when you couldn't pay attention, you were talking about the new job, and how you loved what you were doing now, and feeling that it was *really yours,* and a result of choices you had made on your own, and you looked proud of yourself."

"Yeah."

"So, you looked okay, and then something happened, after I started talking. What did I say that . . ."

"You didn't say anything," she interrupted. She looked agitated. "I didn't even hear what you said."

"Theresa, I feel like you know more than you are saying to me."

"You *looked* happy for me . . . you were just taking in that I was proud, and you looked pleased for me, and it was uncontrived and natural, and you probably weren't even aware of it."

"Ah, you saw that in my face . . . and something happened."

"I was touched that it mattered to you, and felt grateful that I could bring this to our conversation, and then just felt this big 'whoosh' you know, and I got a little dizzy, and my hands got kind of tingly, and then numb."

"I have the sense that there's more in that 'whoosh' than meets the eye, so to speak. It touched you that I shared this triumph with you."

"Yeah, I guess it's that old thing of feeling close to someone and how I have to work up to allowing someone to know me."

"What else?"

She regarded me with a rueful eye. "In those moments I feel . . . I'm getting a little dizzy again."

"You're fine, a little dizziness is all right in here."

"I feel really affectionate toward you, and sometimes when I feel that affection . . . I have this sense of panic, almost. It scares me."

"It scares you that you feel so connected with me." I knew what was going on now, and as I gently coaxed her to continue, I wondered why I had not fully known it before. "Tell me more about that sense of panic.

It is not that you just feel affectionate toward me because you have expressed that to me before."

She looked at the floor, then out the window across the field where the water tower stood next to the train tracks. The train was going slowly by, birds were diving down to snatch bits of grain from the deck of a car. A man hung off the last caboose, swinging his hat for the traffic to resume as the red and white bar blocking the traffic swung back up. "Is that a passenger train?" she asked.

"Sorry, it's a freight train; it's not for you."

"Too bad." A long silence. "Okay, I'm going to give this a try." She closed her eyes for a moment and took a breath. Was she shaking slightly? "I've been having these dreams," she said, opening her eyes, but turning her head and looking out the window as she spoke. "I've been having these dreams that you and I are, you know, sexually involved. And they're really real feeling, and I wake up in a panic because I have this terrible feeling of shame, and that I can't undo it, and I think, 'great, now I've irrevocably screwed this up too . . . the one place where I might have some chance of getting my life back.'" She seemed to be hardly breathing. There was a long pause, but I didn't sense that she wanted me to respond to what she had revealed. She turned her gaze from looking out the window and looked at me. "Sometimes, when you are so tuned in to what's going on for me," she continued, "it's new, you know, and I feel this affection for you, and then I get panicky."

"Theresa, I can see that talking about this is difficult for you. Hang in there with it. Say more about that panicky feeling when you feel a sense of affection for me. It seems to come up, you said, when I seem to be particularly attuned to you and we share something."

"Yeah, you know, those moments of grace. And I sometimes want to back off from that, 'cause it's just so right there, and the sense of panic follows that affection."

"But you mentioned these sexual dreams you've been having that seem to be related to this sense of affection but also to the sense of panic . . ."

"Yeah, because that sexual part is sometimes right behind it . . . that feeling of connection and affection, and that's new . . . I mean that the sexual feeling would follow, or be combined with the affection part. I just feel like I don't know how to handle that. I feel like I'm going to mess it all up . . . that I *have* messed it all up."

"By telling me this, you feel as if it's all messed up."

"Yeah, now it's out there." She sounded dejected.

"If you are feeling connected and affectionate with me, and there's that sense of sharing, you sometimes feel sexually attracted to me . . . that's when you get dizzy."

"And I try to shut that off really quickly because I don't want that here," she interrupted, her speech pressured. Suddenly she was agitated again and looked like she wanted to climb out of her own skin. "At the first sign of it, I kind of shut off. I think that's where that sense of distraction comes from. Sometimes my hands get tingly and kind of numb."

"So that's where that dizziness and numbness come from too, as you try to shut those feelings down, when you are feeling *both* affectionate and sexually attracted." This reflection, and the fact that her disclosures did not alter my calm and receptive demeanor, seemed to help her recover her composure.

"Yeah! That's a good point. If I just felt one or the other, I might know what to do with that. If it was just the sexual part, I could say, I know how to deal with that 'cause it would be over here," she made a pushing aside motion with her hands, "but combining that with this affection makes it seem really dangerous," and as she said this she thumped her chest resonantly above her heart with her open hand. I smiled inwardly at the directness of this gesture. "I mean these dreams have me all freaked out," she said, a helpless look on her face. "And I've been trying not to think of that when I come in here, so when it asserts itself when we're together, I just kind of pretend like it's not here." I had never seen so many emotions pass over her face in such quick succession as she revealed the different facets of her conflict.

"You know, Theresa, I think that maybe I too have been feeling that there's some sexual energy in the room and have unwittingly sent you a message somehow that we shouldn't talk about this like we are right now."

"How so? My heart is going like mad right now!"

"But you're not dizzy . . . we're talking directly about this."

"Yeah, that's weird. I'm not dizzy at all!"

"How about your hands? Are they tingly or numb?"

"No."

"That's important, remember that. Anyway, I think I was the one who called these special moments that happen in here between us 'moments of grace.' That kind of puts it in a spiritualized frame of reference. It apparently only captures one dimension of what is happening in the room. I wonder if we have *both* been colluding to ignore something we have both sensed but kept out of awareness."

"But they are moments of grace too," she objected feelingly. "There is a spiritual quality to that sense of sharing."

"Yes, there is, and I don't want to discount that. But you are also having some erotic feelings that are also a part of those moments, and that's important. It's something you are trying to ignore or repress, and you seem to be saying that that's where the dizziness and distraction is located."

"Well, I can't have those feelings in here!" she said, again suddenly animated and distressed. "I don't want to lose everything this has meant. I mean it's crazy. I'm feeling this where I least want to." She paused to collect herself, then said, "And you're *not even my type!*" There was a brief silence in response to this jarring segue, and we both laughed. Some of the energy of the moment seemed to diminish.

"Of course you can have those feelings in here, remember?" I said smiling. "You can have all of your feelings and impressions in here, and none of them are wrong or forbidden. But all of them are also open to explore."

"But this *always* messes things up for me!"

"You ascribe far too much power to your erotic impulses. Anyway, it's not what you feel that screws things up but how you act on those feelings. We both know that sex between us is not possible, and in terms of our work together, not desirable. You are well aware of how the two types of relationships are mutually exclusive."

"Yeah, that's why I can't understand why this has come up here, and in my dream life. I mean, are you saying that it's okay for me to have these feelings toward you, because of the safety of this relationship?"

"That's exactly what I'm saying. I'm also saying that like all the other feelings you've had in here, including other feelings about me, that they're important and meaningful, and I'm sorry that I might have sent you a message that they are not allowed."

"I don't think you sent me that message, but I'm happy to share any blame! God, my mind is racing . . . but I'm not dizzy or distracted! I'm all here! I feel a sense of relief, but I don't know why. I thought that if we talked about this . . . I don't know. I had a sense of dread about it. I wonder how you're hearing this. You're a man, right?"

"Last time I checked. What, do you think that because I'm a man I couldn't maintain any perspective here if you brought this up? Theresa, for a moment I want to set your fear about these thoughts and feelings aside, and tell me why you would hate to give them up. How are they important to you? What would it feel like if you lost them?" This was a pretty big shift, and probably a little premature, but it also communicated that I was sincere about her being allowed to bring all her fantasies, feelings, and thoughts into our relationship.

"You're liking this, right?"

"I know it may sound like that, but because you are feeling so much trepidation about telling me this I think maybe you are not speaking to the other part of it. What about your dreams and sexual feelings toward me speak something important to you?"

"Yeah, I didn't mean to be flippant." I waved her statement away with my hand, and tilted my head in an intent listening attitude. She reflected silently. "I don't know, but as you say that, as scared as I am, I do think that something valuable is there. I would feel a loss because, I have to admit, it's nice to feel a kind of aliveness too. I have been so muted and only half there. It feels new. But it's because it's in here . . . I don't know. Maybe on some level I both fear and hope that you feel some erotic attraction toward me. You don't have to respond to that," she said jokingly.

"You are afraid that I would feel some erotic attraction toward you . . . that would feel pretty dangerous?"

She pondered this. "I thought so, but now that you've said it, somehow it doesn't seem as ominous." She sat, seemingly absorbed in contemplation of this.

"Where are you? It looks like you were pondering that just now."

"Yeah, I realize that I'm afraid of my father's quasi-sexual stuff, and also of messing up this relationship between you and me, but these are two different fears with different causes. I shouldn't fear it if you felt attracted to me because I trust you to have your feelings but also to be honest with me and take care of this relationship. I think I just peeled those two fears apart, and now I don't need one of them."

"That's a great insight to have."

"Wow, it feels like a different kind of 'whoosh,'" she said, a look of excitement in her face, "like a relief. I feel like I can ask you about it and be okay with whatever you feel."

"Then let me tell you how I feel. I feel a lot of affection for you. I often feel very close to you and that we have a deep sense of sharing. I really value you and our travels together in here. I'm not aware that I'm feeling an erotic attraction for you. Has there been anything about my words or demeanor that has made you feel otherwise?"

"No, but now that I've asked you, I feel like that part is maybe something that is connected to how I fear that something funny is in the air with my dad, yet I have liked that I'm the special one with him. Just as I have wanted to feel important to you."

"Ah." I paused. "You mentioned that you feared and hoped that I might feel an erotic pull, how is it to hear from me that I'm not feeling the same erotic attraction here as you are? I wonder whether your ego's not a little dinged on hearing me say I'm not feeling that?"

"You know, somehow it's not. Perhaps because I hear what I really want to hear, and perhaps most fear not hearing: That you care for me . . . and as I say it wondering if you've felt a sexual attraction seems frivolous. It somehow makes it easier to contemplate your question about what in this is important and valuable to me." She paused, took a deep breath and exhaled. She closed her eyes, and I watched her face.

After a moment, a sad look took shape there, and I said, "A sad look just passed over your face, talk to me."

"I was just thinking that so much of life has passed me by, and my marriage turned to shit, and my relationships with my father and men have been problematic for a long time. And in here is the only place where I have had a really good relationship with a man, or at least the most important place. And here is the one place where it can't be sexual, but it's the one place where, because there is so much understanding and communication, it *should* be sexual . . . you know. Not that I want it to be in reality, but that I wish I had a relationship like this on the outside where affection and sexuality and spirituality were all part of the same relationship. That seems to be the feeling in the dream. I guess that's it; I want what I've experienced in here with someone else out there. Wow. I can't believe I just said that. I mean," she said, rare tears springing into her eyes, "that I really want that. I can't remember having, or even wanting, that feeling for a very long time. It's a sense of passage into something new."

"Isn't it wonderful that it's when you are feeling close to me and a sense of affection for me, that *that's* when you feel this upwelling of sexual desire. My god, Theresa, I think your sexuality and your spirituality may be coming together! I'm not even your type, but you are experiencing in our relationship here what you want out there. Something in you that has been long dormant has been brought back to life in the safety of this kind of relationship; in fact, I'll bet that it's precisely *because* you feel there is no possibility of sex between us that you have been able to reconnect your feelings with your erotic impulses . . . because it's safe. And your fear that your sexual impulses could destroy it all didn't come about. You can own those impulses and still be safe!"

She had listened intently to my unfolding interpretation, and tears had begun rolling down her cheeks when I emphasized how *wonderful* it was that her affection for me was connected to her sexuality. We sat together for a while in a "moment of grace," and each of us smiled, knowing that the other was thinking the same thing. Theresa broke the long silence saying, "I don't *happen* to be feeling any erotic attraction to you right now, even though *it would be okay* if some fantasy followed my affection for you!"

"Okay, I'm glad we've got that straight," I bantered. How *do* you feel right now?"

"I have that sense that I sometimes get when I dance or do yoga, like I'm completely focused and in tune with my body and my breath . . . like I live right here in this moment and this pulse. Like I'm all here."

"You look like you're all in one piece right now. That's a nice place to be."

"Yeah, it is. But I also feel a sense of something waiting . . . like I want to carry this into the rest of my life, and see how that changes things. I don't really know what that will look like, but I'm curious, you know, I don't know . . . to make it real out there. Sometimes it's hard to hang onto it out there. I tend to forget things that are so clear to me in here. But the two worlds are much closer together now."

"And will become closer still."

"Yeah," a long pause. "So, you don't have a brother do you?"

In the sessions immediately following, Theresa continued to speak about her erotic dreams and feelings toward me, but after a while this changed to exploring the world of her relationships in the rest of her life. She was surprised that sexual traumas she had experienced in her marriage were again brought to mind. She recalled periods of dissociation in sexual encounters when she could not reconcile her hostile and powerless feelings with the experience of being sexually involved. She felt proud that she had respected herself by leaving that relationship to become more independent, and she explored ways that she could now follow through fully on that impulse in other areas in her life. She described how she longed for some new "outside" opportunity to "practice" a deeper integration of her erotic and emotional self. It was as if in talking to me about her sexual feelings in our relationship enabled her to work through a fundamental conflict in a safe environment and consolidate something within her own identity.

Eventually, Theresa's erotic feelings toward me no longer possessed the same energy as before. Her feelings became not only available, but also eventually ordinary. After the first conversation about it, Theresa no longer experienced the distraction or dizziness that she had felt in previous sessions. The exploration of the themes in her dreams (which quickly diminished and then ceased) further illuminated Theresa's movement toward the integration of love, sex, spirituality, and trust. Though she could identify her relationship with her father as the primary and formative context for her conflicts around these issues, more than ever before, she took responsibility for how she chose to play these conflicts out in her own relations with others. She felt free, she said, to look toward initiating relationships, especially with men, with a greater confidence and self-awareness of what she was about. In fact, she was eager to try her newfound wings and enthusiasm.

Theresa ended her moratorium on dating and began accepting invitations from men. She quickly found the old seduction routine emerging in the interactions, but not from her. She was bored with that dance. Her criteria were different now, she said. Now she wanted a relationship with a man that had dimensions to it.

"So we're sitting at dinner, and he says, 'I'm not looking for anything difficult. I'm tired of difficult women.' There was a kind of patronizing feel to it, like 'this is how I want a woman to be.' I picked up my bag and said, 'good luck with that,' and left. I just walked right out, dinner half finished! It felt really good to know instantly, 'this is a dead end,' and 'this is one of the jerks.' You know, I could just see what this guy was all about."

Theresa's relationship with her father was also improving. As she set new limits and changed the rules, he was forced to respond, and though wary, she felt a reemerging affection for him as she felt more secure in her increasing independence from him. She said one session, "As I get my own life more and more, I think, 'What was I so afraid of in him?' I think I blew some things out of proportion because I hadn't done my own work by getting my own life. He seems to have almost shrunken physically, it's weird!"

One session I had the windows in the office open. It was the middle of spring, and a cool breeze blew down from the mountains and across the plowed fields beyond the city. The air was filled with the sweet smells of cultivation and the songs of returning birds. We both seemed at a loss for words but were comfortable and familiar with one another's silences.

"I've been thinking about it," she said, "I think I'm finished for a while, coming in here, I mean. Something is complete this time around, and it's as if I need to do some more living before I come back and begin again."

"It's been quite a journey, hasn't it?" I said, smiling.

"Yeah it has, and I know this is just one part of the trip, but I'm not going around in circles anymore. Can I come back when I need to?"

"You know you can."

But Theresa didn't come back. Nine months later I got a letter from her describing some of the changes she had realized over that gestation-like period. Over her father's strong objections, she moved to New Mexico to work in a food cooperative. The cooperative connected with a collection of organizations with alternative and holistic interests in nutrition, health, yoga, and personal development. She had met a man, a musician, who shared her vision for a relationship. She wrote, "I'm having to remind myself all the time to keep old fears from sabotaging my present joys. It's a full-time job, but so far, it's working! I remember how terrified I was to let myself even know many of the accessible things that now just seem like my particular 'soul work' to be in a relationship. Now I feel like I can mostly get back to all the parts of me, and at the same time hold this other person in my heart. It's quite a balancing act. I'm grateful that you were there to be my guide."

I was grateful too. Like most clients with whom I have felt a sense of deep participation, I felt privileged that Theresa allowed me into her inner world and that we became important to one another. The client often does not realize that, in this sense, the validation works both ways. I, too, feel fulfilled when a client allows me to participate meaningfully, and to help make a difference that matters. I, too, part with more than I brought to the encounter.

CASE TWO DISCUSSION
Transference and Countertransference

TRANSFERENCE IS A phenomenon that emerges in all therapeutic relationships. A therapist responds to client transference regardless of whether he or she recognizes it as such or accounts for its emergence from within a favored theoretical orientation. My work with Theresa illustrates the importance of recognizing the many ways in which clients enact not only their unconscious conflicts but also their characteristic ways of relating to others and their ways of interpreting their interior and exterior worlds.

The traditional view of transference involves the oft-observed phenomenon that clients import into their relationship with the therapist feelings, conflicts, and expectations that seem to pertain to important other figures in their life. The idea is that the client *distorts* the immediate relationship by attributing to the therapist characteristics, motivations, thoughts, and emotions that are expressive of the client's unconscious structural conflicts and history of interpersonal trauma (Brenner, 1973). Because of this phenomenon, the client begins to respond to the therapist in idiosyncratic ways that likely reflect how the client responds to other important figures. This can, of course, be confusing to the therapist who cannot see a basis in reality for the client's perceptions and behavior.

It is this gap between the therapist's and the client's perceptions that alerts the therapist to the emergence of transference material. The therapist experiences the client's perceptions of him or her as distortions of reality that are based in the client's past rather than grounded in the present relationship or behavior of the therapist. The manifestation of this "transference neurosis" gives the therapist important insights into the client's historical and structural issues. The therapist begins to understand the client's specific projections and the unconscious conflicts that these projections represent. The therapist also forms a view about the interpersonal world the client "comes from," and how the client experiences him- or herself and others. The particular qualities of the transference reveal the client's characteristic defenses and anxieties, which are the client's response to unconscious conflicts. If there is sufficient identification with the therapist and his or her aims, an alliance forms, and the therapist can collaboratively explore these aspects of the client's experience.

In this traditional model of transference, *interpretation* of the underlying unconscious conflicts is the intervention best suited to help the client gain insight and increase awareness. The more conscious of inner processes the client becomes, the less energy and activity will be invested in defenses like projection and the less the client will distort the therapist's intentions and expressions. The interpretation of the client's transference and the "working through" in the therapeutic dialogue of the issues that the transference represents move the client toward greater self-awareness and integration.

Like most concepts that originated in early analytic theorizing, the idea of transference has evolved. Clinicians have moved away from early formulations based strictly on Freud's idea that the therapist is a "blank slate" upon which clients project their unconscious conflicts. Although descriptive of some dimensions of the phenomenon, many modern theorists feel that the traditional model does not do justice to the client's legitimate experiences in the therapy relationship. Modern conceptualizations emphasize the interpersonal process and meaning making *between* therapist and client and attempt to account for the contributions each person makes in participation with the other.

The traditional model assumes that the client's transference is a distortion of what is real, which implies that the therapist has access to an objectivity or a reality that the client does not. Thus, for the working-through phase to be successful, the client must ultimately accept the therapist's view of the meaning of the transference as illuminated by the therapist's interpretations. But can a client's transference really be *exclusively* an unconscious projective manifestation of conflicts based *solely within* the client, and only with others in the past? In other words, can transference be understood apart from the present interpersonal process in which it takes place? The therapist, while hopefully gaining a dimensional understanding of the client's process, still has no access to an objective platform from which to make such assumptions. The client's transference distortions may be influenced by this present relational event with the therapist. As a participant-observer, the therapist is bound by the processes of mutual influence that characterize all relationships in which different subjective worlds come into contact with one another.

A potential problem exists when the traditional idea of transference is not contextualized by what we know about interpersonal processes and the principles of mutually influencing systems. The problem is that the client may sense that to make progress he or she must move closer to the *therapist's* understanding of what is valid and correct, potentially giving up important areas of legitimate self-experience. If the client must tacitly accept the therapist's transference interpretations without reference to how the client's experience emerges from the client–therapist encounter, parts of the client's inner world may become squelched and lost to view. As discussed in the case of Chloe (see Case 4), this creates a situation that may evoke the client's resistance or, if the client does not rebel, a "cure by compliance," as the client is inclined to accommodate the therapist's version of reality at the expense of his or her own (Stolorow & Atwood, 1992). In this sense transference and resistance are interrelated processes. The degree of resistance correlates with the transference activity being shaped by the quality of the therapist's empathy.

The idea of a cure by compliance is important for all models of intervention regardless of which dimension (cognitive, unconscious, behavioral, and so on) of the client is being addressed. Many people seeking therapy come from a history of development in relationships in which they were forced to make choices between remaining faithful to themselves or conforming to others' demands to an excessive degree, accommodating an "alien" reality to avoid interpersonal discord. For a child growing up with caregivers who are insufficiently attuned to the child's legitimate strivings, affects, and needs, the choice is between giving up these parts of the self or disrupting the essential relationships the child relies on for survival. Faced with such a choice, the child will almost always choose to preserve the important relationships and disown the parts of him- or herself that seem to be unwelcome or threatening to important others. But these forbidden aspects do not really go away. They represent essential core elements the child needs to be whole, and they are secretly preserved. Necessary but forbidden, these sectioned-off affects and strivings become the source of enduring inner conflict as the child grows into adulthood.

Clients with such an interpersonal history are particularly susceptible to a cure by compliance as they have already learned to disown or delegitimize their own thoughts and feelings. If the client's resurrected needs and strivings are appropriately reemerging in response to the therapist's accurate empathy, but the therapist fails to sufficiently understand or recognize the client's current experience of the therapist, the therapy may reenact the client's traumatic history. The essential point is that the therapist must guard against assuming that transference interpretations are unrelated to their own subjective processes, or that they are divorced from the client's legitimate subjective experiences of the therapist. Both client and therapist participate in a relational field from which neither one can remain detached. This is true even if the therapist naively attempts to maintain a "neutral" stance. Transference is inseparable from the mutually influencing relationship between client and therapist.

It should be apparent that when viewed systemically these transference phenomena transcend theoretical orientation. Whose frame of reference provides the starting point for change is relevant in any approach. For instance, a cognitive behavioral approach emphasizes that the client should substitute distorted ways of thinking and acting in favor of the therapist's model for what is real, adaptive, and productive. However, if insufficient attention is given to how the client's problems emerged from legitimate and valued constellations of self, then the therapist's well-meaning interventions confirm to the client that his or her disowned, shameful, or sectioned-off areas of self-experience should remain cloistered and hidden.

The second contemporary model of transference seeks to account for the above-mentioned criticisms of the traditional model. It rests on the idea that each person exercises a capacity to create an inner "working model" of reality. This model includes perceptions of self, others, and the world in general and is constructed from the individual's history of making meaning of experience. This constructivist position supports the idea of transference emerging from the organizing frames of reference that predispose the person toward certain interpretations. These organizing frames of reference are not ordinarily the focus of conscious awareness but are latent assumptions. They are "just the way the world is," the cognitive architecture for that person.

Piaget observed that each child is a "little scientist," developing and testing hypotheses at every turn (Piaget & Inholder, 1969). By the time the child reaches adulthood, the countless learning events have developed into a cognitive architecture, or schema. These interpretive models are constructed to represent experiences that stand for the real world (Bruner, 1990). But a person's internal map is a cognitive and experiential representation of our unique experiences. There is no one-to-one correspondence (as there is with a road map) between our individual map and an objective reality.

The client entering therapy brings a learning and experiential history that is both a source of stability and also of distress. Recognizing some features of the new situation with the therapist as similar to relationships in the past, the client will impose similar ways of making sense and meaning on the uncertain situation therapy represents (Stern, 1988). This form of transference is really an interpretive bias that the therapist experiences as the client not recognizing the unique features of the new situation or relationship. It is as if old learning is getting in the way of the new potential, keeping the person from responding with flexibility. The client does not form an accurate perception of the therapist and fails to recognize the new relational opportunity because of "hardening of the categories."

In contrast to the traditional definition, the contemporary definition of transference includes *all* of the client's perceptions and emotions toward the therapist, not just those springing from conflicts embedded in the dynamic unconscious of the client. Because the client's frames of reference are ordinarily not explicit and open to examination, part of therapy involves exploring how these underlying schema serve to organize all of the client's experience. As the schema become manifest in the new relationship with the therapist, the therapist assumes that these stand in for prototypic responses of the client in general. Making these underlying organizing principles the focus of awareness and intentionality is a central goal in therapy. Referencing and making overt the interpersonal process between therapist and client can best serve to achieve this awareness. As the therapist seeks to empathically engage with the client and understand the client's inner world, both look for a mutual ground of understanding and connection. But invariably there are many instances in which the client feels that the therapist's empathy has failed. It is often the ways in which the subjective worlds of therapist and client do not intersect easily that provide the greatest potential for therapeutic illumination as differences in interpretation and experience are made explicit.

Of course, the therapist also brings to the therapeutic meeting a set of personal organizing and interpretive principles that are just as subjective (though hopefully more thoroughly examined) as the client's. The therapist seeks to help the client recognize repetitive patterns of perception that likely influence all of the client's relationships, but this can only be offered from the therapist's subjective view of *what is happening* as their worlds collide and the mutual encounter unfolds. The therapist does not get to merely prescribe.

Countertransference, the reactions the therapist is having toward the client, can also be conceptualized along the traditional and contemporary dimensions I have outlined. The therapist may have unresolved conflicts that become unconsciously projected onto the client. Just as with client's transference, these unconscious conflicts may derive from the still charged remnants of past relationships, traumas, or developmental periods in the therapist's life. Something in the current relationship with the client may evoke these hidden parts of the therapist's inner world.

At another level, the therapist may simply be experiencing the client through perceptual frames of reference of which the therapist is not fully aware. These interpretive sets are not necessarily emotionally charged or derivative of the therapist's unresolved issues but are reflective of the therapist's way of perceiving others based on his or her unique interpersonal development and history. When a supervisor asks a therapist trainee, "What is your countertransference toward this client?" it is often this second definition of transference that is being referenced. The supervisor is asking, "What feelings, thoughts, and reactions are available to you as you recall sitting with this person? What sense are you making of the client?"

However, when the therapist finds that he or she is having a powerful reaction to a client that appears disproportionate to the situation, it is likely that the therapist is reacting less exclusively to the client and more to some internal process. Something about the client is evoking regions of self-experience that are ordinarily sequestered from the therapist's view. When the supervisor senses that the student therapist appears to be responding to the client from a suddenly reactive and emotionally charged perspective, the question "What is your countertransference?" asks the student therapist to set aside attempts at rational explanation and to wonder what associative links might exist between current feelings and other dimensions of the therapist's inner life. This dimension of countertransference is usually more difficult for the therapist to excavate and examine because it also involves the process of repression, not just an ability to shift perspective and accommodate an alternate view.

Theresa's case reveals that in reality these different dimensions of transference are not distinct and separate but rather are interactive and embedded in one another in the client's self-experience and expression. The unconscious schematic frames of reference and the dynamic unconscious processes are intertwined in the experience of the person. In Theresa's experiential world, for instance, men are described as sex crazed, unreliable, self-absorbed, and exploitative. This view constricted the kinds of new opportunities available to her as she negotiated the terrain of her interpersonal life. For her, this was simply "the way the world is," her interpretive map drawn from a long history of interpersonal events.

Theresa transferred these expectations to some degree into all new encounters, including those with the therapist. She doubted that I, as a male, could really be of use to her or that I would prove trustworthy. For example, her interpretation of my arriving late to our appointment meant that I was unreliable. Her resentment over being "powerless" in the face of my authority to negotiate an acceptable meeting time was an initial transference manifestation of this interpretive set. She hesitated to reveal aspects of her life for fear that I would punish her. Most important, she expected that I would certainly be susceptible to, and desirous of, seduction, and that the appearance of her erotic feelings would certainly cause this to occur. These transference reactions emerged from real events with me, not exclusively as projections from within her.

But underneath the terrain represented by Theresa's interpretive map lay dynamic conflicts with their origins in early developmental frustrations. These frustrations stemmed primarily from an emotionally incestuous, sexually tinged relationship with her father. Theresa learned early on to fear the association of intimacy and sexual feeling because her father was not "safe" to practice with. His own frustrations made him too likely to seek a gratification that felt "not quite right" to her. Her father's narcissistic demands that she be available to facilitate his needs squashed much of the movement Theresa made toward differentiation and autonomy. But Theresa had adapted, and her later sexual conflicts and acting out expressed her unconscious ambivalence around issues of control, sex, and intimacy. She gradually brought these legitimate but frustrated developmental needs into her relationship with me.

When I stifled a yawn or shifted in my chair, these seemingly inconsequential behaviors activated powerful transference fears that touched on these archaic core injuries. My behavior meant to Theresa that I must be bored with her, that she was not "special" or worthy of care. Later, when I became a real person to Theresa, not just "any therapist," she began to idealize me as a child does a parent. I was "the only man she could talk to," ideally empathic, and she began to desire my approval. These desires were based both in her sense that there was potential in the current encounter to restore her to greater wholeness and expressive of the archaic unrealized needs she brought to this encounter.

At one point I revealed to Theresa my own countertransference desire to gratify her need for reassurance. I wanted to tell her she was exceptional, extraordinary, and I wanted to soothe her longing. I feared, however, that this direct gratification would recapitulate her old patterns of relating on an "evaluation basis." In making my own processes explicit, I was aware that I was more directly influencing the relational event. I knew that our subjective worlds were being made explicit to one another in a way that illumined the transference as it constellated in the current moment. In other words, I explored the transference with her rather than gratified the transference desire. Also, this exploration in the context of our relationship heightened the trust between us. My disclosure was much more reality-based than merely giving her a sham respect, or interpreting her longing in reference only to her disappointment with her father.

Well into the therapy Theresa disclosed that she had not only been hiding from me but also actually not experiencing things she feared would *disillusion* me: "I thought that if I value all the things I want to be, all the things I'm working on in here, that this other part won't even exist . . . it will be gone. But last week I found out it's not gone." When

Theresa revealed this piece of transference (which is the flip side of ideal-izing me), I realized that a cure by compliance can almost be an implicit demand of therapy, that sectors of the client's world can become hidden from view in the transference. As the client seeks to embrace new thoughts and behaviors, it is natural to want to eschew old self-defeating ones. But it was Theresa's growing faith in the reliability of my attention and assurance that I would not treat her as her father had that enabled her to risk my disillusionment and show me parts that she herself wished to disavow. This is always a turning point in therapy, and it is at this point—when old ways of being conflict with new opportunities—that the strongest transference conflicts become manifest.

Theresa was aware that all her other relationships, "especially with men, expressed some part of this piece of never having really gotten away, but needing to be close." Her ambivalence about differentiation and intimacy manifested most in her erotization of a variety of needs and conflicts for which sex cannot possibly substitute. Frustrated in her attempts to address these issues in their rightful place, she collapsed her struggles in love, intimacy, control, and autonomy into a singular effort at adaptation through sex. Her seduction plan became the method by which she sought to redeem her losses, but she ended up fur-ther losing herself.

When Theresa became erotically attracted to me, two important transference processes were happening. The first is that she sought to express her dynamic conflicts with me in the same way she had with other men. If she could seduce me, then she would have dominated and controlled me in a way she had been unable to do with her father. In this sense, I was still a stand-in for her father, as were other men. But she was more aware of her sexual ploys through our work together, and she distrusted her manipulative impulses.

The second process expressed in Theresa's erotic transference with me more directly involved her emerging archaic needs and thrust toward growth. Her sexual attraction partly emerged in response to her percep-tion that I was proud of her—that I was spontaneously and genuinely celebrating her success and appreciating her. She felt grateful and affec-tionate toward me. These feelings gave rise to a sense of intimacy and connection with me and then to erotic feelings. This was the first time she could remember that her erotic feelings had been linked to feelings of affection. This was an effort at synthesis, integration, and growth. But she so valued our relationship that she couldn't allow this unwelcome and "destructive" erotic element, and so she attempted to repress it, causing the conversion symptom of dizziness.

Theresa had made real progress. Her feelings of intimacy and affection were now partly connected with her sexuality. The therapeutic relationship had given her a "corrective emotional experience" in which old feelings and traumas were present but not played out in the same way as in the past. Again, exploring the transference in the context of the current relationship legitimized the client's experience as well as illuminated its genetic roots in the past.

I think I must have unconsciously sensed Theresa's emerging erotic transference and been a little uncomfortable, for I characterized our moments of connection and intimacy as "moments of grace." This language certainly spiritualizes any erotic energy that is present and sends the message to the client, "Let's not go there." In other words, my countertransference may have helped prevent certain self-states from emerging in her. It is no wonder that Theresa, in addition to ascribing destructive powers to her erotic feelings, would have to develop a conversion symptom if she sensed that the expression of her erotic attraction would be unwelcome to me. Again, this illustrates that transference and countertransference are phenomena that emerge as the subjective worlds of client and therapist collide.

Reframing Theresa's erotic feelings as appropriate to her work in therapy eventually allowed her to normalize and integrate these feelings further. She realized she was using our relationship to do the work she needed to do, that her erotic attraction to me was part of her learning to feel close to someone with all her faculties available, and that it didn't need to destroy, control, or manipulate the relationship. Though she both hoped and feared that I would have erotic feelings for her, she also came to trust that the strength of the therapeutic relationship could contain them and not result in their inappropriate expression. Theresa came to experience a sense of self-possession and trust in her own ability to contain all of these powerful and sometime conflicting thoughts and feelings. She came to know what was of value for her in relationships and longed to generalize this newfound sense of self in her outside world of family and relationships. This enabled her to differentiate from her family as never before.

Carl Rogers (1951) said that when we speak of transference and countertransference we are sometimes just playing with the world of real relationships. But as any person who seeks to know another understands, ghosts often dwell in the attics of our minds and hearts. They are the shades of old loves, old terrors, and old losses. Understanding transference is an attempt at making them visible again.

Fighter Pilot

. . . in the partial darkness he imagined he saw the form of a young man standing under a dripping tree. Other forms were near. His soul had approached that region where dwell the vast hosts of the dead. He was conscious of, but could not apprehend, their wayward and flickering existence. His own identity was fading out into a gray impalpable world: the solid world itself which these dead had onetime reared and lived in was dissolving and dwindling. . . . The time had come for him to set out on his journey westward. Yes, the newspapers were right: snow was general all over Ireland. It was falling on every part of the dark central plain, on the treeless hills, falling softly upon the Bog of Allen and, farther westward, falling softly into the dark mutinous Shannon waves. It was falling, too, upon every part of the lonely churchyard on the hill where Michael Fury lay buried. It lay thickly drifted on the crooked crosses, and headstones, on the spears of the little gate, on the barren thorns. His soul swooned slowly as he heard the snow falling faintly through the universe, and faintly falling. Like the decent of their last end, upon all the living, and the dead.

—James Joyce

I looked down at the polished gold pocket watch that the old man placed in my palm. The cover was beautifully and elaborately embossed with filigree. I pressed the winding mechanism and the cover flipped open. The second hand ticked away, the black minute and hour hands hovered over an ivory face, the hours marked in gold. I noticed that the hands indicated the correct time, five minutes before the end of our last session.

"How can I accept this?" I inquired with my eyes, looking back into his bemused face. His features became suddenly stern, his gray bushy, spiking eyebrows frowned over the piercing blue eyes, slightly red and rheumy around the lids. He tilted his gray head toward me and said, "Don't argue with me, son."

"Yes sir," I said softly, emphasizing the second word. "It's very beautiful." The lines around his eyes crinkled as his stern expression changed, and his gaze again shone with an approving fatherly light. He wasn't about to say thank you with words, and he wasn't about to let me prevent him saying it with this gift. I reached out my hand and he shook it in his firm grip, but he patted me on the arm affectionately with his other hand as he walked past me. He paused at the door, nodded a parting, and walked down the hall and out of the building. I walked over to the window and looked out. A few flakes of snow drifted down from a light gray cloud cover. I watched as he got in his car. He opened the door of a burgundy Cadillac. As he lifted one leg stiffly in, he looked up and saw me watching him and dismissively waved an arm in my direction. I could imagine the look of disgust on his face, and I laughed out loud. He closed the door, started the car, and drove away. I looked down at the ticking watch. I knew its history, its story, and it truly was a beautiful thing.

———

"Look, son, I'm here for one reason, and one reason only, and that's because my son of a bitch doctor told me I had to come. If I hadn't been with him so long, I wouldn't do it. But I respect him. I don't believe in this, and I don't need a head doctor. I told him I'd come one time to get him off my back, and that's it. So we're just talking."

"Well, Mr. O'Connell, I'm all for you doing what you want. Since you're here now, can you at least give me an idea of what's bringing you in?"

"Don't be coy, son. Mercer said he already talked to you, I don't know what rubbish he told you. How old are you? Are you old enough to be out on your own? Damn doctors get younger every year."

"I'm 43!" I said, not knowing if I should be amused or irritated. "Dr. Mercer told me a little, but I'd like to hear your perspective."

"Forty three . . . don't look it. *What* did he tell you?"

I had just come from a powerful session with another client, and the sudden shift in tone between her and this bullying and crotchety old man had me a bit disoriented. "Well, he said you have been depressed for some time but that you refuse to take any medication for that. He told me that you had been in a car accident, that your wife was in the car and had been banged up pretty badly, and that you were having some trouble with that."

"What kind of trouble?" he demanded to know.

"That you are experiencing some anxiety about driving. In fact that you couldn't drive anymore because your anxiety about getting into another crash is pretty severe."

"Anxiety," he said dismissively, and I had the impression that the word itself offended him. "So he told you I'm *afraid* to drive. Did he tell you the accident was my fault?"

"Yes, he also said that you felt pretty bad about hitting the other car, and that a girl in that car had to be taken to the hospital, that you were pretty upset about her being injured, but that she only had a broken arm."

"Only?" he said. "It *was* my fault. The policeman gave me a ticket for failure to obey a traffic sign to make sure I knew it. Did Mercer tell you my wife has Alzheimer's?"

"Yes, he did mention that. He also said that you haven't had much help in caring for her but that you recently found her an assisted living arrangement at a small facility. Is that right?"

"That's right."

"Mr. O'Connell, how did you get here today?"

"I took a cab," he said, shaking his head once, as if he still had to get his mind around that idea.

"Were you nervous . . . afraid, about riding in the cab?"

"No."

"It must have shaken you up pretty badly to be in that accident; you want to tell me about it?"

"You doing your thing now?" he said, as if to say, "I'm onto you."

"Like you said, we're just talking." A wry smile played on his lips for a moment, but then he began telling me about the accident. He had run a red light and broadsided another car in the intersection. His wife suffered multiple facial lacerations and some bruises. Mr. O'Connell was bruised but mostly unhurt. Other motorists stopped to help, but in the interval he had become terribly upset, especially since the other driver, a teenage girl, had become hysterical. Those who had stopped to help quickly took control of the scene, and the ambulance had arrived promptly. I could tell from his narrative that his feeling of helplessness in the emergency deeply affected him. I thought, this is a man who is used to being in complete control. He seemed ashamed to have caused the accident and injured his wife and the girl.

"You know *why* I ran that red light, son?" I shook my head. "Because my wife, Annette, was trying to open her door and get out of the car while it was still moving. I don't know what she was trying to do, or why she wanted to suddenly get out. She had popped her seatbelt off and was reaching for the door handle." He shook his head.

"It does seem like you really needed some help at this stage of her illness. It's hard seeing someone you've always known slowly fade away from you. They're still there, but not really," I said, fishing.

"I found a good place in Woodstock. She'll be okay there," he said, not biting. "I just need to get back in the saddle so I can drive up there and see her."

"So you feel like there's no other reason that you should not be able to drive?"

"Of course not," he said, in an offended tone. I still occasionally fly my plane when I can get someone to mind Annette."

"Oh, you're a pilot."

"I was a fighter pilot in World War II. You heard of that one?"

"I *think* I have . . . didn't they just turn that into a movie?" [*Saving Private Ryan*]

He smiled. How pleasant his face suddenly became, as if some other person had been hiding there. "Did you see that movie?" he inquired.

"Yeah, I did."

"You know the problem with that movie? All those soldiers . . . those boys looked too old. We were all just kids, 18, 19. They should have put some kids up on the screen."

"In what theater did you fight?" I said, trying to be clever. He got the joke, tilted his head to let me know he was ignoring it, and responded to the legitimate level of the question.

"Europe. You don't want to hear about that. That was a long time ago." I shrugged and lifted my eyebrows, as if to say, 'I'd like to hear, but if you don't want to talk about it.'" He did not respond. I decided I couldn't be too subtle here.

"Tell me about this depression Dr. Mercer mentioned. He said that you've lost interest in just about everything, that you can't sleep, that you're not doing any of your hobbies anymore."

"I don't want to talk about that." He didn't want to talk about anything.

"You want me to show you how to not be bothered by driving?" I said, trying to gain a foothold in the conversation.

He looked at me skeptically. "Sure."

Well, that was something at least. For the rest of the session I mapped out for him a schedule for a simple systematic desensitization plan, walking him through each step for the week. I had never before used such a straightforward, problem-solving, behavioral plan with a client; almost all of my work involved at least *some* investigation into the client's inner world.

"Let me get this straight. On Day 1 you want me to just sit in the car for 20 minutes and not start it. Then on Day 2 you want me to only start it."

"Yeah, each of those five times a day. Then on Day 3 I want you to back to the end of the driveway, and then drive back to the front of the driveway, until you're bored."

"I'll be bored before I'm finished with the first one."

"Good. Boredom is good when you're doing this; that's what we're after. If at any point you begin to feel nervous, stop and go back to the previous step. Day 4, go around the block 10 times. Go a little further on Day 5. Day 6 you find the nearest intersection with a traffic light and go through it five times. He looked dubious about it all. "Did you learn how to fly in one easy lesson?" I countered his look. "When you taught new guys to fly, did they do it all at once?" I challenged.

"I'll tell you what. Some boys would come back from the tough missions and hardly be able to fly at all." That seemed to give him a reference point, a handle for his own struggle.

"There you go. You had a bad crash. It takes a little time to work back up. Then, next session," I said with a grin, "I'd like for you to drive to our meeting here."

"Next session," he said, with a bemused expression in his eye. "You an Irishman too, son?"

"I have some of that."

"I thought I caught a whiff of bullshit in here," he said with a wink.

"You sure you didn't track it in yourself?"

"Ha," he said tilting his head, which I noticed had a slight but persistent tremor, "I might 'ave, I might 'ave."

The next session Mr. O'Connell drove himself to the appointment. "Things must have gone pretty well," I offered, as soon as we had seated ourselves. "I saw you drive up." He waved his hand dismissively.

"I had to jump straight to Step 4."

"Driving around the block. Good." His scowl returned; my encouragement appeared to irritate him.

"I will admit that I had a little trouble getting out farther. No one cuts you any slack anymore. No one has any goddamn manners! Would it cost them anything to let you merge?" I put up my hands in a go figure gesture. "Anyway, I drove around the neighborhood a lot. Neighbors must have thought I was nuts. Then I went a little farther each time, and after a couple of days it was no sweat."

"You just needed to get back on the horse, no big deal."

"No big deal," he repeated.

"So let's do something about this depression," I said, uncharacteristically directive and challenging. I thought I might have a little credibility now, but that he would again roll right over any subtlety.

"Like what? I'm not taking any pills."

"Okay, no pills. First tell me all the things you used to do that you don't do now. Stuff you took pleasure in that has become flat or stale to you."

"I believe the phrase is 'how weary, stale, flat and unprofitable seem to me the uses of this world.'" He saw me lift my eyebrows. "What? You think you're so smart, college boy? A few of the rest of us went to school too. Some of us even taught a little."

"Ah, you were a teacher?"

"I was a lot of things. After I graduated from Yale . . . you heard of that one?"

"I *think* I have." This was beginning to become a pattern.

"That was after the war . . . G.I. bill. I taught high school English for a while. After that I got into business. There's a lot more money in business you know," he said with a conspiratorial nod.

"You did well?"

"I did very well. I retired 20 years ago, and I'm still doing well. By the time I was your age, I had a million dollars. You made your first million yet?"

"I think I'm suddenly feeling discouraged with my career choice," I said.

He laughed. It was a full, uninhibited laugh, and his face lit up with pleasure. "Don't worry, there are more important things than making money," he consoled.

"So every person with money has told me," I countered.

He laughed again. I was pleased. For us to achieve anything we would need to find some kind of rapport, and though the age and "stage of life" gap between us was great, this felt like a beginning.

"So you did well," I prompted again.

"I did well. I had a good life. My daughter gave me two grandkids.

They live in Denver so we only got to see them two or three times a year. My wife and I got to travel all over Europe. Every year we'd take a trip. We even took a trip where we camped all over East Africa once. She was an avid traveler. She had languages so that made it easy.

"It sounds like a very full life. I was struck that you said you 'had' a good life, not that you 'have' a good life."

From under the bushy gray eyebrows he gazed at me with his piercing blue eyes, and I suddenly felt, by the intensity of his gaze, as if he had me lined up in the crosshairs of some invisible gun scope. He started to speak, paused, then said finally, as if taking his finger off some inner trigger, "I suppose that's a legitimate observation."

"In some ways it feels as if there's nothing left, that it's all behind you. And something about being in the car accident has brought that to the fore." I shut up, thinking that I might have already overdrafted my relational account.

"Do you know what it's like to outlive your usefulness?" he asked irritably. "No, of course you don't," he answered his question without pausing. "I've had a life full of good things, and I'm no stranger to difficult situations. I always handled it, and I never let my fear get to me. So, yes, causing that accident shook me up. It wouldn't have flustered me in the same way in the past, I can tell you. And then, to not want to drive. You have to understand son, I've been in scrapes in my life that would make your hair stand on end, especially in the war. Well, never mind about that. Anyway, it's been hard taking care of Annette, especially as she's gotten bad. That's all I'm going to say about it, so there's not much to talk about, and there's nothing wrong in my head. It's just hard getting old. Don't get old, that's my advice to you."

"I'll keep that in mind. My Dad says getting old is not for sissies."

"He's right about that. Look," he continued, "it's simple. Try taking the woman you have lived with your whole life to some institution because half the time she's forgotten who you are. *It's as if your whole life never even happened.* You'd wonder too if other things are worth doing."

"I get that. I think I would feel that nothing seems significant if my partner of many years just forgot it all," I hazarded. This seemed to keep him going.

"What am I going to do, work in my woodshop? I won't travel without her. It seems pointless, though I do occasionally travel in the states to watch shows."

"What kind of shows?"

"Watch shows."

"What kind of shows do you watch?" I persisted.

"Is this your Abbot and Costello routine?" I shook my head, lost. "'Who's on first?'" he said inquiringly. I shook my head again.

"Okay. Try and follow me here, and I'll say it real slow so even someone with Dr. in front of his name can get it. I collect antique watches. Mostly gold pocket watches."

"Ooooh," I said, "you go to watch shows."

"You'll be okay, son. I probably have just over 200. Just the really good stuff. No junk." He reached into his jacket pocket and pulled out a gold chain on which hung a polished gold watch with gold filigree on the cover. It spun slowly in the air between us as he handed it to me. I took it, turned it over in my hand and pushed a button, and the case sprang open.

"I have two of those," he said, nodding toward the watch. My father gave me both of them, and one I carried with me all through the war . . . every mission. Never missed a tick. I kind of thought if that watch could keep running that I might just keep ticking myself."

"This is very beautiful," I said sincerely. And in that moment I was struck by just how lovely a thing it was, a work of perfection and elegance. It had a sense of weight and heft in the palm. The black hour and minute hands hovered in the thin space over the crisp dial, and below was a separate much smaller circle and dial where a tiny hand ticked off the seconds. He seemed suddenly subdued, pleased with my pleasure. He offered a few comments about its history and construction.

"May I wind it?" I asked. I don't know why I wanted to wind it.

"Just take it real easy. Don't keep going if you feel any resistance."

I turned the knob and felt the spring within tensioning. There was something pleasurable in the clicking action. I smiled as I felt some tension, and stopped turning, imagining the delicate works inside the gilded exterior. I smiled and handed the watch back to him.

"I can understand why you would want to collect these watches. There's something satisfying about having to flip open the case to look at the time, and to wind it to keep it going. It's so elegant. Do you have any shows coming up that you want to attend?"

"No, I don't feel like going anywhere. I have enough. Enough money, enough things, and now with Annette settled, plenty of time on my hands. That's all there is to it."

His statement, "plenty of time on his hands," struck me. I wondered if he caught its metaphorical value. The watch was still in his palm, gears ticking away. Clearly, with his wife no longer in his care he suddenly had a lot of time, and also, in the big picture, very little life time left to him. He seemed to be aware of both at once. He seemed to imply that his life was finished, but that he was still alive. There was nothing to do but fill up the space of his remaining days, but he could not discover anything that was pleasurable or meaningful to him. His wife was lost to him. He was now the only keeper of their history together. No longer was it *between* them, a shared life. The accident had proven to him that he was no longer in control. His powers had faded. He was no longer the fighter pilot with courage in a crisis and firm hands on the stick and trigger. Was this why he overcompensated with this pushy, gruff, irritability; his attitude that others must be merely tolerated? What was worse than the accident was his failure to know how to handle it after it had happened. What if I could get him to reflect on these themes, I wondered. What if I could encourage him to explore the experience of being near the end, find something of value here at the finish when everything else had receded and fallen away? But how, with such a defensive front, to begin?

"Plenty of time on your hands," I repeated his words, to see if I could spark something around these ideas.

Nothing.

"So there's not much in your life that you really feel like doing," I said, trying to salvage something . . . anything. No response. Just his piercing steady gaze under the tangled brambles of his bushy gray eyebrows and a slightly bemused expression on his wrinkled face.

"I wonder if we talked some about what's happening for you with Annette being hospitalized and you feeling that normal activities just aren't very pleasurable anymore . . ." I trailed off, thinking that this sounded awfully clinical. It felt as if we were back again to a kind of stalemate. I'd lost him again.

"Well, I'm going to tell Mercer you did okay son. He's not a total nincompoop after all. I'm back in the saddle, driving the caddy . . . no sweat," he said reaching for his jacket.

"We have a little time left," I said, realizing that this would be our last session and that my tack was all wrong. Damn! I had never worked with the elderly before, and my sense was that this guy was tougher than most!

"Oh, that's okay, I have some errands I need to run now that I'm driving again," he said with a wink.

"Well, I'm a little disappointed you're leaving," I said, standing as he stood up from the couch. "I was looking forward to seeing your watch collection." Where did that come from? Why was I so interested in being helpful to this irascible old man?

He turned a searching gaze onto my face. "You serious . . . you really want to see it?"

"Yeah." I was about to say something like, "I know that's been an important activity for you," but said instead, "The one you showed me is magnificent, I'd like to see some more."

"Well, I suppose I could bring a case of them for you to take a look."

"That'd be great."

————

The next session when I greeted Mr. O'Connell he said, "I guess you can call me Mike, son." He had two large wooden polished cases with black handles. I pulled a coffee table up close to the couch. He set the cases down on the table. I sat down beside him on the couch as he opened one of the cases to reveal row upon row of antique pocket watches.

"How about that!" I exclaimed sincerely impressed, seeing the neat rows of shining gold discs, some of them intricately worked with great artistry. He took a watch and handed it to me, explaining where it had come from, its maker's status in the history of timepiece manufacture, its rarity and collectibility as well as its approximate value. As he selected each piece he explained its unique features and charms. A few had inscriptions inside the faceplate, a message from someone long dead to someone long dead, as if the timepiece retained a little of the original owner's life. But the message was now divorced from the lives that gave it meaning. The hands stood still over the dial where once they had faithfully measured off a life in what must have seemed like endless revolutions. Mike opened the back of one watch to reveal the gears and wheels and springs all compacted into a Newtonian, orderly, and predictable universe. I wound the knob and watched the gears and wheels spring into motion.

"Do they all keep time?" I asked.

"Many of them keep accurate time. I suppose they all could if I had them calibrated by a watchmaker."

"It's not important to you that they keep time accurately," I said, somehow surprised by this information.

"It's not important to me. I keep the one I carry calibrated."

"It's just the beauty of the thing itself that most intrigues you."

He smiled.

With all the watches scattered about, and absorbed in their examination, I lost track of the time, and my secretary buzzed me to say that my next client had been waiting for 10 minutes. Together we put the watches away.

"These aren't even the best that I have," he informed me. "I keep those under lock and key in a safe place. Would you like to see them?"

"Yes, I would."

"I'll bring them next time," he said, surprising me again.

———

The next session was a repeat of the previous one, examining the watches, except that he brought a watch collector's book and we referenced a few of the watches and recorded their information. The following sessions similarly were spent cataloging the watches. I felt a little guilty about getting paid for sitting around getting an education about antique pocket watches, even though I was enjoying the process. It was now our sixth session, and I resolved to earn my pay by nudging Mike closer to something that resembled therapy. But he quickly brushed aside any prelude to these intentions, and instead we pored over the collector's manuals he brought. He had shown me how one could inventory, catalogue, and value the timepieces. I searched for identifying features on the watch itself. "Your eyes are better," he asserted. We both looked it up in the various books and wrote the appropriate notes in a new three-ring binder he had divided into decades of time.

———

"Mike," I said, in the following session as we sat together on the couch, unable to find any information in the book on a gorgeous French watch, "I don't feel like I'm earning my keep. We're supposed to be doing therapy in here, but all I'm doing is helping you organize your collection."

"I thought you liked learning about the watches," he said, turning toward me and looking a little crestfallen.

"I *do* like learning about the watches," I said sincerely, "I'm having lots of fun, but I don't like accepting money for doing therapy when I'm not."

"That's because you lack imagination. No wonder you haven't made your first million yet."

"Humor me here. We're supposed to be helping you get past your depression," and even as I said it, it sounded stupid to my ears.

"*I feel better,*" he said, turning toward me on the couch. "There. Is that what you need to hear. Do *you* feel better now? You said I should take pleasure in something, and I don't know why, but I'm taking pleasure in this," he said sweeping his hand over the cases. "Now if you don't want to do it, if you want me to quit *therapy*," he said, and I could hear that he was working me, "I'm not sure what might happen. I might do a harm to myself. You want that on your head?" His eyes widened questioningly, and he tilted his head expectantly. I looked at him skeptically, and his eyes narrowed with a mischievous glint.

"How did your wife ever manage to live with you for so long?"

"It's one of the great mysteries," he said, turning back to the watch.

"Okay," I persisted, "humor me . . . talk while we work. Tell me about your life."

"What do you want to hear?"

"Whatever you like, start out at the beginning."

"I was born."

"Maybe not that far back."

"Okay, how about I tell you how Annette and I met in France during the war."

"That sounds good."

And so he began with the first of many stories. She was a "great beauty" born of an English mother and a French father. The Germans had "rolled over the French in about 20 minutes," but after the liberation of Paris, Mike met Annette while he was on leave. He told of their brief courtship and their pledges of love to one another, and how he would return to her when he could. He was summoned back to duty. He secretly thought that he would never see her again, not because he questioned her faithfulness, but because he never expected to live through the war. He was in the thick of it, escorting and protecting bombers, conducting strafing missions, attacking German lines, taking fire all the time. The casualty rate among fighter pilots was high, he said. He lost a lot of friends. He didn't want to talk about that. Annette had told him that he still dreamed about it because he talked and groaned in his sleep. But he "couldn't remember" the dreams, he dissimulated. As he spoke I occasionally asked him a clarifying question to make sure I understood but made no other therapist type observations or interpretations.

Once, he related, he was almost shot down and though wounded, managed to nurse his P-51 Mustang back to the airfield. That was a tough one, he said, one of the few war experiences that really shook him to the core. "I was hit pretty badly, and I wasn't sure if I could make it back before I ran out of fuel and blood. It was tough to later climb back in the cockpit after that, but you've got no choice; you have to do what needs to be done." I was reminded of his recent traffic accident, his trouble driving. So, he was referring to himself when he had said that after tough missions "some of those boys" had trouble flying more missions. Because he was wounded, he got to go back to Paris. He went to Annette's house, but it stood empty. He searched Paris, but could find her nowhere. "I was a kid, so full of love that I thought my heart would break because I thought I would never see her again. I had lost a lot of friends, and thinking that she was gone . . . but it probably saved my life."

"Saved your life? How do you mean?"

"Those guys that had lots of people back home, or a girl, they just hurt too much from missing them. They played it safe sometimes. That's okay if you're on the ground, it's good, I guess. But you play it safe as a fighter pilot and you're not going to last long. You have to fly full out like there's no tomorrow. After I thought I'd never find Annette, I flew like a demon. I didn't care."

"Because you never thought you'd see her again," I said smiling.

"Right."

"But you did see her again."

"After it was all over I went back to Paris. Some of her letters had caught up to me by then. And there she was, at her parent's house that had been deserted when I had gone there before. She was right there waiting for me. That was a happy day, I'll tell you. After the war we moved back to the U.S., and I went to college and she became a teacher."

I looked at him appreciatively. "What a great love story." I never would have imagined he could show that underneath the gruff exterior he was really sentimental.

"Well, everybody starts out with a love story . . . then you get married," he said, trying to disqualify the tenderness of the moment.

"Marriage wasn't all it was cracked up to be?"

"It was fine. It was real life . . . ordinary life, not all the drama, like in wartime. You really interested in this nonsense?"

He seemed to be humoring me. But as the sessions went on and he told more stories of his life, I could see that he needed less prodding, and a little later didn't even need an invitation. We sat, side by side, identifying, cleaning, and cataloging the watches, and I could see that he now enjoyed telling me of his life. He spoke of specific battles and sorties. Mike seemed to remember all of these vividly, where enemy planes came from, the specific maneuvers of attack and evasion, the number of planes that went down. He affectionately explained the wonders and idiosyncrasies, the flying and attack capabilities of his P-51 Mustang, "the old bitch."

Once, many years after the war, Mike attended an air show where a sister plane to his P-51 was on display. The pilot who owned the plane invited Mike to sit once again in the cockpit. Mike declined. It felt too much like a souvenir, he said, apart from him. The guns were missing, of course. Out of the context of history and battle it was not the same plane, the extension of his own body . . . the enclosure that was his weapon and lifeboat in the air. Too many years had passed, and he was content to stand under the wing and remember. He spoke of the camaraderie the pilots shared, explained that in a brief time and extreme circumstance you could form a bond that lasted a lifetime. But many of his old buddies were dead now, all of the few closest friends were gone. He didn't want to talk about that.

In the next session he changed the topic of his stories, and reminisced about postwar life with Annette, of ambitions achieved and even of dreams unrealized.

"I thought I might like to be a writer at one point, kind of a Thomas Wolfe meets Ernest Hemingway."

"What would that look like?" I laughed.

"I don't know . . . a thoughtful adventurer," he mused.

"What happened to that dream?"

"Oh, I wouldn't call it a dream . . . just a notion, you know," he said, handing me a silver watch. "See if you can polish that little discoloration off of there," he said, giving me a polishing cloth. "I came to the end of it when my first stories all came back to me with rejection slips. Never a single hit. Not even a crumby magazine."

"Yeah that's tough."

"Good thing though . . . I'd hate to see what rubbish I was trying to inflict on people. There was this one story though; damn, I wish I still had it."

"What was it about?"

"It told the story of a time that I was lost over Germany at night. I had become separated from my squadron. I didn't know if I was flying into a world of trouble; the Germans were still strong in the air after the Battle of the Bulge. I thought I might fly right into a German squadron. It was scary as hell, and then something happened," he shook his head.

"What? What happened?" I asked intrigued.

"I started climbing and broke through the cloud cover. I thought I wouldn't be such easy pickin's up there. The sky above me, it was as clear as water, with all the stars filling the whole sky, reaching right down to the farther horizon. It was a helluva sight and a feeling I will never forget." He stopped fiddling with the watch in his hand. "I was in an airplane that was low on fuel, lost over a landscape I couldn't see because of clouds below, but all above me was speckled with stars. And I was flying through it but felt like I was going nowhere, like I was just suspended, hanging from the sky, like one of those stars, like I could go on like that forever. You know what happened then?"

"What?" I asked, absorbed in his narrative.

"I felt a sense of peace. Right there, lost and a mile high—nothing between me and the ground but gravity and air. I mean you get hit and God ain't gonna reach out his hand like a cloud and palm you back down softly. You tend to go down burning if you're a pilot. But right then, somehow that didn't matter. I thought, it's all right, it's all right," he repeated. He paused, then said, "I thought, no matter what happens in my life, if I even have a life, I've been through the worst of it, and *I can take anything*. Just a sense of peace in that moment." He shook his head. "I wish I'd kept that story. That was the best one I ever wrote. It's been a lot of years since I remembered that," he said reflectively. "It was a long, long time ago."

"As you describe it, if feels like it's very fresh, like it just happened."

"Some things are like that, I guess. Other things, even important things, just fade away." I could see that he was drawing something from the "peace in that moment" as he remembered this experience.

Mike narrated more stories from his life while we continued the work with the watches. I recalled with irony how often I had steered clients *away* from storytelling because it sometimes detracted from the immediacy and potential of the therapeutic encounter. Now, here I was, encouraging Mike to tell stories from his past because I didn't know how else to engage him.

By then, though, I understood that something important *was* happening in our time together, and that it had mostly been below my radar. My expectation was for Mike to reflect on his inner world of thoughts and feelings, to directly explore his reaction to the institutionalization of his wife, to get to the roots of his depression. I also wanted

him to explore how the car crash may have evoked traumas and memories that he had never fully explored, traumas that related to those
extreme situations he had lived through as a warrior where his life had
sometimes hung by a thread. He had said, describing his war days, that
"there are some things you never really get over." But he had prevented
any further inquiry, especially into how these events might still filter
down through the years and into the present.

I realized that I had wanted Mike to conform to *my* method. But
didn't I always preach to my students the maxim that the "real master
responds to uniqueness." Here I was stuck in my "categories" for how
therapy must proceed. But Mike insisted on doing things his way, as he
always had. He wasn't in the least intimidated by "experts," or by any
mystery that many new clients suppose infuses the methods and process
of the profession. There was little chance Mike was going to more
equally share control of the relationship with me. But Mike engaged me
in a way that he found acceptable. Our work with the vintage pocket
watches, and my interest in them and his stories, seemed to give him
pleasure. I remembered how exciting it always was for me when I
brought someone new to sailing out on my boat, and how much pleasure I received from witnessing their delight in discovery as they learned
the ropes. Mike seemed to experience something similar with me.
Wasn't one of my intentions to address his anhedonia? What was wrong
with him renewing his interest in something right there, with me?

———

As Mike's storytelling took on a rhythm across the sessions, I realized
that another process shaped our time together. I had forgotten the
importance of *life review* in the later stages of development across the life
span, probably because I had never lived them myself. Mike grafted this
process onto the immediate activity of cataloging the watches. My
expectation that he look into better understanding himself, his personality and conflicts, was the imperative of youth, and especially of middle age. Mike was telling me, "That's all finished for me, but I can look
back and reflect on my life. I can distill out of time and experience all
the generative, valuable and poignant impressions that string together
as the meaningful story of my days." I realized that his storytelling put
him in touch with all of the emotions that pertained to those experiences and that he was handing his stories on to me, bequeathing the
experience and history of them into my keeping. If there was no one to

remember them, did they really exist at all? Telling the story of his life helped him to realize it in the present.

I could also see, as Mike weaved his narratives, that these memories did not necessarily represent some objective or factual drawing of events as they "really" happened. Rather, the distinct pen and ink edges of the pictures from those times were colored in with retrospective thoughts and emotions; they reflected a constructed world made from the process of looking backward. As I listened carefully I saw that *memory is also a creative process,* that the narrative that took shape in Mike's dialogue with me was infused with the meaning he had created, *was creating as we spoke.* He saw his life through the lens of having already lived it, and he needed to reconstruct those memories into a meaningful pattern.

There was nothing "untruthful" about this reconstruction. I suppose that all personal history is revisionist as one ages. As one travels farther along the road, the angle of view changes the perspective on the same scene. How differently one's life must appear when, after traveling toward a destination with an endlessly receding horizon, the line between the sky and land suddenly rises up to meet you. Could he have become aware, when I was not, that something valuable had been happening all along? Is this why he had said to me that I "lacked imagination?"

As Mike's stories became more consolidated into a life narrative, our activity of working with the watches became an apt metaphor, unspoken but constantly present between us. I felt as if together we were *polishing time.* Mike summoned up his memories and strung vignettes and stories together, meaningfully cataloguing the events of his life. Along with his stories of those extreme and heroic days of war, he told of ordinary life. He recounted his travels with Annette. Once he told of a dog he had dearly loved, "the best dog in the world" (it was the only time I saw his eyes mist up . . . as if *that* was a loss he could allow himself to fully feel and share). There were stories of things he thought he might have done if the flow of his life hadn't carved out a channel that constrained the rushing waters of choice and aspiration and dreams.

At times Mike was congenial, and at times irascible and gruff, though by now he wasn't fooling anyone. It was as if he wanted to remind me that although he might be enjoying our time we still weren't doing "therapy," at least not on my terms. As long as he could tell himself that he was getting a "good helper" with his collection, he could convince himself that he didn't need my help as a therapist. That admission he would never make, and I didn't want him to. If the thought that he needed to see a therapist so near the end of a life well lived was intolerable to him, then I was happy to collude with him and pretend that we were doing what he allowed us at the beginning, just talking.

———

Identifying, cataloging, and polishing the watches was three-quarters finished. One session Mike startled me with a story that impressed me with its sensitivity, poignancy, and openness. The story reminded me of the Robert Frost poem, *The Road Not Taken.* He and Annette were vacationing at a ski lodge in the Swiss Alps in the mid 1950s. Mike seemed to just want to describe the scenery and the fact that he had been an avid skier in his younger years. But in the middle of his narrative he became lost in thought, as if he had forgotten I was there. He looked up after a few moments, snorted, and handed me a polishing cloth, trying to cover for the break in flow.

"Uh, uh," I said.

"What?" he looked at me skeptically.

"You were lost in thought . . . what were you thinking about?"

"None of your damn business."

I put the watch down, sat back on the couch and folded my arms in a gesture meant to convey that "You don't tell, and I don't work."

"It's private. Don't you people know that it's a good thing to have private thoughts? It used to be accepted, even admired that a person didn't go around confessing to everyone."

"Fine." I persisted obstinately, not moving. Giving him a little of his own medicine, I thought.

He shook his head. "Goddamn Irish. If I wasn't one of them, I'd get rid of the lot." (I'm no more Irish than Scottish, English, and Native American, but Mike seemed to want to believe that I was Irish. It was an interesting bit of transference that I didn't feel the need to interpret or refute.) "All right . . . One day . . . ," he capitulated.

I picked up the silver watch again, absently using my fingernail with the cloth to get the tarnish out of the creases.

"I was up in the ski lodge. It was at the very top of the mountain with a commanding view of the whole valley, truly spectacular. Annette was off somewhere or other, I don't remember why or where. I was sitting there just looking out when I turned and saw this girl. She stood by the window, taking in the view over the valley. The light up there was really something, and it came through that window and lit up her hair. She must have been in her late 20s; I would have been in my 30s.

She had just come in from off the slopes. There was something about her face, she had a round, fair face and blond hair . . . she was Swiss, and she looked over at me and smiled. That smile . . . it was as if the whole room suddenly collapsed into the one thing. I just got up and went right over to her. I was a Young Turk then," he smiled. "I bought her a drink, and we sat at a table talking and looking over that beautiful snowy scene below. She didn't speak much English and I less German. We could barely understand one another. I guess that was part of the charm and the humor of it. We pantomimed and gestured a lot. We laughed and spent the whole afternoon talking together . . . or trying to. Sitting there, alone with her, some kind of understanding came up between us. I think I felt as close to her as two people can be."

He looked into my face. "You're wondering if we became lovers." It was a statement, not a question, but it was accurate. I just held his gaze. He shook his head reflectively, "No. We didn't. I won't deny that I thought about it, felt a strong pull toward finding some private room together, and I know she was thinking about it too. It was like some beautiful possibility hanging in the air between us, and that was okay, just to leave it there. I wanted that moment to last. I wanted to just . . . I don't know, fly away from that mountaintop straight up into the air where there was no one else. But, of course, it couldn't last. When we parted," he shook his head, "I almost kissed her . . . I was aching to kiss those lips. But I just held her hand for a long time and we said goodbye. That's all. I was married to Annette, and I loved her too." He looked up at me realizing that he had just said he loved a woman whom he had only just met, shrugged, and said, "It's strange. Maybe that sense that you know someone, that you've always known them is just an illusion; you don't want to tax it with real life. But I'll tell you what," he said, furrowing the gray brow and looking directly into my eyes, "I still remember that girl's face as clear as a bell . . . as if it were yesterday."

The sense of wistful regret lingered in his face for a moment. Not regret that he and the girl did not become lovers, but regret that the choices of life accrue and prevent the possibility of other things, the regret of not being able to live more than one life at a time, and the regret of roads not taken. "I don't know why I thought of her just now. Sometimes I wondered," he said shaking his head as if he still couldn't make sense of it, "sometimes I wondered what happened to her; 10, 20 years later that beautiful face would pop into my thoughts. I'd think, 'Where in the world is she?' Can you account for that?" he challenged.

"No, I can't. Sometimes the ways of the human heart are too mysterious."

"Well, that's probably the smartest thing you've said yet. I guess now she's a fat old Swiss grandma with no teeth," he grinned mischievously.

In another session Mike remembered a fellow flyer who had been shot down and died in the war. Patrick, like Mike, was from Boston, and he also still had family in Ireland. Perhaps their Irish heritage was what drew them together. After the war, when Annette and Mike traveled in Ireland, they went to visit Patrick's grave. It was a hard thing, Mike said.

"Were you two especially close?"

"Yes, we were. Back then, and under those conditions, you form friendships with a few of the guys real fast . . . usually the guys that have been around as long as you have. But this was different. Patrick was one of the new guys, and I just took to him. I was always watching out for him when the squadron flew. He was like a kid brother, you know. I felt real bad when I heard he went down."

"You weren't with him on that mission?"

"No, I was grounded because I was wounded. I wasn't flying then. I guess I always felt real badly about that."

"What, that you weren't there with him?"

"Uh huh. If I hadn't been . . . " he stopped. He shifted in his seat, saying nothing. It had never happened before that Mike stumbled across such powerful and conflicted feelings that he couldn't bluster his way through them.

"I had the sense just then that you feel somehow responsible about Patrick's death. Do you?" In the moment, this felt like a very bold inquiry.

"I guess I've always felt a little responsible, even guilty." I was surprised that he responded. He seemed suddenly open and vulnerable.

"I had told him I'd look out for him," he said. "Then, when the time came, I wasn't there for him. He was just a kid, you know?" There was a kind of implied appeal in his question. I nodded. "I guess I couldn't help it," he said reflectively. "I guess looking back now, I was really just trying to encourage him, fill him with confidence so he could do his job. There's really not a whole lot you can do when you're actually up there and things get bad. Maybe I always took my promise to him a little too literally, but I've always felt bad about not being up there with him when he got into trouble. But, you know, a lot of guys went down," he said, shaking his head. I could see that he was once again pondering the extraordinary circumstances of those days and reevaluating his perspective.

"I had the sense just then that you have always felt you wished you could have protected him, that you've felt guilty about that, but that now, looking back, you realize that you couldn't have done anything, that you were really trying to fill him with confidence."

"Yeah, but back then I meant it. I guess when you're young *you make promises you can't possibly keep.* You think you have these incredible powers, that you're master of any situation. But then life teaches you differently. Then you get shot or something, and suddenly you realize, some things are bigger than me. After the war, I always wished I hadn't told him I'd watch out for him, as if I let him down. But now, I guess it's all right. I did the best I could for him. I didn't have anything else for him other than what I gave him. I sure missed him. He was one of those guys that could take you to a whorehouse and convince you it was a church. He was full of himself, and a real talker, always smiling. You know, I feel, talking like this, that I'm a young man trapped in this old man's body. I remember so much about the feelings of those days. They were terrible, but they were also some of the defining moments of my life. But getting old, you realize you just have to let yourself participate with it. I guess you can't fight it, and there's a kind of acceptance that you have to get or you're in big trouble. Patrick, that boy, did all right. The truth is, there was a time I was a little jealous of him. He gave it everything, and his last act was, well . . . it was something. He didn't have to live on past those days and make it all mean something. In some ways that's harder. That was a sappy part of that Private Ryan movie, but you know, it's true too."

"So you living through it, making it mean something, that kind of redeems his loss."

"Yeah. You know, there's a whole squadron of guys that I can hardly remember. I look at the pictures, you know, and I wonder, did I know that guy? They're like ghosts. Other guys I remember real well. Looking at those pictures of us all lined up in the squadron, I see how young we all were. It makes me know how old I am. I guess I'll get to see 'em soon eh?" he joked, wanting to move back away from the powerful feelings that I had come to realize ran underneath all of his stories. "Some of the fellows are left. I used to see them at the reunions."

"You don't go to the reunions anymore?"

"No, I haven't been in years. They're kind of boring actually. They pack you in a bus and show you the sights like a bunch of old farts that need their hands held."

"Yeah, but maybe you should go again, see all the guys you used to know," I said conversationally.

He paused reflectively, "Maybe I will. If I move us out to Colorado to be near my daughter, I'd be closer to the next one. I believe the next reunion's going to be out there somewhere."

We were at the end of inventorying the watches. Mike had 206 gold and silver pocket watches whose estimated value totaled more than one hundred thousand dollars. In our 18 sessions together, Mike and I had cleaned, identified, and catalogued them all, recording the information in the now full three-ring binder. As we worked on the last two, I wondered what we would do without this background activity to structure our story time.

"I'm selling the plane," Mike announced toward the end of the session as we sat together putting the watches back in the velvet-lined case.

"You won't miss it?"

"I will miss it, but I can't fly alone anymore anyway. Truth is, I haven't flown it for two years. It's time to let it go. I'm thinking of moving too. My daughter wants Annette and me to come live near her so she can see us more often and so we can be near the grandkids. I don't know if it's a good idea."

"You don't want to be out there with them?"

"I'm stuck in my ways. I'm not sure I want to move, or move Annette. She's in a good facility. But it would be good to be near my daughter and the kids . . . if she can handle it. I'm an ornery old bastard you know."

"No!"

"I know it's hard to believe, as sweet tempered as I appear. Well," he continued, "since this is our last visit I want you to know that you've been a good worker." There was that humorous look in his eye again. "Expensive, but good," he clarified. "I'm going to tell old Mercer that he did all right."

"Our last visit? So this is it? You're bailing out?"

"This is it." He stood up, and worked his way around the table. I latched the cases and put them in the middle of the floor. I realized how skillfully he had avoided any discussion of "termination." I thought of all the buddies he had lost and how he rarely wanted to talk about those losses.

"Mike, I just want you to know . . ."

"Don't start in with that," he interrupted, heading off any overt expression of mutual sentiment. "Listen, I have something here for you." He lifted the gold chain that attached to the watch that he always kept in his pocket. I knew that it was one of two that his father had given him. It might have even been the one that he carried with him during the war, but in that moment I didn't want to clarify. He unlatched it from the chain and pressed it into my palm.

"How can I accept this?" I inquired with my eyes, looking back into his bemused face.

His gray, bushy eyebrows frowned over the piercing blue eyes, slightly red and rheumy around the lids. He tilted his silver head toward me, "Don't argue with me, son," he commanded.

So I didn't.

CASE THREE DISCUSSION
Narrative and Constructivism

AS MIKE DESCRIBED his reaction to his wife's memory loss from Alzheimer's disease he said, "It's as if a whole life never even happened." His lament struck me as particularly poignant. I tried to imagine what it would be like if all my friends were dead and my most intimate partner had faded away and slowly "forgotten" our life together. What if I were the sole bearer of the tale of my own life, and all the characters within it had passed into the half-light of memory, taking something of the truth of it as they receded? "I have plenty of things, and time on my hands," said Mike paradoxically as he wondered how to fill his days with something of value now that the springs of his life were winding down. Would his own inscription, like those engraved in the gold that we had polished, be preserved within some context of meaning, or pass into an unknowing and indifferent hand?

Mike had given me his stories, the narratives that our time together had conjured out of a well-lived existence. With me he surveyed the terrain over which he had traveled, remembering and revising from the perspective of time passed. When he handed me his father's watch, it was really the narrative of his life that he was bestowing on me and wanting me to value. Like each of us, Mike needed a "witness," an audience to validate his tale, to help him evoke its emotions again, infusing it with meaning. He wished to create an inheritance by the telling so that in some small way it would survive him. As I write this, I guess it worked. I'm sharing his story, dear reader, with you.

In my clinical work I range pretty freely in terms of how I approach any particular client, though certain underlying assumptions about therapy organize my approach. These assumptions will, I hope, manifest across the cases. One of these organizing ideas that I hope is especially apparent is that we each create our own reality as we respond to the existential "givens" of life and participate with others in a relational world. Each of us has the sense that our view of self and the world represents some objective reality or "truth" that is "out there" and universal. But this is an illusion. Our truths are "in here" and, hopefully, open to revision. With regard to social realities, we each construct a subjective model of the world and ourselves within it.

A central tenet of postmodernism, and of its offspring constructivism, is that at the social level there are no "Platonic" absolutes or universal truths, no body of knowledge or reality that is *apart from the perceiver.* Each person lives in a subjectivity that forms in participation with others, especially family, as well as the larger culture. In contrast, the traditional "modernist" view (upon which much of science is based) locates the therapist in the role of "expert" and as having access to a reality that the client needs to get. Constructivist theorists assert that the only reality relevant and accessible to the therapeutic inquiry is *subjective reality*—that of the client, the therapist, and the psychological field created by the interplay between the two (Stolorow, Brandchaft, & Atwood, 1987). In this intersubjective model, these authors argue that the idea of an objective reality is really an instance of a psychological process termed *concretization*—a symbolic transformation of subjective experiences into configurations the person believes to be objectively perceived and known. Attributions of objective reality, in other words, are concretizations of subjective truth. Still, you might want to refrain from running with scissors.

With regard to social realities, the meaning that each of us creates as we string together the myriad incidences of "concretization" in our participation with the larger world forms the narrative of our lives. This is the story we tell ourselves about ourselves, which carries the "truths" that stand in for a history of integrated experiences and impressions. The methods and assumptions of the (modernist) scientific method seek to uncover existing facts through reductionist methods that "reveal" essential truths. There is no doubt that this is a powerful method of knowing. But as Maslow reportedly said, if all you have is a hammer, the whole world looks like a nail. With regard to the human sciences, methods grounded in participation, not objectivity, give us access to phenomena not otherwise available. Postmodern and constructivist approaches to therapy tend to reference the humanities, not physical science, for their operative methods. Narrative approaches emerging from this orientation emphasize the creation of contextual meaning through process, not the search for facts or scientific "truths."

Combs and Freedman (1994, p. 270) outline six interrelated ideas that characterize postmodern thought as it applies to psychotherapy:

1. *Realities are socially constructed.* This is the core idea of social constructivism. Each person develops within the larger social context (family, culture) that shapes identity, thinking, feeling, and worldview. As Mair (1988) observed, each of us is made in the image of the master story that we serve.
2. *There are multiple possibilities for how to describe and classify the "reality" of any situation.* Anyone who has ever sat at a family dinner knows this one.
3. *Knowledge is performed, not found.* This is reminiscent of Sartre's statement that the only truth is action—what one does. Knowledge is not outside the process of participation but is a product of participation.
4. *Knowledge is constituted through language.* Language is the medium through which we construct reality. Language also includes gestures and pictures—all signs used to convey meaning. Words are not passive carriers of fixed meaning but are imbued in the structure of their use with the subjective meanings of the narrator.
5. *Realities are organized and maintained through narrative.* We combine the distinctive pieces of language molded experience into a meaningful whole or narrative that expresses our subjective reality: the story that extracts the essential elements and preserves them in context. Narrative organizes, maintains, and shares our experience, making it a part of the larger social narrative (Brunner, 1986).
6. *There are no essential truths.* Disappointing, I know.

Social constructivism concerns itself with how family and culture provide themes that shape the kinds of narratives that emerge within these larger systems. These themes are embodied in the culture's laws, religions, and institutions, as well as in its shared mythology, motifs in art, literature, and film. This story is greater than the individual: "The telling of our storied experiences allows others to take us in and gives us a future beyond ourselves. We are articulated by these themes, permeated and formed into relevant beings in the image of the story" (Mair, 1988, pp. 127–128).

Constructivism at the level of the person concerns how each person crafts a subjective reality out of the myriad experiences of life with others and the world. As a person's concept of the world grows, he or she organizes future experiences according to that concept. We make distinctions based on socially and personally constructed frames of reference that continue to organize and punctuate reality (Keeney, 1983).

Narrative in therapy concerns itself with how those subjective truths are "storied" into an organized collection of meanings structured (and partly attenuated) by language. Language is the means by which a person comes to know and create the world, and our construction of reality is contained by the language we use to create it (Brunner, 1986). Perhaps Shelly anticipated this idea in postmodernism when he proclaimed, "Poets are the unacknowledged legislators of the world." Put simply, reality is what we make of it (Watzlawick, 1984).

As a person makes sense of his or her life, memories are organized into stories, and the stories of discrete events and experiences weave together to form a life narrative. These narrative themes constitute a personal mythology that serves as an interpretive filter through which the person makes sense of new events. Clearly, then, a client's narrative is more than "just a story." Narrative gives one access to how the client's inner world is constructed or organized. The story is like a travelogue describing the terrain, the topography of the person's interior landscape.

One way in which we consolidate a reality is by telling our stories to ourselves as we behave in sync with our narrative. We live in the body of our conscious and unconscious narratives (Kershaw, 1992). We get a certain kind of job, marry a certain type of spouse, engage in certain causes and recreations, and so forth. As we "tell" our different stories through action and thought, we contact different aspects of our own reality. We structure what is allowed to happen and constrain or free our potentialities depending on how flexible and accommodating the narrative is to modification. What meanings are contained within the story that allow or disallow certain ways of being, feeling, thinking, and experiencing others? How does a narrative contain the structure of conflict and tension that either propels a person to change and resolution or keeps that individual stuck in a lifeless storyline? There are many ways to tell the story and many ways in which the therapy relationship can change it.

The meanings embodied in the story and the language that carries that meaning never remain static in the therapeutic dialogue (Anderson & Goolishian, 1990). Therapist and client are in the process of creating new history on the way to change. In other words, they become co-authors of new stories that influence the unfolding future narrative possibilities. The therapist cannot predict specifically how participation with the client will turn out as the client imagines new story lines. It's like writing a novel; the characters reveal themselves in the process of their creation. "As we interact with clients, the system is engaged in a mutual, recursive process of perturbation and compensation and, ideally, through this new process new, more satisfactory contexts or realities are co-created" (Becvar, 1997, p. 160).

Each person "stories" his or her life to give it structure and meaning. The therapist tells a story about the client's story, a metanarrative, that helps not only to understand the client's narrative but to create opportunities to change it (Kershaw, 1992). A person's stories give access to and describe a different realm of self-experience. To help the client see the dimensions of his or her reflection as it constitutes in the relationship, the therapist holds up a mirror of the client's narrative. When the client is trapped in a story that inhibits the possibility of change and growth, the therapist can help the client to "re-story" the narrative. Again, the observer is part of the observed as the therapist participates with the client to discover a new narrative emerging from the dialogue that is expressive of the client's inner strivings.

There is no single way to accomplish this goal, no one technique that suits all clients. Often the constraining narratives that clients use to story their lives have very tight plot lines! As Milton Erickson (1994) observed, "Each person is a unique individual. Hence, psychotherapy should be formulated to meet the uniqueness of the individual's needs, rather than tailoring the person to fit the Procrustean bed of a hypothetical theory of human behavior" (p. 1).

In my participation with Mike, I came to understand that he was recreating his life with stories, and I think it surprised us both that we found a medium through which we could both participate. As he conjured up memories from his past, he evoked the feelings and meaning these narratives had possessed for him before, but he also infused the narratives with new emotions and meanings that emerged from the perspective of looking back. He was telling and revaluing the story of his life. Evoking these emotions with me as an audience gave Mike access to parts of his self-experience that would not have been available to him if not for the facilitating language of the therapeutic relationship. This process in itself was an antidote to his depressive malaise and life crisis. It was as if this life review allowed Mike to realize that he had lived his time well and, at some parts, even heroically.

As he told the stories, he not only created new meanings but stumbled across some charged memories as well. When remembering his war experiences especially, he sometimes prevented any further inquiry, saying, "I don't want to talk about that." I knew that he sensed that some of these wounds were too big and too private to share directly and that he wanted only to refer to them obliquely. He was too old, he said, to open that door. He chose to carry these memories with him intact, almost as if he wanted to preserve them from becoming desanctified by too direct an explication. Some experiences deserve to remain wrapped in the shroud of mystery. He was honoring his dead.

Some experiences that Mike related seemed to have a parallel process, a metaphorical equivalence, to challenges he was facing currently. These challenges involved losing his wife to Alzheimer's disease, the loss of his own power, and his crisis of value and meaning as he felt more alone in his final years. He told the tale of flying his plane high above the cloud cover and ascending into the sudden blackness filled with stars. He described how he discovered an almost sacred sense of timelessness and peace, even with the ever-present threat of death from enemy aircraft. As I listened to him, I sensed that telling this narrative put him in touch with the same inner resources he had drawn on at that earlier time. When he intoned, "It's all right, it's all right," I heard him not only remembering his feeling of trust, come what may, in that extreme situation high above the German countryside, but invoking his powers to meet his current life battles.

Mike needed a way to "reframe" the unacceptable idea that he was coming to see me for therapy. So we created a new story between us that better fit with his larger narrative and the ways in which he saw himself. There was no room in his personal mythology for a "head doctor," which was fine with me. We were just polishing and cataloging his timepieces (his pieces of time). We were only researching and organizing his valuable collection, not carefully arranging the store of his valued memories and emotions. He wanted, he said, to "tidy up" his collection and to assess its value before he died so that it could be a legacy. He certainly did, in ways that we both came to see as the real value of our meetings, but about which we had an unspoken agreement not to comment directly.

It occurs to me now that Mike agreed to return after the first two meetings only when I took an interest in his *person,* not his *problem,* when I expressed a desire to see his watch collection. Soon after that, I also went from being "son," to being Eric, and he to being Mike. With the activity surrounding the watches to diffuse too direct an acknowledgment that we were now in a relationship, other dynamics were allowed to emerge. There was Mike's transference that I must be Irish (I became "son" on a different level, since *he* was Irish). There was also the loss of the young Irishman, Patrick, whom he was supposed to protect and for whose death he still felt somewhat responsible. Sometimes I felt like I substituted for Patrick in hearing the *rest* of the story of Mike's life after Patrick died. I subtly tried to find a way to re-story Mike's guilt over surviving Patrick. Our reframing that someone had to live to make Patrick's sacrifice worthwhile and that Patrick had received the glory that, at one time, Mike had sought, made a small contribution to incorporating losses that sometimes seem larger than the stories we can tell about them. It is, perhaps, where narrative leaves off and poetry begins.

Mostly Mike did not need to re-story the past or to tell a better narrative that would give him more freedom, fulfillment, or choice. Mike needed a witness to validate the story that was already behind him, to evoke its impressions, emotions, and meanings, so that he would know how to approach the narrative leading to its conclusion. In some small way, he was reclaiming his past, owning it fully. He gave me (and himself) his stories, and he wanted me to have something tangible so that they would not be lost in time—the gold watch, the one his father had given him, the one (my story tells me) that he carried with him through the war.

✂ ✄

Truth Is a Razor

A child draws the outline of a body.
She draws what she can, but it is white all through,
She cannot fill in what she knows is there.
Within the unsupported line, she knows
that life is missing; she has cut
one background from another. Like a child,
she turns to her mother.

And you draw the heart
against the emptiness she had created

—"Portrait," by Louise Gluck

They fuck you up, your mum and dad.
They may not mean to, but they do.
They fill you with the faults they had
And add some extra, just for you.

—"This Be The Verse," by Philip Larkin

The truth is, I don't really like working with troubled teenagers, and Chloe came into therapy under circumstances that every therapist dreads. The 18-year-old daughter of divorcing parents, she didn't hide the fact that she didn't want to see me or any other therapist. Her last therapist forewarned me that she was being "forced" by her parents to seek treatment. She was, as they say, "acting out," and it was, apparently, my job to do something about it.

As a colleague once observed, "Nobody gets out of their family alive." A bit of an exaggeration, but one that's recognizable, to some degree, to most people. Of course, psychotherapy often involves, directly or indirectly, some exploration of family pathology as it filters down in time through an individual life, into present thoughts, emotions, and relationships. Everybody inherits. The psychological inheritance each person receives from one's family affords the dowry for that person's marriage and is bequeathed to the person's kids, and the whole great cycle continues. It's part of the mix of life. And it's often the stuff of therapy, especially for kids who are in the thick of it like Chloe.

Chloe was having more trouble than most kids surviving the travails of early adulthood. One can never reduce into a single set of identifiable causes why one kid fails to thrive while another somehow manages to get to adulthood with minor injuries. I quickly discovered that Chloe certainly had her share of disappointments. The problem here, for me, was that the few troubled teens I had worked with seldom had a language to articulate their misery, or a motivation to communicate it to anyone who looked remotely like their parents. And language and interest in exploring one's inner life are the oxygen that psychotherapy needs to be vital.

Chloe was another casualty from the domestic frontlines, the everyday terrors of family life. Somehow we were supposed to find words together that made growing up more tolerable. Somehow, presumably, I could persuade her to find some motivation for therapy, and she could discover a desire for change.

But I should have found out more about Chloe before I accepted her as a client. I should have known that it was a setup for failure. I should have referred her to someone who enjoys working with troubled teens. I chided myself for vanity. I accepted Chloe as a client because at the time I was a postdoctoral resident and a therapist I respected recommended me, and I was flattered. A poor reason, and one for which I did not want my new client to suffer. Others warned me about clients like Chloe. Chloe even warned me about clients like Chloe. When I insisted that her reluctant mother let Chloe make the arrangements for our first appointment, Chloe said on the phone: "I don't care when we make it. It doesn't matter anyway; no therapy is going to make me any less messed up. It's a waste."

Now, here she sat in the waiting room, slumped in a chair with her eyes closed, Walkman headphones blasting so loud I could hear the music from where I stood. I spoke her name twice but failed to penetrate the percussion of gangster rap pounding away like a sonic sledgehammer: "Brain stem music," a colleague once called it. I was about to reach down and touch her hand when, sensing me standing in front of her, she opened her eyes. Without moving, she looked me over skeptically. I watched her critically sizing me up, assessing my appearance in my black blazer over a blue tee shirt, dismissing me as irrelevant before we had spoken our first words. She must have felt me forming a first impression of her too: taking in the eyebrow piercing and nose ring that seemed imposed on her attractive face, the uncombed black hair with the orange streak falling over her pale shoulders, which were partly covered in a black tank top. On the white skin (out of place in Southern California) of her right shoulder perched a tattoo of a black crow, its beak pointed toward her ear. She reluctantly dragged the headphones off her head and acknowledged my introduction with a grunt, sullenly following me down the hall to my office.

We paused briefly as I stepped aside and motioned for her to enter the room ahead of me, a minor convention on my part intended to imply to the client, "You take the lead from here." Chloe sensed some intentionality in the gesture, paused suspiciously, then walked deliberately across the room and sat in my chair. I sat on the couch without a word, tilted my head and looked, slightly bemused, into her alert face. In response, she crossed her legs, leaned forward, put her index finger to her chin like a Hollywood therapy cliché, looked straight into my eyes, and said, "Hmm." She unwaveringly held my gaze for a moment, then suddenly rose from the chair and started inspecting the contents of the room. She picked up a piece of pottery, turned it upside down to look at the bottom signature, put it down. She wandered a few feet and stood in front of a framed watercolor hanging on the wall.

"This piece sucks," she asserted.

"What don't you like about it?" I asked.

"I don't like anything about it. The colors don't work. It's flat, it's static, it's supposed to be abstract but it's just bad."

"I couldn't agree more," I said honestly.

"If you don't like it, why do you have this shit on your wall?"

"I share this office with another person."

"Is he a good therapist? . . . 'cause his taste in art sucks!"

She turned to see my response to her question, so I put a dubious expression on my face and shook my head side to side doubtfully. Chloe turned her face away to hide the ghost of a smile. "Ah," I thought, "that was easy." The therapist I shared my office with was actually a talented woman therapist, but Chloe was right about the art.

"This print's good," she announced looking at a silkscreen. "Most shrinks have cheap posters on their walls, or stupid sayings: God grant me this and that bullshit, and the wisdom to know bullshit from horse-shit." She wandered over to an oil painting and stood silent. "This one's really good," she announced, standing in front of the desk over which it hung. Another long pause: "Did you paint this?"

"Why do you think I painted it?"

"Goddamn therapists. Because your *name* is painted on it in the corner."

I was somehow surprised that she bothered to know my name. "No, my mother painted it. It actually hung in the Corcoran Gallery in Washington, D.C.," Chloe put on a disdainful face in response to my naming the city, "for an art show. It won a competition there. She painted it in 1957." I was about to say, "So, you really like art," antici-pated her scornful rebuff, and kept my mouth shut.

"Are all of her paintings this abstract expressionist stuff?"

I was again surprised, this time that she could name the school. I noticed, with a bit of scruple, that I was suddenly more interested in her. "Most of them; a few portraits and landscapes too."

"It reminds me of a Kandinsky I saw at the Met . . . *in New York City*. This is one of hers too," she said, walking to the painting over a side table, "but she didn't sign it."

"Good eye," I said, and hoped I didn't sound patronizing. She didn't react. I took that for a good sign. Silence, as she lingered looking at the painting closely. I liked that she could stand there in front of a painting, saying nothing. It didn't feel *entirely* passive aggressive, and I thought I might be able to make allowance for her lack of civility. I was going to need to find areas of connection with Chloe for there to be any possibil-ity of productive therapy.

"Well, let's hope the son is as talented as the mother," she said with an air of resignation. She walked over to the couch where I sat, and stood there in front of me impatiently.

"What?" I asked.

"Well, you'd better get into your shrink chair," she said exasperated.

———

I was her third therapist in six months. I called her last therapist, whom she refused to see anymore, to ask his impression of Chloe. He seemed to need to talk about it. He said that their work together had not been productive and that she was a poor candidate for outpatient work. Actually, he said, "That kid is really messed up, and she needs a lot more than outpatient work. After the first few weeks, she didn't show up half the time. She doesn't want to come, and she lets you know it every session she does come." As he recounted the brief history of his association with Chloe, I heard "borderline personality" mentioned a couple of times, along with a few other vaguely diagnostic observations. As I listened, I reminded myself that the "borderline" diagnosis often seemed to be more expressive of therapist frustration than client's psychological organization. I braced myself for tough going. He agreed to send over her file. "Good luck," he said. "Let me know how it goes."

"Hmm," I said. When I was a kid, I saw an amateur boxer get the crap kicked out of him by a kangaroo in a carnival sideshow. I think the boxer was supposed to go one round with the kangaroo without falling down to win $50. He seemed to feel pretty embarrassed about it until his buddy climbed into the ring and went down even faster.

"Well, I'll send that file over, let me know how it goes," he said again.

Two days before my first appointment with Chloe, I read through her file, trying to piece together what was happening in her life. I expected the usual disjointed collection of documents and therapist's notes and observations. Often I choose not to read a client's file before the first meeting, preferring to form my own impressions of the person without being influenced beforehand.

This file was different. The first time Chloe's parents took her to therapy, her therapist performed a thorough evaluation of the family situation. She recorded each member's impressions and view of the family's troubles, along with some penetrating observations about the parents' relationship, impending divorce, and their relationship with Chloe. Chloe had an older sister who had recently left for college, a younger brother in grade school, and a younger sister in junior high school. Apparently, Chloe's parents expressed little tolerance for the idea that their daughter's problems bore any relationship to either the disintegrating family or their personal relationships with her. They pointed to the fact that her younger siblings seemed to be managing in school and had few behavior problems. Her parents had been unwilling to engage in any sessions that were not specifically related to "solving Chloe's problems."

In the notes, Chloe described her mother to the therapist as "cold and controlling." She said that her mother used to be fun to be around when she was a child, but that "she has turned into a bitch," and that she had "closed in on herself." The therapist had observed that the "mother has strong traits of obsessive compulsive personality disorder, is very rigid and defensive." The therapist noted that Chloe's mother seemed to have catalogued every injury ever received from a marriage she appeared unwilling to leave or attempt to improve. The father, a successful stockbroker, seemed to the therapist as "more emotionally available to the kids" but "ineffectual." He "appeared emasculated" by his marriage which he, too, seemed unable to improve or leave. He resented his lack of influence in the family and claimed to welcome an "impending divorce." He had disengaged from sharing any interests with the family, but he spent a lot of time pursuing numerous extramarital affairs of which all in the family were aware and which spilled over into open conflict. Chloe's mother had "accidentally" backed into a car she thought belonged to one of her husband's mistresses in a parking lot. It turned out to be the car of one of her husband's clients. "It doesn't matter," she reportedly said, "he's probably doing her too." The prevailing climate in the house was one of conflict and hostility, an ongoing sniper war where everyone kept their heads low until the next chaotic skirmish broke out. Neither parent wanted to accept an offer of either family or marriage therapy.

In my brief contacts with Chloe's parents, I discovered nothing to disqualify the former therapist's impressions. Chloe's mother had practically dictated her expectations for how she wanted therapy to proceed and the results she expected for her financial investment. My immediate response was to be sympathetic to her concerns, but to explain to her that I would need to speak with Chloe directly about setting our first appointment. She objected to this arrangement, relenting only when I gently insisted. To her demand that I report to her the progress of our work (after all, she was paying, she said), I explained that Chloe was 18 and, therefore, controlled the terms of confidentiality, though I encouraged her and her husband's participation and involvement after I had a chance to talk about it with Chloe. They had "been that route before," she said, and neither parent wanted to consult with me directly in the therapy setting. It was her contention that Chloe simply needed to "snap out of it" and "stop making herself the center of attention."

As is often the case when one child becomes the lightning rod for the family's charged atmosphere, no one wanted to look at how Chloe's problems expressed what was unspoken between family members. One clue to Chloe's distress was that her behavior became progressively more problematic once her older sister went away to college. This sister, who had been defiant, rebellious, and "out of control," had apparently channeled enough of the family electricity to insulate the others from some of its effects. With her gone, Chloe somehow became conductive, and the behavior problems of which her parents complained became expressive of her own and the family's ills. And those problems were significant.

Chloe had surprised everyone in her family, her parents reported in the file, by transforming from a compliant, attractive, "no trouble" third sibling, into an oppositional, irresponsible, sloppily dressed, self-destructive "terror." Though she had always gotten good grades and stayed involved in sports, music, and art, when she entered high school she had begun "hanging out with the wrong crowd." She often stayed out all night at parties. The police arrested her twice for underage drinking, as well as once for petty theft when she stole a carton of cigarettes from a convenience store. She was indiscriminately sexually active ("acting like a slut," her mother said), had stolen money from them, and seemed to have no plans or goals beyond wanting to move out of the house, which her mother opposed. Her mother expressed a desire to have Chloe live with her "after the divorce." As it turned out, the divorce had been "impending" for four and a half years, and even a separation had yet to take place.

The most notable aspect of Chloe's changed behavior by far pertained to the destructive and injurious acts she practiced on herself. In the past 10 months she had begun cutting her arms, wrists, and thighs with a razor blade. At first, the cuts were superficial. Over time, they became deeper. In her attempt to conceal her behavior from others, she treated the lacerations herself with butterfly bandages. But as her cuts became more severe, they necessitated her seeking emergency treatment on three occasions, requiring sutures to close these deeper cuts. A few months prior to her entering treatment with me, she attempted, and very nearly succeeded, in committing suicide by swallowing a fistful of tranquillizers. A friend found her unconscious and brought her to the emergency room where doctors pumped out her stomach.

The more I read, the more I regretted accepting Chloe as a client. She did seem highly unsuitable for a course of outpatient treatment. She was volatile and unstable, and, even more important, she was unmotivated. Her actions indicated that she possessed little of the self-reflective awareness upon which effective therapy depends. Her past involvement with therapy seemed to indicate that she was probably not able to form a working relationship with a therapist. Without this relationship to serve as the vehicle for productive change, there was little chance of progress. She was very possibly suicidal. What she really needed was a group home or a day treatment program where her behavior could be more closely monitored.

On the other hand, I chided myself, she was in need and floundering. I might be able to do some good. Perhaps I could facilitate her entry into a more suitable setting. In any case, I had already agreed to see her. What kind of therapist attitude, I asked myself, would I want my own kids to face when they finally present themselves in therapy to recover from their years of growing up with *their* parents? That clinched it. I would meet Chloe and see what could be done.

Now, here she was, judging the art on my walls and criticizing by her incivility my lack of art with her. This kid was tough. Not just difficult to relate to, but tough in that I sensed something hard and committed at the center of her anger. It was more than brattiness. It was something that could only have emerged in response to real pain, and therefore it deserved respect. She was sitting on the couch now, and I was in my chair.

"So, what, I gotta talk, right?"

"That's the idea."

"How's that supposed to help? It never has. Why would you want to listen to all my crap . . . so you can get paid a hundred bucks an hour?"

"Partly because of the hundred bucks an hour, but also because I'd be interested to understand you better. I'm interested in people, in what's important to them." The first shots were fired.

She paused, "The art in my house is all shit. My parents think it's really cool and modern, but it's the kind of junk you see hanging in corporate offices. They think because they paid a lot of money for all these pictures that they must be worth something."

"You're an artist then?" I asked, glad she was starting to talk.

"I do art. I wouldn't call myself an artist yet. But I do a lot better than that," she said, derisively waving her hand toward the ugly watercolor.

"That's a relief."

"Yeah, not as good as that though," she said quietly, pointing toward the painting over the desk. I let her see by my expression that I acknowledged the praise and was impressed by her ability to make the distinction. Here is something to work with, I thought.

"Maybe you'll let me see your stuff sometime." This was a risk, and premature, but the whiff of angst from unrecognized artistic efforts is a palpable scent. I also knew from her file that her parents disapproved of her desire to pursue an art degree in college. Now they would approve, I imagined, of anything that would keep her out of the hospital.

"Mmm," she responded noncommittally.

"Only if you'd like to, of course," I continued, "sometimes art is like dreams, you can tell a lot about what's going on with the painter from the painting."

"That sounds like crap."

"Actually, it's not. I used to own a gallery, before I was a therapist." These two observations were not really related, but I was looking for points of contact. It was also an exaggeration I felt entitled to make. I actually owned a picture framing store that also sold art prints and paintings.

"Really, where?"

"In Virginia."

"Psheew," she said dismissively, as if art couldn't happen in Virginia. But I could see she was becoming curious.

"Where did your mom go to school?"

Now we were getting somewhere. Chloe was interested in something. There was little chance of her launching right into her own struggles and concerns. It would be a slow testing to see whether I was even worth talking to further.

"She went to American University."

"Is that a good school for art?" She said it flatly, but it was the first time she had spoken without an edge of criticism or hostility.

"My mother went there a long time ago. I don't know whether it's still a good school or not."

"Hmm," she said.

"I guess you were interested at one time in going to school for art?" How could I have said it . . . a beginner's mistake. I had gotten this from the file, and I wanted it back before it was out of my mouth.

"What, did that asshole shrink tell you that?" she asked.

Teenagers always feel threatened when you glean information from secondary sources, especially when they are as fragile and suspicious as this one and feeling the oppression of authority in all aspects of their lives. Chloe had apparently had many battles with her parents over this issue.

"I guess I picked that up from Dr. Hale," I said.

"Dr. Hale," she said disdainfully, "He's an idiot."

"It's annoying to realize that people are discussing you when you're not there."

"Yeah! No," she contradicted herself, "I mean it's no big deal. It's not a secret or anything. He's just an idiot." She sat stewing, and I had the impression that she was angry for allowing herself to respond off guard and affirmatively to my comment . . . as if my empathic comment *mattered* to her.

After a moment she looked up at me, snorted, and said in a resigned tone that implied that she might as well give this idiot a chance, "I used to think about going to school for art, but I don't think about it any-more. Hale made a big deal out of it, like I had given it up, and needed to confront my parents or something, because they thought my doing art was stupid. Like I needed some kind of intervention, like you would do for a drunk. That was the least of my problems," she muttered.

"There was a lot more important stuff to worry about," I said. As she rested her arm on her thigh her sleeve had slid up, and I noticed for the first time the lines of razor scars and a large flesh colored band-aid near her wrist. She must have sensed that my glance had taken them in; a moment later she unconsciously shifted her arms, folding them to turn the marks from view.

"Have you heard about my family?" that intonation again.

"Only a little. When we first talked, I asked you if I could get your file from Dr. Hale, and you said you didn't care. That had some stuff in it from past sessions, but I'd much rather know about it from you. What's it like? I get from your look right now that it sucks."

"That's an understatement."

Chloe surprised me then with a vivid description of life in her family. She talked angrily about her parents "fake" divorce. "You couldn't blow them apart with a canon. Who else would they have to make miserable? They're like those guys that tie themselves together by the wrist and then whip out the switchblades." She said that she would be in favor of them following through with a divorce, but she seemed resentful about it. She talked of the loss she felt when her sister left for college. "We don't talk as much now because she's so far away. She always worried about me, but she had to get away, just like I'm going to get away soon." But she acknowl-edged that she had no clear idea of what was next for her. "I know I'm screwed up, but every time I try to get my shit together, stuff happens and I can't deal with it. It's like I want to screw up, but I don't really." She spoke of her "clueless" former therapists, and derisively described one's attempt to get her to construct "affirmations" that she could recite to her-self to "increase my self-esteem." Though she remained aloof, and the tone of her voice remained hard and cynical, Chloe made an effort to tell me her story. Just as important, in contradiction to my prejudice, she knew how to use words. She was articulate in her unhappiness.

As we both settled into the session, my worries dissipated that Chloe would completely dismiss me as irrelevant, and I became absorbed in her narrative. She spoke of her parents' imposed expectations about her future and how they were indifferent to what had been her most cher-ished interest: art. As she described how the family had slowly disinte-grated, through the cynicism I thought I heard a hint of longing and remorse when she described her early loss of emotional connection to both of her parents.

I was struck by Chloe's vivid impressions. "My mother never has a real conversation any more . . . her face *is like rubber.*" These impressions argued that behind that cynical defensiveness there was a sensitive observer. "They are both either way too far into my stuff or not around at all. For a long time, I was still close to my dad. But then he got weird, and I had to cut him off."

After she said this, Chloe must have picked up on some slight change in my expression or an enhanced alertness that I did not intend to convey. I thought later that she was extraordinarily tuned in to subtle signs and distinctions in expression. Responding to this change, and without seeming to be covering up anything, she continued, "I mean, it wasn't anything perverted. It was just, like, he always told me I was his favorite kid and that I understood him more than my mom, and shit like that. I used to kind of like it, that he wanted to talk to me."

"It felt good to have your dad need you; you felt special."

"Yeah, But after a while it was like he was just kind of glomming onto me, and I got kind of disgusted. My sister told me she felt the same way before she went to college."

"It seems like you felt it was too close in the wrong way, like he was turning to you for support he should have been getting from your mother. It's hard to feel like parents are being parents when that happens."

"Yeah, exactly," she said, and then paused reflectively.

She seemed to have forgotten to reject my offerings and fend me off, and I thought I understood a little more about why she needed to keep me, and others, at such a distance. How, I wondered, would her conflicts around her father's using her to meet his own needs play out with me as our relationship deepened?

I was pleased. This was the basic stuff of rapport building, using reflective comments to communicate to the client that the therapist understands the dimensions of her inner world. And Chloe was responding. As the session progressed, she seemed to accept the opportunity to have a listening ear. I noted the contrast between my initial impressions and my perception of her now that I felt that I could be somewhat effective. This might work. We hadn't talked about her cutting herself or her suicidal feelings, but that would come in time as our relationship developed and she came to trust me.

With any other client, I thought, I would have addressed the issue of suicide and self-harm immediately. I would have secured her agreement to call me if she ever felt desperate. Most clients would find that kind of directness and support helpful and reassuring. But I sensed that Chloe would have rejected these offers because they would imply that she wanted or needed my support and help. I would allow the relationship a little time, and then address her self-injurious behavior when she believed that I could be of help.

I secretly prided myself on my empathic skills and thought of Chloe's other therapists with sympathy. No kangaroo was going to kick *my* ass. "Affirmations!"—Ha! This kid had an incredible sensitivity to anything contrived or phony. She was smart and had a keen ear for nuance. Given a climate of support and respect, she just might be able to use therapy to get her life together.

Of course, Chloe had little awareness that she had contrived a cynical persona to protect herself from what might be painful contact with others; a persona that kept her from getting what she needed the most. But she was very perceptive, almost paranoid, in her monitoring of cues from others. A talent, I reasoned, that she developed from her long history of anticipating disappointment in her relationships. What this kid needed, I told myself, was someone to really "get" what she was suffering as she tried to tear herself away from a toxic family environment and launch herself into the world with her own thoughts, ambitions, and sense of identity.

The first session had gone much better than I had hoped. She was talking. As I ushered Chloe to the door, I wondered if she would follow through on what we had decided would be weekly meetings.

"So, do you think you can tolerate coming here each week?"

She didn't respond directly, but paused and said, "I know I gave you crap on the phone, but I appreciate that you told my mom to keep her big nose out of it."

"I didn't exactly say that."

"My point is," she said, irritation creeping back into her tone, "you let her know this would be none of her business."

"Well, you're 18 and legally an adult, and I feel like the only way this can work is if you're willing to do it and it's confidential. I told your mom that I won't report to her on our conversations . . . that it has to be between you and me. She wasn't too happy about that," I added gratuitously, looking for a little extra mileage from this exchange.

"But she's paying."

"Yeah, and that means that she is supporting these sessions," I said opening the door, "but the conversations you and I have stay in this room."

"Cool," she muttered as an expression of consent, "I guess I'll see you next week," she said, stepping out.

"Cool," I said, as an expression that I acknowledged her consent. Chloe rolled her eyes, pivoted, and walked down the hall. "Hey, you think you invented 'cool,'" I said, standing in the doorframe, "my generation invented 'cool' before you were even *born*," I called after her.

"Whatever!" she said disdainfully over her shoulder, as she passed through the double doors and out into the street.

Over the next five or six sessions, Chloe continued to slowly open up. She talked about her conflicts with her mother, her disintegrating relationship with her boyfriend, and her frustration about trying to find a decent job that paid enough so that she could get a place of her own. At a deeper level, she was able to talk about the storms of emotion and despair that seemed to overwhelm her when she felt she could no longer cope with the many frustrations in her life. In one respect I didn't care what she talked about, I just wanted her to engage in our dialogue. It was far too early to begin challenging or interpreting the particular configurations of her self-expression or how she made sense of the events and relationships she described. She seemed willing to have me track her closely, tolerated my asking questions when I didn't understand, made efforts to help me get her impressions and feelings. We verbally sparred a little as she exercised her talent for cynicism and I offered my sardonic replies in return. She liked these minor contentions, and I understood her desire to engage me on this level to mean that she was feeling an increasing connection with me and needed to create some temporary distance to protect herself. I would explore its meaning with her later. I was developing a working relationship with Chloe. Things were starting to get better, and I had yet to make a real interpretation.

My confidence got a reality check a short time later when I noticed a new bandage on Chloe's arm. It looked as if she was attempting to conceal it under a long-sleeved shirt, but its edge was visible beyond the cuff. I waited to see if she would mention it. She didn't. Toward the end of the session I asked a few leading questions that would provide an easy segue for her to explore the subject. She knew what I was up to but didn't respond, deftly steering the conversation elsewhere. I persisted.

"I'm noticing a bandage on your arm today. Do you want to talk about that?"

"I have been talking about it," she said folding her arms, her tone becoming suddenly hard.

"I mean, do you want to talk specifically about the cutting part . . . about how that happens?"

"Not really."

"Not really?"

"Not really!"

"How about if we talked about some things that you might do that would help you explore what's happening before you cut yourself . . . that would get more directly to what is going on for you."

"What, like *journaling*," she said derisively.

"Well, that might be one way, but maybe it's not for you. What about the idea of putting up a blank canvas and going at it."

"Going at it? You mean ripping it up," she taunted.

"You know what I mean . . . more directly expressing your emotions through some other medium than slicing your arms."

"Oh. Yeah, I think I want to slit my wrists . . . no wait. Why don't I go do some painting instead. Let's see, a little yellow and blue, a beautiful scene with a happy sunset. . . . We'll all feel better!"

"I was imagining more of a Jackson Pollock kind of process."

"Oh, yeah, there's a model of mental health for you. That did him a lot of good, didn't it?"

"I get the impression you don't want to talk about this today," I said in a way that so emphasized the obvious that she cracked a cynical smile.

"I *knew* there was a reason they finally let you play with the other children." Chloe was referring to a childhood incident I had illustratively related to her in which I had subdued an older bully by knocking him over the head with a toy wooden musket.

"Maybe we'll talk about it some other time. I hope your arm is okay," I said lamely.

"Maybe we will. I've got it under control," she said.

The next three sessions went well. I felt that Chloe and I had developed a tenuous rapport and that my initial prejudices about her were mostly wrong. I observed that she was increasingly able to make use of what therapy had to offer her. Of course I also saw what her other therapists had termed her "borderline personality" traits. She was impulsive, emotionally labile, had little tolerance for frustration, and was self-injurious. She tended to idealize or repudiate others and think in all or none, black and white terms. She was prone to the kind of "fragmentation" under duress that let me know she had big holes in her internal architecture where important relational experiences and self-supportive structures should have been built. But I also saw Chloe in more human terms as a sensitive, perceptive, and fragile soul who protected herself by developing a hard shell.

Chloe's interpersonal history had afforded her little opportunity to develop the kinds of internal strengths and abilities that would have helped her regulate and channel her passionate feelings. Now the barricades she had built around herself precluded her gaining these skills and strengths through the give and take of reciprocal relationships. Yes, she was unpredictable, and her emotional storms flip-flopped between being impulsively expressed outwardly and being turned back on herself in destructive binges of abuse. Her self-loathing was palpable, but I felt that Chloe also possessed some firm ground at the center of her shaky life. There was something solid in her, like the core of a planet whose outer atmosphere is all a tempest. At that core, she knew that she deserved the same things all of us want: to belong, to be loved, to love someone, and to find a place in the world to cultivate her unique calling in terms of talent and interest.

As I got to know Chloe better and felt her investment in our work increase, I began to think of a treatment plan. My goals for our work included the following:

1. To make an agreement with Chloe that she would make no suicide attempts and that she would sign a "contract" to that effect.
2. To help her stop her self-mutilating behavior by getting her to see how this worked against her own interests and progress.
3. To further a therapeutic alliance that would help her to explore the conflicts underlying these behaviors and come to greater self-understanding, differentiation, and integration.
4. To help her articulate the effect of her family's current dynamics on her sense of self-efficacy. (Chloe was adamant that she wanted no "joint" sessions with her parents.)

These seemed like reasonable goals, and I wanted Chloe to see how they expressed my growing care and concern for her. I tried gently to win her support for them as guides for our work together. I felt certain that I had enough rapport with Chloe to suggest some ways that she might more adaptively respond to her periods of despair than the self-destructive cutting she had committed in the past. But Chloe resented the whole idea of the "goals for therapy" discussion, and I had to put the suggestions in the background of our sessions together because I did not want to further disrupt the fragile alliance between us.

Four weeks later, however, I noticed that Chloe had been cutting herself again. I again invited her to talk about what had caused her to use so extreme a method of expressing her anger and despair. I encouraged her to consider other ways to communicate that she was in distress. I made it clear that I was always available to talk with her if she felt in danger of hurting herself. I tried to help her understand that if she fully engaged in what we were doing she would not need to resort to using her own body as a medium for this anger that turned back on her, that she would be able to use words to discharge it directly. But to this appeal on my part she responded with either cynical taunting or sullen silence. In the following weeks she seemed more distant and inaccessible. She questioned whether therapy was useful. Nothing had really changed in her life . . . not that she expected it to. She didn't know why she bothered. How, I wondered, had things changed so rapidly in our sessions?

As the weeks wore on, this change continued. The more distant and disengaged she became, the harder I tried to listen to Chloe closely. The more I steered her to be immediate and direct in the sessions, the more she resisted my interventions. I wondered again whether it was *because* there was the opportunity to get closer to me that she found it necessary to create misunderstanding, that her resistance reflected her fear of being hurt by me as others had hurt her. I invited her to explore this theme in light of the change in the tone of our sessions and asked her to reflect on what she felt happened to disrupt the rapport of previous meetings. She remained evasive. She only said in response to my asking her to reflect upon our relationship that it was "Okay, I guess."

After this discussion our sessions seemed to get back on track for a while. So, we muddled along, and I thought that at least she experienced me as someone trying to care for her. And occasionally she would use our session to ventilate her frustrations and anger. Secretly, however, I wondered whether I really was doing Chloe any good. I had noticed in the previous weeks that I sometimes felt a nagging anxiety about our upcoming appointments. I realized that I increasingly contemplated our meetings with a kind of low-level dread or displeasure.

Taking care to preserve Chloe's confidentiality, I talked over lunch about her case with a colleague to get some new perspective. It helped to tell the story of my work with Chloe, and I realized as I spoke that we had made some progress.

"So how do you feel when you're sitting with her?" he asked, ordering coffee and lighting a cigarette.

"Depends on the session. Sometimes I'm relieved when she's just talking. Sometimes I feel really engaged with her, the hour flies by and I'm very gratified with our session."

"But not recently." He took a drag from his cigarette, and despite blowing the smoke out of the side of his mouth, it drifted back over the table.

"I'm still trying to eat here, okay?" He took another long drag, blew the smoke downwind, and then put out his cigarette.

"Thank you. No, not recently. Mostly I feel ineffective and like I'm talking to someone from Paris."

"Why Paris?"

"Because Chloe is condescending and abusive when I don't understand her language."

"Ah. So what happened before things changed for the worse?"

"I tried to help her come up with some alternatives to her self-destructive behavior."

"Ah. So she's manipulating you with this cutting thing, huh."

"I don't think so. She tries to hide it from me."

"But not very well."

"No. But she never brings it up, and when I do she wants to change the subject."

"This is the one who is suicidal?"

"Well, she had an attempt some time ago . . . not recently," I said. He looked dubious.

"I don't know. From everything I've heard it sounds like she might be manipulating you with the cutting. She's got you going, dancing to her tune like everyone else. She's a borderline. She gets off on you having to pay attention to it. Maybe it's a power thing. Has she ever come on to you?"

"No. And how is it that just saying someone is borderline sounds like you are making an intervention and not merely a diagnosis.

Actually, it sounds more like a sentence: 'I now banish you to the borderline.' "

"Wait 'til she starts following you home, and you'll wish you could banish her somewhere."

"This is not helpful."

"I'm just saying, first of all, you don't like working with teenagers; second, she's got you dancing; third—I forgot to bring my checkbook, can you cover this? Thirdly, I forget what thirdly is, except that I think you're doing great with her. Hang in there. At least you have managed to establish a connection with her. So far that's further than anyone else has gotten."

"Yeah, thanks a lot. Don't even think of lighting that," I said, pointing with my fork as he took another cigarette from the pack.

Two weeks later Chloe was sitting on the couch looking disengaged. She stared out the window. "You seem not to know where to begin today," I offered.

She shrugged, "I don't have anything to talk about." A long pause. "I mean, what the fuck is the point anyway? All I do in here is complain."

I had noticed that her use of profanity lessened over the weeks as she became more comfortable and articulate in our meetings, and it increased when she was frustrated and struggling. Something had happened. I studied her for a moment, then said, "Chloe, would you mind rolling up your sleeve."

She sneered and pulled back her sleeve. There were no new cuts. "See," she said, "nothing up this sleeve either."

"Do you want to tell me how and where you hurt yourself?"

"No . . . but that's very impressive doctor," she said patronizingly.

"It seems pretty important to talk about."

"Why's that?" she said folding her arms.

"Why's that? Because, if you are cutting yourself, I need to know about it. We need to do something about it so you are not hurting yourself."

"Like what?" she sneered.

"Like why don't you start by telling me what happened to upset you so much?"

"You want me to feed you a line of crap like I have been?"

"You've been feeding me a line of crap?"

She stared sullenly at her feet. No response.

"Then why don't you tell me the truth now."

"Truth is a razor," she said angrily, lifting her head and looking into my eyes. A long silence as she held my gaze.

I suddenly felt nervous. "What the hell is that supposed to mean?" I surprised myself by asking her, breaking the silence. Careful, I told myself, don't let your frustration upstage her and take up too much space.

"Never mind, you wouldn't get it."

"You're right; I wouldn't get it through mind reading."

"Fuck off."

"Look Chloe, I can't help unless you talk to me about what's going on with you."

"Maybe I don't want your 'help,'" she said, making quotation marks in the air with her fingers.

"Okay, let's back up," I suggested. "Something has happened to upset you since I last saw you. Would you be willing to at least fill me in on what has happened?"

"Is it that important to you?"

"Yes."

Chloe spent the rest of the session giving me a detached, emotionless inventory of events that week. She had had a big fight with her mother, and they had screamed at one another. She thought her boyfriend was probably being unfaithful with someone who was a mutual friend. She had a job interview at a beachside clothing store; she didn't know how it went. She recited this catalogue as if they were dates in history, not pertaining to her, without even her ability to give words to her anger, unhappiness, or outrage. I thought I would have to content myself with this much for now. She had at least told me she had not needed stitches for the wound on her thigh. Things would get better, I reassured myself.

Things didn't get better. In contrast to the alternating self-disclosing and defensiveness of earlier sessions, Chloe became increasingly defensive. I tried to discover what could have disrupted our fragile therapeutic alliance once again. I had passed no judgment, made no unreasonable demands. I had been supportive of her obvious struggle to differentiate from her parents and come to terms with her disappointment in their shortcomings. I also wanted to help her give up her self-destructive behavior, which was clearly now hindering her from engaging in therapy with an open and straightforward disposition. But she continued to refuse to contract that she would not injure herself or inform me of any suicidal intentions. I considered "forcing" her to accept these conditions by threatening to terminate therapy if she could not accept these rules. But this felt so much like a recapitulation of her existing issues that I was certain she would quit therapy.

Most important, her refusal to contract with me about her cutting still did not feel like she was trying to manipulate me. She never wanted to talk about her suicide attempt or her cutting. It was an area she seemed to prefer not to bring to my attention at all. Now she was making a stand about it. I chided myself; I should have insisted on her agreement to some basic conditions in the very beginning. This would have avoided putting us in the untenable situation of my using termination of the relationship as a cudgel for compliance. But would it have mattered, I wondered? Chloe would not have abided by any rules that were not to her liking anyway.

"Chloe, it seems like we have lost our way here," I offered one meeting, "and I'm wondering what to do about it. For the past few weeks you seem to not want to be here at all. I'm at a loss, so I'm hoping you can help me out, because I'm not sure what you need to make this work." No response. "I mean it seems like we were getting along pretty well, but that recently you haven't wanted to engage with me in our talks together."

"You sound like my dad when you say that."

Ah, I thought, I was wondering when that little piece of transference was going to appear. "I sounded like your dad when I said that," I reflected back to her.

"Yeah, '*you never talk to me anymore,*'" she imitated her father. "'*I don't even know you anymore, you used to be such a good girl.*'"

"So, when I ask you what's happening between us here, it sounds *exactly* like your dad whining that you don't give him what he wants . . . that you don't gratify him anymore by giving him attention."

"No, not exactly like it."

Good, she heard the part I wanted her to. The Polonius technique, "by way of misdirection, finding direction out." I wanted her to explain to me her way of constructing reality, not the other way around.

"He wants me to be all loving and his little girl, and listen to his complaining."

This was more than she had given me in weeks. "There must be something I do that makes you think that's what I want."

"I don't think that's what you want. You're not whiny. You don't want to complain to me, you want to hear *me* complain. Figure that one out."

"What might I want from you then that reminds you of what happens with your dad?"

"How the hell should I know . . . to be a good little patient I guess."

"Oh, okay, it feels like I might be judging you or implying that you could be doing this better?"

"Maybe . . . I don't know . . . or, shit. Maybe you just have expectations or something. You're the one that's supposed to understand things here, and know what to do. But you can't make things any better for me."

There was a lot here. "I might have some expectations of you, and that feels a little like your father wanting something from you."

"Yeah."

"And it seems like I should be able to know a little better what I'm doing . . . to give you some answers or something. Your father hasn't protected you and neither have I."

"Yeah! But how could you protect me or understand my life. What you want from me is . . . I don't know . . . I mean look at you sitting in your shrink chair; what do you know about what I have to deal with?"

"I agree, Chloe, I can't protect you."

This conversation was a double-edged sword. All kids seem to have a need for a fantasy involving idealized, all-powerful caregivers, protectors who can keep them safe. It's a good fantasy for a while. It gives them a sense of invulnerability so that they can throw themselves into new experiences. But as kids develop more of a sense and structure of self, they have to gradually give up this illusion of invulnerability and protection. They have to accept a more realistic version of caregivers who are flawed, but important and sustaining. At some point we all realize that our loved ones cannot protect us from our own life. I would have seen it as a positive sign if Chloe developed a little of that idealizing transference toward me. It would have signaled that she was looking to our relationship to address some of those losses.

In Chloe's case, her parents' troubles subverted this legitimate developmental imperative. The climate of hostility and conflict and her caregivers' narcissistic use of her to meet their own emotional needs added to her pain. It had become apparent in our sessions that Chloe was like the third leg of a three-legged stool; each of her parents turned to her for gratification they could not get with the other, triangulating her into their relationship. As long as she complied, responded to each of their needs and allied against the other, the family was more stable. After her sister left for college, however, Chloe became the sole gratifier of her parents' needs. But she had had enough, and surely this was one piece of her burden, and a key to her "transformation." The family legacy of chaos stripped away too fast the illusion that she was safe and protected. Now Chloe's fantasy, her lurking transference hope that I might be that idealized powerful other, was faltering, just as it had faltered with her other therapists. It was a truth that Chloe needed to accept for her to eventually take responsibility for her own life, but I could see that she resented me for it.

"Why do you want to talk to me anyway?"

"We've met for a few months now; why do you think?"

"No bullshit questions in response to questions, just give me a straight answer."

"Okay, because I like helping people look at their lives. It's important . . . and at the risk of scaring the crap out of you, because I've come to care for you, and I want to help you become whole again. My guess is that it might be hard for you to hear me say that."

She shrugged.

We sat in silence for a long time. It was a lot, and I didn't want it diluted by too much talk, even though I wanted to explore her reference to my "expectations." I waited, but Chloe did not speak. The silence deepened.

"Our time's almost up," I said after a while. "Is there anything you want to say before we end?"

Chloe shook her head and left without a word.

For a few weeks, Chloe again seemed to reengage in our sessions, but I felt something missing. It was as if her faith in what we were doing was crumbling. She held back, appeared elusive and diffuse, and I could tell that she struggled outside of sessions to hold it together. Though she found a job at a clothing store in Pacific Beach, she seemed increasingly depressed. Her relationships at home got worse as she made preparations to save money and get a place with her boyfriend. Her parents approved of neither the idea nor the boyfriend. Chloe bristled at the suggestion that I could suggest a therapist who would meet with all of them to mediate their disputes.

One session, she again sat sullenly. I noticed she wore a loose long sleeved shirt. "Chloe, may I see you arm please?"

She shrugged but made no effort to show me. I leaned over and gently lifted the sleeve above the wrist and saw a new bandage there. "Why do you have to make a big deal out of it? It's none of your business," she said in a resigned and exhausted voice. She crossed her arms. "Don't worry about it, it's not too deep, and it's not what I want to talk about."

"Too bad," I said. "You are under my care, and I have to know that you are not in danger of harming yourself . . . and clearly you are in danger."

"You don't know anything," she said.

"So you tell me something. Why do you do this to yourself?"

"Because it feels good, stupid!" she said with sudden force.

I was taken aback by this eruption of energy. "Yeah, right. Look Chloe, you are in trouble. These past few weeks you seem really down, and I'm concerned that you are going to seriously hurt yourself again. I need for you to agree that you are not going to cut or harm yourself in any way if we are going to continue working together."

"So you want to make me quit coming here then? Fine!" She stood up.

"No, I don't want you to quit, but I'm not going to be held hostage by your refusal to play by my rules."

She looked at me surprised, and then bitterly. "It has nothing to do with you!" and pacing muttered, "stupid, stupid, stupid."

"Chloe, I need to make sure that you are not going to hurt yourself. To do that I could have you hospitalized," I threatened calmly.

"For how long," she said disdainfully, pausing to turn toward me, "I've been there before, you know." She clenched her fists, and her face contorted as if trying to find words for her frustration. I stood up and soothingly motioned for her to sit down, but she turned and walked out the door. It was the first time she had left a session before the complete hour.

———

I contemplated my options. I could call her parents and let them know that I was worried she might be in danger. This would be a justified breach of confidentiality. But I was certain their response would exacerbate, not stabilize, the situation. I could have the police pick her up and hospitalize her. At least then she would be in a controlled setting. There was also the option of a crisis center. I called them, and they said, yes, they had a bed. The sound of it made me pause. It would be an involuntary commitment. It would probably mean the end of our therapy. I thought of her two previous therapists with a different kind of sympathy now. Strike three, I reflected bitterly.

I decided to wait an hour and think about it. I reflected on our initial sessions, and the success I thought I had creating an alliance with Chloe. Now I wondered if she really used her sessions merely as a forum to complain. Was she incapable of any real change, just as she herself asserted? I knew that I anticipated our appointments with increasing displeasure. No, I had begun dreading our meetings. Chloe was resistant and entrenched, so caught up in negative self-image and expectations that others wanted to manipulate her that it rendered her unable to muster the kind of self-reflective capacity necessary for effective therapy. Despite the opportunities before her, I thought with irritation, she refused to even look at how her self-destructive acts undermined everything I was trying to achieve with her. "Because it feels good," she had said. Ha! A cynical and aggressive rejection of my help.

This was the problem in working with troubled teens, I told myself. Adult problems may be solidified, but at least adult's frontal lobes are fully developed, I muttered to myself sarcastically. And what do you expect from her borderline tendencies, I asked myself? Despite my best efforts at entering her world, understanding her as she wished to be understood, she let me know at every meeting, directly or indirectly, that I had failed. I paced about the office, reviewing in my mind the diagnostic criteria for borderline personality disorder: Unstable relationships, check; idealizing and then demeaning important others in a polarized fashion, check; volatile and unstable emotional shifts, check; suicidal and self-harm behaviors, check; poor impulse control, check.

One thing made me decide to wait it out. Though I thought Chloe must be the most resistant client I had ever seen, and though I felt as if she often deflected any interventions other than those expressive of basic empathy, she had said that I would "make her quit coming here." It implied that I would have to force her to not come, and indeed, in five months I could not recall her ever missing a session! She was always on time, slouched down in the same chair in the waiting room, her Walkman blasting away to "make sure the other crazies don't talk to me." She must be getting something from our sessions, I thought, if only the experience that I could tolerate and not abandon her. Further, during that time, though she had cut herself, she had made no actual suicide attempts. This was surely a kind of commitment in itself, this *action* on her part that said clearly, "I will be there." I decided to have faith in that history and to see if she would appear for her next session.

It was at this point in Chloe's therapy that something happened in my own life that changed my perspective on her struggles and made me mindful of the subjective frames of reference I brought to my sessions with her. My work with Chloe occurred during a year of postdoctoral residency in Southern California. Years earlier, I had needed a change in my professional life; something new to keep me interested. Though lucrative, I sold the picture framing and art gallery business, and with the wife and kids, packed up and moved to San Diego to complete my doctorate in clinical psychology. It was something I had worked on for a decade as I juggled the various obligations of life. Neither my then wife nor I had jobs waiting for us, but with the proceeds from the business, some inheritance, loans, and whatever employment would surely be available we thought we could keep the wolves away. It had worked out pretty well.

However, by the time I became Chloe's therapist, stresses were high as I contemplated what was next. Finances were strained to breaking. Years of grad school grafted onto the other obligations of family took their emotional toll, and my own kids weren't doing so well in school. I felt overwhelmed. I had that sense of fragmentation and diffusion one experiences when emotional resources are completely depleted. Now, sadly, it looked as if I might have to sell my one remaining asset to make ends meet: my old 30-foot sloop, which had been my project, my pride, and my solace in rough times and rough seas, sailing the Chesapeake Bay and now the wide Pacific.

She was the family boat, and my father and I had invested a lot of "sweat equity" to bring her back to life. Years before I contracted with a trucker to haul her cross-country on a tractor-trailer from Virginia. As the trucker handed me the bill in California, he must have been comparing the cost of the move with the worth of the old boat when he remarked, "You sure must love this boat." "It is a wonderful madness," I replied. I hated to think of selling her, yet there seemed no way to afford her. I had discussed it with my wife, and she, with patience and reason, marshaled the facts into lines so straight that they appeared in my imagination like a phalanx of Roman soldiers. We had arrived at the rational solution. It made sense, in light of current circumstances, to sell the boat. I sadly agreed and decided to post an advertisement at the chandlery. However, when I left the chandlery the next day, it was not after having posted a notice for the sale of the boat, but with a new anchor that cost $468 (plus tax). And I felt better . . . a lot better! I went home to share my joy with my wife. She was somewhat less enthusiastic.

Why, she asked, would I purchase an anchor for $468 (plus tax) when I could not even afford the boat it was supposed to hold? I explained to her the beauty of the anchor, that this was an anchor that could hold you in any storm, could keep you off the rocks in the fiercest gale. I even showed it to her, invited her to see how its form so beautifully followed its function, to see it as a work of art. How could she not appreciate the necessity of protecting and securing me and my boat with a strong, invincible anchor? In California, I explained, the holding ground is different: sand, rock, and coral. It's different terrain down there, not like the Chesapeake mud in which my father and I had anchored. In California, when the wind picked up or the conditions got nasty, I sometimes woke on the boat to discover the anchor dragging and the boat drifting out to sea or toward some danger on shore. *I needed this anchor.*

She thought I was missing the big picture. She began making highly rational arguments to my increasingly irrational and defensive justifications. The more she pushed me to admit that I should not have bought the anchor, the more beautiful and necessary that anchor became, and the less I felt she understood me. This debate went on for some time. About the point in the argument where the anchor was beginning to possess magical powers for me, she delivered the coup de gras with, "You're in denial. We're going to have trouble paying our rent this month unless you charged 'that thing' on our credit card!" "So what," I countered, "we can live on the boat!" It disorganized me when she started accurately throwing around psychological terms and I had not had time to regroup. She threw up her hands. On the way out of the room, she said, in one final, accurate, interpretation, "Well, I guess sometimes an anchor is more than just an anchor!" I had not realized she had picked up so much while editing my dissertation.

That night I slept on the boat, feeling hostile and resentful. I knew I had been feeling adrift and ungrounded, as precarious as a boat hitting the rocks. Sailing had always been my best way of pulling back together and soothing my own fragmented soul, a connection to sustaining experiences of time on the water with my father or my children. To hell with what made sense; I didn't want to sell the boat! I had considered replacing the traditional old sloop with a smaller, cheaper modern boat that had no wood to varnish, one that did not need so much care, but there was no room in my imagination to put such a vessel. It just was not me. Irrational and self-undermining as it seemed, buying that anchor for the boat made me *feel* better. My boat was in order, well fortified for anything the weather might throw at me. As I sat pondering in the cockpit, seeing the anchor attached to its chain up on the foredeck in all its functional and self-defeating beauty, I thought of Chloe.

If Chloe had not quit therapy with me . . . if she showed up for our session one more time, I decided I would take a gamble. I decided to share with Chloe my experience of buying the anchor: How it was so irrational, and made me feel so much better when I had felt overwhelmed. I also decided to tell her, and here was the risk, that I now understood why she felt the need to cut herself when she felt completely overwhelmed. Far from being ultimately self-destructive, for her it was an attempt at coping, of temporarily pulling herself back together, of getting the overwhelming and unbearable feelings outside of her. Cutting was Chloe's way of externalizing her despair. Physical pain has the startling effect of focusing one's attention on the immediate situation, much different from the pervasive and diffuse threat of impending self-disintegration.

The more I thought about it, the more I believed I understood why Chloe refused to sign a suicide contract as a condition of working together. That would be like getting her to agree that her pain was bearable. Maybe she wanted to *communicate* to me that her pain was unbearable. Why else would she not just capitulate like other clients who understood it as a reasonable request? Could it be that for Chloe it was so central, and yet so without any clear structure that she could express, that she had intuitively held her ground against my intrusion? If so, I wanted her to know that I could see that she had refused to disqualify the message that she felt she could no longer contain her pain.

As I reviewed my history with Chloe, I also realized I had been unwilling to explore how Chloe's self-cutting was, paradoxically, her attempt to achieve a sense of wholeness in response to the experience of fragmentation. The colloquialisms for this are descriptive: A person says they are "falling apart," "going to pieces," having a "breakdown." I remembered, when we first met, Chloe's own description of herself as a "basket case," which is how one advertises a machine that had been disassembled for repair, but never fixed and reassembled, its parts thrown in a basket in disarray. If cutting served Chloe's efforts to prevent a sense of complete disintegration, could her cynical assertion that it "feels good" actually have been true for her? Could truth, indeed, be a razor when all else resolves into a thin red line, like the shape of the letter "I"? A single act that both records and expunges the terrible inner terror and brings consciousness back to a single point here-and-now? Yes, truth could be a razor when all else seemed lost and she could find no other way of hanging onto the fundamental experience that she inhabited her own skin.

How irrelevant my suggestions must have seemed to Chloe. Especially since these suggestions were, like her other therapist's "affirmations," merely prescriptions from me, and not a product of our mutual exploration and dialogue. She must have sensed that part of my wanting her to sign a contract was so that *I* could feel comfortable and in control, acknowledging only that harming herself would hurt *me.* My attempts to persuade, and later to coerce, her to give up cutting for more "adaptive" methods of coping communicated to her that I did not understand her inner world where cutting *was* adaptive. The situation reminded me of Rollo May's (1979) observation that neurosis is not a *lack* of adjustment; in fact, an adjustment is precisely what a neurosis represents. The client's "sickness is precisely the method that the individual uses to preserve his being" (p. 95). My attempts to take her cutting away from her also communicated that I could not accept that she lived in an experience in which self-injury is actually a move toward cohesion. Was that why she said that maybe she didn't want my "help"? Because I had never demonstrated an interest in exploring the utility, even the value of her cutting, she assumed that her inner world was too unpleasant a place for me to enter—that I could not accept it. *And she was right.* I did not want to enter deeply into a world with Chloe in which irrational cutting was a step toward feeling better. Maybe Chloe's actions, I thought now, said to me that it is better to hurt and be alive.

I was concerned that Chloe would scoff at my story and not accept it on its own merits. I worried that she might feel patronized by the qualitative difference between my buying an anchor for my sailboat and her slicing into her own flesh. But I also wanted her to see that, at least, I was ready to accompany her to wherever she might need to take me in her inner labyrinth. Her resistance had been in response to my unwillingness to fully meet her on her own terrain in a world I could not accept. She feared being hurt by me as she had been hurt by others who were important to her, others whose disappointment that she would not conform to their "expectations" meant, for her, the loss of her meaningful connection with them. I knew I didn't have to play by the conventional rules that govern other types of relationships. This was therapy, and the normal economy that regulates how people stay connected did not apply. It startled me to realize Chloe feared being injured by me despite my efforts and what I thought of as my empathy for her. I was the one who wanted her to change for the better, the one who wanted to help pull her out of the mire of self-hatred and despair, the one who didn't want to get his shoes muddy.

I hoped that she would realize that I now saw that she had been willing to come to me, every week, on time, but that I had been unwilling to completely come to her. Most of all, I just wanted her to allow me to have another shot at understanding her the way she wanted to be understood, not the way I wanted to see her.

As I walked down the hall to the waiting room and turned the corner, Chloe was slouched there in her customary chair, her Walkman blasting. I made an effort not to smile in relief. Normally I prefer to let the client start the session, but this time I asked her if I could begin. Chloe sat silently at first listening carefully. She actually smiled cynically at the part about how buying the anchor made me feel better. But as I narrated the escalating argument between my wife and me, where her rationality only served to further increase my distress, Chloe's face became serious and dark and she nodded in recognition. I had prefaced the story by saying that I had had some stuff happen that gave me a different perspective on her cutting herself, and she had snorted skeptically. Now, as I was ending the narrative, she needed no interpretations about the parallels; she was way ahead of me. She just put her face in her hands and cried for a long time. It was the first time I had seen her cry. Then, partly to remove herself from that moment of vulnerability, she offered, "It's about time. Did you think that signing that stupid paper would really keep me from offing myself if I really wanted to?"

Things changed after that. It was as if there was something between us that remained unnamed but which is at the core of any successful therapeutic relationship. To any objective observer, it would appear that this was the point at which the real work of therapy began.

Chloe wrestled with the problems in her life. She struggled to grow up faster than she would have liked, trying to negotiate difficult changes without the inner and outer resources that could have supported her. And her self-referential view of relationships and events had to transform to accommodate others in the world . . . me included. She was, of course, just at the beginning of her journey of self-awareness, and many other struggles emerged as therapy continued. To me, however, the real work of therapy, and the most healing aspect of our hours together, was the emergence of that ineffable substance that infuses the spaces between the borders, connecting them across the chasm.

Carl Rogers (1969) spoke of this reaching as a kind of universal experience, when a person realizes he or she has been deeply heard and the moistness in the eyes is a kind of weeping for joy. "It is as though he were saying, 'thank God, *somebody* heard me. Someone knows what it's like to be me.' In such moments I have had the fantasy of a prisoner in a dungeon, tapping out day after day a Morse code message, 'Does anybody hear me?' And finally one day he hears some faint tappings which spell out 'Yes.' By that one simple response he is released from his loneliness; he has become a human being again" (pp. 35–36).

I continued to meet with Chloe for about a year. Of course, it was not all smooth sailing. Still, she never again cut herself during that time. She never signed any contracts. I never asked. By the time we ended our meetings, she was applying to art schools. She had moved out of her parents' house, and she had gotten a job that paid her enough to share a place and pay most of her bills. She was partly paying for her own therapy. And she came, on time, every week. There were times, she said to me, when she "couldn't handle it" and pounded on her legs with her fists. I could see that she was making an effort to not cut herself, partly to acknowledge our work together. Toward the end of her therapy with me, after one such episode, she related, "The next day I saw all these giant bruises on my thighs, and I thought this is just stupid, I don't need to do this to myself. There have been lots of times I thought it stupid . . . not too many when I thought I don't have to do it anymore." Hearing her say it brought tears to my eyes. Our work together helped her to internalize our relationship, and she began to be able to contain her powerful storms of affect.

Once, toward the end of therapy, Chloe suffered some serious setbacks that made her feel particularly vulnerable. She felt like cutting herself, but she also thought of our many meetings as representing a kind of track record. She said she imagined us in the customary setting of the office, she replayed our conversations, and somehow this helped her to pull back together. She said that during these times she could summon up my voice and hear it clearly, and she could hear her own voice responding. In that imaginary dialogue, she explained, she could often know better all the different parts of what she was feeling and thinking, finding somehow what she needed to do to help herself. I hope she still can.

CASE FOUR DISCUSSION
Resistance and Empathy

DURING THE EARLY part of our work together, I thought Chloe was the most resistant client I had ever seen. I didn't think her resistance had much to do with me. Primarily, I thought this because I knew that my *intentions* toward her were always to understand and help her, and I thought I was communicating this through a fundamentally empathic demeanor. Before we resolved the disruptions that kept us from deeply engaging one another, she seemed an unwilling participant. I saw her as guarded and defensive, and indeed, she could often be uncivil and insulting. I thought she had little inclination to look too deeply into her inner world, and in that I was most in error. I came to my work with Chloe with a traditional view of the nature of resistance, but my involvement with her taught me that resistance has multiple causes and levels. Some manifestations of resistance are produced by the collision of the client's and therapist's subjective frames of reference.

Sigmund Freud (1917) found that when his clients attempted to reveal their inner thoughts and feelings through free association they often reached a point at which they were unable or unwilling to continue. He surmised that they were resisting making explicit, or calling into consciousness, repressed material that was shameful, repulsive, and anxiety producing. Freud saw resistance as the client's innate protection against emotional pain. On one hand, he considered resistance to be a natural defense against overwhelming abreactions, however he also considered that it was a signal to the therapist that the client had come very close to the work that needed to be done. Freud considered the appropriate intervention to be an interpretation or analysis of the resistance that would give the client insight into the material that was being repressed or denied.

Freud's famous client, "Anna O" (Bertha Pappenheim), gave him his root metaphor for therapeutic work. She referred to the "talking cure" as "chimney sweeping" (Jones, 1953; Shultz & Shultz, 1996). When a chimney flue is stopped up, smoke fills the house, obscuring one's vision and making one's life a noxious environment. The smoke seeks outlets in other areas of the house, in the same way that psychological symptoms are indirect and perplexing attempts to get rid of the energy associated with repressed material. Freud originally saw a client's resistance as a kind of misbehavior, but later he saw it as a necessary part of the therapeutic process. Still, resistance itself carried a negative valence as Freud came to view it as an obstructionist and unproductive client activity. It was the job of the therapist to overcome the client's resistance through analyzing its meaning for the client.

Cognitive therapists took a different view of resistance. Rather than seeing it as a barrier against repressed and painful material, resistance was seen as a way of protecting one's own construction of reality. The idea is that people represent the world in which they live by constructing *cognitive schema,* maps that help the person predict and negotiate the terrain of life. The therapy process threatens, indeed calls for, an alteration of the client's way of organizing and predicting the world. Resistance serves to protect the person from too much change, disorientation, and displacement of old ways of seeing him- or herself and the world (Mahoney, 1988). Resistance serves as a kind of appropriate hesitancy about embracing changes that could unseat core references and old and meaningful systems of value and self-experience (Liotti, 1989). Anyone who has ever worked with victims of a natural disaster has seen the effect of too much change too fast.

Early in my studies to become a therapist, I became aware that what most attracted me about working with clients was not simply the amelioration of specific symptoms but using therapy as a medium for exploring the total human experience. Each client was a particular constellation of the infinite range of possible expressions of living. Each inflected the forces of life, and channeled, emphasized, and even opposed these forces in particular configurations. Existential approaches to redefining traditional analytic concepts appealed to me because the emphasis on holism spoke to my own commitment to remember that it is a person engaging his or her existence, not merely a "patient" who responds to my question: "So, what brings you here today?"

Existential approaches emphasize that to become fully aware of one's own condition means to be open to impressions, thoughts, and feelings, the life experiences that make one vulnerable and exposed to the joys and vicissitudes of existence. One can tolerate only so much existential awareness at once, and resistance in therapy came to be viewed as a protective "block" to this full awareness. As people bump into life events, and the interpersonal failures that cause them to experience pain, they begin to constrict and close themselves off to new opportunities for engagement and participation. Resistance is considered part of the client's "space suit" in an environment that is seen as alien or inhospitable for survival. Bugental and McBeath (1995) argue that the forces within the person that fend off the therapeutic inquiry are the same forces that provide some stability to the client's way of being in the world.

This was certainly true in Chloe's case. She experienced my expectations that she would give up cutting herself as usurping her efforts to remain an intact being, even if that meant staying closed off and insulated. My initial empathic inquiry, which she cautiously welcomed, was supplemented, or perhaps supplanted, by my desire to "help" her discard the only way she knew to achieve stability and prevent a sense of annihilation.

Whether psychodynamic, existential, or cognitive, most approaches to therapy embody the prevailing attitude that the therapist must somehow see to break through the client's resistance. Usually the therapist draws from interventions such as interpretation, disputation, education, or exhortation. The therapist may ask the client to gather evidence against his or her blocks, or use coping imagery, flooding, or shame attacking exercises. The client may be asked to eschew "irrational" thinking for rational processes that have the blessing of the therapist.

In other words, the therapist must muster a set of tactics designed to defeat the client's stubbornness. However, like Chloe, clients often seem ingenious in their ability to devise new ways to resist the best therapeutic maneuvers to overcome their resistance. Resistant client behavior seems, in this sense, to conform to Newton's third law of motion: For every force, there is an equal and opposite counterforce. My work with Chloe taught me that when overcoming resistance becomes a contest the client will always win. I came to see that clients possess their own wisdom as to how quickly they can become open to change and under what circumstances.

Dolan (1985) recounts the story of a man watching a butterfly emerge from its cocoon. Impatient with the slow progress of the butterfly, he decides to pry away the impediment of the shell, thus allowing the butterfly its freedom.

> He fails to recognize the protective nature of the constricting "resistant" cocoon. The butterfly, with the man's "help," is set free in the cold air prematurely. Deprived of adequate time to make the necessary adjustments within the cocoon, it crumbles into a suffering, helpless heap. The therapist must have reverence and appreciation for each client's personal rate of change, idiosyncrasies, difficulties, vulnerabilities, and resources. (p. 3)

Like the cocoon of the butterfly, resistance may temporarily slow a client's progress, but it simultaneously expresses a protective wisdom that can never be fully verbalized by the client. If asked about their reluctance, client's can only say—if they can speak of it at all—that for some reason they are frightened to go further or to talk of certain things. The butterfly's helper would see this as a moment when stronger intervention is required: Tearing open the cover and exposing the interior is considered by many to be the most efficient and useful thing to do. Techniques such as interpretation and confrontation are used to strip the client of old and confining constrictions. Without doubt, if the moment is right and the client is ready to deal with the realization that such measures bring, these techniques can be profoundly effective. The problem is that the therapist sometimes attempts to force the client into a premature insight that may not become fully integrated into the client's experience because the idea seems more the counselor's than the client's. The paradox is that the therapist's efforts to speed up the therapeutic process produce the opposite of the desired effect. As Erickson (1980) observed, knowing the correct treatment is not sufficient; it is equally important that the client be receptive and cooperative regarding the therapy, or the therapeutic results will be delayed, distorted, or even prevented.

Traditional models of resistance include the assumption that although the client's resistance may be in response to something happening in therapy, that resistance is none the less something that occurs *within* the client. Certainly there were dimensions of Chloe's resistance where this explanation seemed to fit. However, in any approach that centralizes the ongoing relationship between therapist and client as significant to the healing enterprise, there is another dimension of the phenomenon of resistance, and it is here that I learned the most from my encounter with Chloe.

In relational and systemic models, resistance is understood not as something that occurs *within* the client but as a phenomenon that emerges *between* therapist and client. Here, the intrapsychic is embedded within a larger context; the person's reality never exists solely within the "bag of skin" as in the traditional model of the individual psyche. Rather, the organization of experience, indeed, the structure we call "self," develops as a result of the ongoing mutual influence between the experiencing individual and the larger world of persons and things with whom the individual is in relationship (Ginter & Bonney, 1993). In other words, my experiences are never wholly contained within me but are coproduced between me and those persons with whom I share psychological space. This idea has roots that spread across many contextual theories and philosophical orientations. What these approaches share is the idea that the client's world can never be understood apart from the systemic context in which it occurs, including the relational processes unfolding between client and therapist. When resistance appears in the course of therapy, it must be recognized as a part of the particular therapeutic dialogue, and the *therapist's contribution* to the resistance must be understood.

For instance, when a client manifests what the therapist perceives as resistance to the therapist's interventions, the therapist is often tempted to conclude that the client is imposing his or her interpretive systems in such a way as to distort reality. I certainly felt this way when Chloe interpreted as injurious my efforts to help her develop more adaptive alternatives to her self-mutilation. After all, the therapist's intent is to help the client. So, when the client responds to the helpful interventions as somehow antagonistic, as Chloe did, the therapist concludes that the resistance must be based on the client's distortion of the therapist or the therapist's activities. In Chloe's case, I thought of her "distortion" of my efforts as transference and experienced it as coming solely from her. I assumed I had nothing to do with this transference distortion, and I ascribed it to the patterns formed in Chloe's screwed up relationships with her parents, patterns that were now being indiscriminately imposed on me. On one level my assumptions were correct. Another dimension of Chloe's resistance, however, had to do with how she understood and interpreted my intentions and activities as potentially injurious. I could easily say (and did say) that her perceptions were illegitimate. However, since therapy involves the unfolding interaction between the client's and therapist's different subjective and experiential worlds (Stolorow & Atwood, 1992), the question arises of whose reality gets to be referenced as the starting point.

It is true that if my internal representations of self and the world do not include the "reality" of a bus moving at a high rate of speed, then it is likely, should I step in front of it, that some self-reorganization will take place. This reorganization will happen regardless of my interpretation of the thing called "bus." Fortunately, most of us agree on what constitutes a bus. Often, however, therapists accord their clinical observations and interpretations the objective reality of a bus, assuming that these observations emerge from some well or storehouse of reality to which the therapist has access and the client does not. In other words, therapists assume the "truth" of their perceptions of the client without sufficient reference to their own subjective meaning making and experiencing. The therapist wants the client to "get" the therapist's more "adaptive," "healthy," "accurate" reality. The therapist may fail to recognize how he or she is influencing the transference of this particular client as both participate in the relational event.

Gregory Bateson's (1972, 1979) observation about inner cartography—that the map is not the territory—is as true for the counselor as it is for the client. When the therapist ignores his own meaning making activity, it may indeed seem to the client that he or she faces the danger of being run over by the therapist's seemingly objective interpretations and interventions. The client, sensing danger, steps out of the way of the bus, and the therapist writes in his notes for the session: "Client demonstrating high levels of resistance." This is exactly what happened when Chloe asserted to me that *for her,* truth is a razor . . . a kind of primitive and fundamental method she used for holding onto some core sense of being. My objective interpretations about her behavior were not "wrong," but they emerged from a reality that was mine, not hers, and it precluded a point of contact between our two worlds. As Erickson and Rossi put it, "Too many psychotherapists take you out to dinner and then tell you what to order" (as cited in Dolan, 1985, p. 6).

Of course, the client must impose meaning making templates on the therapeutic situation and will interpret some of its features as potentially injurious. The relevant questions are "What behavior on the part of the therapist elicits these resistant reactions?" and "How might the client's resistance be in response to the therapist's imposition of his or her own subjective and interpretive systems?" In other words, what is the therapist doing that signals to the client the potential that an already sensitive wound will be injured further by what the therapist intends? Whether or not this client expectation is real, or seems reasonable or rational to the therapist, is not the issue. It is real for the client. The important thing, Chloe taught me, is to understand and illuminate how it seems reasonable for the client to expect that her fears are legitimate.

I did not anticipate that my efforts to help Chloe stop cutting would represent for her an effort on my part to usurp her method of preserving a core area of experience, and yet that is how she made sense of it. The more I tried to get her to see things the way I wanted her to, the more she shut me out. The more I expressed concern, the more she experienced me as intrusive and controlling, just like her parents. Yet she was able to articulate the differences when I invited her to sort out her transference about how I sounded "like her father." It was not that I wanted her to support me emotionally, but I had certain "expectations," and this evoked in her a fear that I would reject her unless she gave up *her* ways of coping and came around to *my* expectations. I did not read a fear of rejection into Chloe's hostile criticisms of me, but that is precisely what she feared most. She sensed an impending retraumatization from one to whom she was turning for assistance in holding onto her life. Clearly, in retrospect, these expectations involved my desire for her to conform to my model of how "healthy" people cope, something she was not yet ready to accept because she was struggling with something much more fundamental: how to contain her existence at all. Chloe wanted me to stay within *her* experiential world, as I had in the beginning, not allow my own anxiety about her "getting better" to impose on her my frames of reference for how and when she should change.

When the hidden and underlying fears and associations of these relational events were made explicit for each of us, they no longer invisibly controlled our interactions. Furthermore, the very process of sorting through it all to find a common ground helped to introduce to Chloe the idea that her perceptions about herself and others were not representative of something true and fixed, but something she had constructed without fully understanding why. Before her therapy she had blamed others—her parents, her clueless shrinks—for the lack of an understanding and helpful relationship that she so desperately needed. After the basic disruption was resolved, Chloe grew less entrenched and rigid in her attitudes, views, and interpersonal behavior with me. As I became more important to her, more of a real person, she became more willing to examine and explore her ways of being in the world and to be open to change and revision. Recognizing and understanding the choreography of the relational dance, I realized, can become one of the most illuminating and powerful aspects of therapeutic exploration. The prerequisite is that the therapist is attentive to, and can make explicit with the client, features of the unfolding relational phenomena in a spirit of mutual inquiry and participation. This exploration and engagement is what sharing my story with Chloe initiated.

Resistance and transference are often two sides of the same coin, because therapy offers clients an opportunity for their derailed developmental strivings to become reactivated in the therapy relationship. For instance, at first Chloe expected that if I were a good counselor I should be able to powerfully and capably handle anything she threw at me. She wanted for me to always be able to understand her perfectly, to be unerringly empathic and perceptive. If I were a truly good therapist, I would have all the answers she needed. As I became aware of these unrealistic expectations, they felt to me like underlying assumptions that might emerge from a child, not an 18-year-old young woman. But Chloe had never experienced the gratification of this childhood illusion with her caregivers. She had been buffeted about, exposed, and stripped of a sense of protection and safety early in her life. Unarticulated but present, this unmet developmental need emerged in Chloe's relationship with me as an unspoken, implicit demand that I, as a therapist, should remediate this deficit by consistently embodying all those qualities of care she had had to give up far too early.

Chloe's frustrated hopes gave rise to powerful feelings of vulnerability and anger, and of being abandoned and ill used every time I failed to ascertain and gratify her needs. I became just another "clueless" therapist who had learned his craft through a correspondence course and who got his credentials through an ad in *Rolling Stone* magazine. Thus, the quality of my empathy in response to the transference meaning of these expressions (and my own participation in their emergence) was central to whether my activities evoked Chloe's resistance or participation.

If the client believes the therapist intends to usurp a core area of experience (such as questioning the validity, rather than the meaning, of the client's need to idealize the therapist), then the client's tentative expression of these hidden developmental longings will cease. These longings will go into hiding, and the protective behaviors the client has used in the past to prevent reoccurrence of traumatic injury will reemerge and manifest as a disruption in the therapeutic alliance (Stolorow, Brandchaft, & Atwood, 1987). For Chloe, this manifested as scorn and distain of me as well as her own self-loathing. In contrast, if the client feels understood by the therapist from within the client's own referential world, these developmental longings will emerge and be accessible, and the therapeutic alliance will be strengthened. The process of recognizing and understanding how these needs and secret desires become revealed and influence one's life and relationships serves to foster integration and to further illuminate the dimensions of the client's inner world. More important, I came to discover that when Chloe understood that I would behave differently than anyone else in her experience and not manifest the same traumatizing reactions, the relationship itself became a healing tonic to her bruised and wounded soul. It is this experience that Franz Alexander referred to as the "corrective emotional experience" (Alexander & French, 1946).

Empathy, in this definition, does not merely imply emotional resonance. Rather, it implies that the therapist must be willing to put in parentheses his own interpretive systems and, like Alice, follow the rabbit of another's self-expression into a unique and personal world. There, as I discovered with Chloe, up may be down, the relations between things may operate according to principles understood only by a Mad Hatter or the Queen or Hearts, and it will be the therapist's job to get to know them well.

Frieda Fromm Reichman is reported to have said that what clients really want in therapy is not so much an interpretation but an experience of something new. This was certainly true of my relationship with Chloe. Yes, we explored the ways in which she was "put together," and this helped her to understand herself better and to be mindful about how she made new choices. But during the troubled times, Chloe kept determinedly coming to meet me every week, not because she hoped I would offer her my insights but because she sensed that she could find something far more fundamental and meaningful. I'm glad she didn't give up on that as I learned to follow a path as thin as a razor past my own familiar reference points and into the place where she lived.

✂ ✄

The Many Chambered Heart

The mind is an enchanted thing
   like the glaze on a
katydid wing
    subdivided by sun
    till the nettings are legion

It has memory's ear
    that can hear without
    having to hear

It tears off the veil; tears
    the temptation, the
mist the heart wears
    from its eyes—if the heart
    has a face; it takes apart
dejection.

           —Marianne Moore

M y third grade teacher, Ms. Steitz (may she roast slowly on a spit over the licking flames of the nether world), was an expert at inducing humiliation. I like to think of her as a *shame artist.* She worked at creating a shame environment the way other artists work with clay or paint. Her classroom was her canvas, and I was her favorite color. For her part, she must have thought I was sent by some malevolent cosmic presence to make her life a torment and to disrupt the ranks of the closely ordered and predictable little world over which she despotically ruled. She was, needless to say, a very unhappy, humorless woman who disliked children and who valued rote learning, obedience, and conformity above all. I was an energetic and willful boy, always into everything. Obviously we were a bad fit.

Ms. Steitz thought that both horses and boys needed to be broken. She had a favorite tactic for any infraction I might knowingly or unknowingly commit: She forced me to stand in front of the entire classroom and place my nose in a small chalk circle drawn on the blackboard. While I stood there silently, my back to the class, she went on with her lesson. I was forbidden to take my nose out of this circle or to turn around to look at my audience. I remember that she always drew the circle a little high, so I would have to tilt my head upward to place my nose in the circle, as if I was expected to lean out . . . to *long* for my punishment. I despised her, and I couldn't wait to be rid of her come June.

Even though I kicked the dust of Ms. Steitz's presence off the soles of my shoes and moved on to the fourth grade, at the time I did not realize that her repeated administrations of humiliation would linger. Her shame bugs had bored their way down into some secret part of my imagination and left a larva of doubt. I had plenty of inoculating experiences at home to protect me from these emotional bumps and bruises. In a home full of boys we took delight in overt conflict; things happened fast, parental justice was swift and fair; there was not time enough for guilt or shame. But something remained of those very public injuries, and I avoided any situation that held the possibility for public humiliation.

Ms. Steitz's larvae didn't fully hatch until years later when I found myself in new situations that echoed standing up in front of others with the possibility of embarrassment. I would find myself in front of a live audience of hundreds, musical instrument in hand, ready to express myself the way I knew I could but for my heart pounding wildly in awful anticipation. Or, even later, giving a talk and feeling a rising anxiety that constricted my throat. I rarely avoided these situations, choosing to battle through these anxiety-producing activities, but I could trace the lineage of my performance anxiety. Though there must have been many other contributing experiences that shaped the "reality" I had constructed, they all collapsed into the screen memory of that primal social humiliation. It took me many successful trials to mostly master that anxiety.

One incident that year sticks out in memory from the hundred unremembered incidences of psychological classroom carnage. It was an experience that I think saved me from allowing Ms. Steitz to take up even more space in my budding psyche. I'm once again standing in front of the whole class with my nose in a chalk circle on the blackboard. I am forbidden to turn around to see who among my so-called friends is snickering at my ignominious subjugation. But as I stand there, nailed to the cross of that blackboard, my friends gambling over the contents of my raided lunch box, a moment of clarity comes to me, an epiphany, bestowed by a merciful providence to preserve me. I think, "dammit, I don't deserve this; there's nothing wrong with me!" And in that moment, in defiance of the commanded silence, I begin to sing!

I am trying to be a smart-ass and show my friends that I'm not really intimidated or humiliated, but I still look back on it as a moment of triumph. I sing *Love Me Do* by the Beatles. (A classmate maintained that I also shook my butt in time with the syllables of the "Pleeese" part, but I deny it.) Everyone snickers, and Ms. Steitz roughly grabs me by the collar and hauls me off to the principal's office. (Ms. Steitz got hers; she got fired the following year at the insistence of the other teachers who were disgusted by her tactics with the children.) I think now of the lyrics of that song, and it makes sense that I chose it. I look back, and I like that little kid. His healthy indignation and anger worked to keep the shame of those isolated experiences from reaching its tentacles deeper into my adult psyche. The angry part that said "I have no reason to be ashamed!" was preserving something important; it was ultimately much louder than the voice Ms. Steitz wanted me to hear. I did have to repeat third grade the following year, though, because I was deemed "emotionally immature."

Somehow these old reflections and associations, not conjured up for many years, returned to me after my first meeting with my new client, Dory. As she told her story, I found myself asking the question: "What if Ms. Steitz died and somehow became reincarnated as Dory's superego?" Oh, well, I think, at least maybe she will have chosen the right therapist.

Dory sat across from me, perfectly upright, legs symmetrically clamped together underneath the knee-length skirt of her business suit. Below the helmet of brown hair, cropped straight at the jaw line, eyebrow length across her forehead, her face was set in an attitude of alert expectancy. She seemed to be watching me for a sign for her to begin a presentation. A leather-covered organizer lay open on her thighs. Her hands grasped the organizer on each side, at the ready. I could see that she was ready to call this meeting to order.

I always note my first impression of a new client because I assume that what that person evokes in me is likely to be similar to how others perceive him or her. It gives me a first shot at understanding that person's interpersonal world. We had introduced ourselves in the waiting room. She had stood up, raised her forearm at a right angle to her straight posture, and offered her thin hand to initiate a handshake. It was a curt, professional handshake, a perfunctory contact of flesh. One instantly understood that nothing could be inferred except the fact that nothing should be inferred.

I already sensed that I was in for it. Here was a woman, I thought, whose formal outer demeanor was constructed along the principles of a siege wall. Releasing the contents of her inner world would be like storming the Bastille. As I ushered her into the room, she took a seat on the couch and assumed this closed but ready posture. I had to suppress a smile. Despite her stiff presentation, I somehow liked her already. There was something, I don't know, *committed* about her personality, however much trouble it probably caused her. Maybe I just enjoy people whose character quirks and idiosyncrasies set them apart and make them interesting. I could see that she wanted to get down to business and assume control of this uncertain and uncomfortable situation. I had a mischievous impulse to suspend this moment of uncertainty, to delay her launching right into whatever was written on those pages. Did I just want to see if she could manage to be spontaneous?

"Dory . . . now that's an unusual name," I said.

Realizing that she could not yet begin, her hands released the organizer, and she crossed her arms across her chest as if to put herself on hold. "Yes, my grandmother's name was Dory. It's a name that comes from the small boats that were built in New England where my mother's side of the family came from." She said this dutifully, as if it were her stock phrase for anyone asking about her name.

"Ah, it's very poetic," I said. But I thought that the lovely, sweeping, graceful lines of a little Gloucester dory had little in common with the right-angled impression this woman conveyed. She reminded me more of a rectangular and utilitarian rowboat. "Well, what's bringing you in to meet with me today Dory?" I asked, quickly abandoning my delaying impulse.

Her arms unfolded and her hands went back to their place on the organizer. Now she knew what to do. "I've been having a lot of anxiety, and this happens in a number of places in my life. First, I've been worrying a lot about things at work that really are not that big a deal. I mean, I find myself being concerned that maybe I haven't done a good enough job on something when I really know that I have. I lie awake thinking about it, and it takes me a long time to convince myself that, no, everything's okay. That's just an example. It happens with other things beside work.

"One very strange thing, this is different, is that I have been worrying a lot about someone being in the house when I get home. It's strange because the house is locked up and nothing is out of order, but I have to go all through the house to make sure nobody's there. I mean, I even look in the bathrooms and closets. It's weird." She paused, indicating that I might be permitted to speak.

"That must be very unsettling. After you go through the house, are you satisfied that no one is there, or do you have to check the house again?"

"I'm satisfied, after I look, that no one is there," she said nodding once. Tilting her head and looking at me over her glasses, she continued "But I need to check as soon as I get home. I get home before my husband. If my husband is away on business, it's worse. Then I sometimes worry during the night, and sometimes in the morning when I wake up."

"So you don't keep checking over and over, but it's worse when your husband is away." I was checking off diagnostic criteria in my head.

"Yes, that's the second thing. I have a sense of dread that something awful is going to happen to him when he's away traveling. I worry about him all the time," she said with sudden feeling that seemed out of place with the rest of her demeanor.

She looked like she was about to move on to the next point. "Say a little more about that," I encouraged. "What kinds of fears do you have for him? What might happen?" I had a sense that there was something juicy in this topic . . . something *messy.*

"I don't know. When he flies, I have this little niggling doubt that his plane might crash. Or when he drives on a trip, I worry that he might get into a car accident or something. Just that he may not get home. Stupid stuff." I thought, these seem like pretty strong abandonment fears, and I made a mental note to listen for these themes in future conversations.

"There's just a real sense of foreboding until he gets home," she continued. "He's kind of a bad driver; that's probably what I worry about most, and he never wears his seat belt. He calls me every night when he's away, so that's good. But it's strange. I mean I don't worry about my daughter. She's away at college. She calls once in a while, you know, just to check in. But I guess it's because she doesn't travel much. I feel like she's safe at school."

"Okay. So it seems that this fear has more to do with your husband. So you just have the one child, and how long has she been away at school?"

"It's been almost two years since Sherry left."

"How long would you say you've been struggling with all these anxieties?"

"Oh, Jeeze, I don't know, my whole life! But I guess it really started getting worse about two and a half years ago. Now it's just ridiculous."

"So you've always been kind of an anxious person, but it seems much worse now. When your husband travels, you have these thoughts that something might happen. Has there been anything, like an accident, that would start you thinking this way?"

She shook her head. "Nothing. It's not like something awful really happened so that it makes sense."

I was going to ask her how she felt about her daughter leaving for school and leaving her and her husband alone in their house, but she headed me off.

"Another thing," she said moving on with her list, "is that I used to be able to speak in front of people pretty easily; that's part of my job, making PowerPoint presentations. But in the last year I've just gotten more and more nervous about public speaking. It's actually something that I do pretty well, but I've lost some of my confidence about it. My voice shakes a little, and I think people can see it. It's embarrassing."

"It really does seem as if you've been struggling with a lot of worry. Do you have any thoughts or feelings about what might be going on for you that this public speaking fear is happening?" She shook her head, no.

"But another thing," she said, plowing ahead, "is that I'm really concerned that my boss thinks I'm not doing a good enough job now. Like he can see that I'm off my game. He's just so good at what he does, so articulate and smooth, and I feel like he can see that I'm not as good at what I do as I used to be."

"You feel as if he's noticing it. Has he ever expressed that to you . . . given you any indication that he is displeased?"

"No, he gives me great evaluations, but I know that he sees it. He's got to see it. We have to present to business groups and make pitches all the time. We work as a team. If I'm not doing it right, it could cost us." She looked down at the organizer, then put her hands flat on the pages.

"Is that everything on your list?" She smiled. It was the first sense I had that she *could* smile, and a *little* of the tightness went out of her face.

"I'm a big list-maker. I know it's obsessive . . . ahhhg," she shook both hands in front of her, as if she had been plugged into an electrical outlet. "But what can I say," she continued, "making a list makes me feel better. Anyway, that's not everything, but it's the important stuff. I've got some health problems, but I'm dealing with that. I'm just so tired all the time. I've got this chronic fatigue for the last couple of years, and they haven't pinpointed what's wrong yet."

"Dory, let me ask you a question: Why now?"

"Why am I coming here now?" I nodded. "I don't know. I guess all these worries have gotten worse, but I can't figure out why. Alex, my husband, wanted me to come. He's been pushing me I guess."

"Ah, you feel a little pushed by him. What might be some of the reasons he would like you to come?"

"Well, he has his own agenda," she said, rolling her eyes as if I would know from that gesture what she meant. She wasn't sure that I saw this, so she rolled her eyes again.

I raised my eyebrows. "You just rolled your eyes; I'm not sure what that meant."

"I guess I didn't say it before. It's on my list too. He thinks . . . well," she took a deep breath and exhaled, "he thinks that I'm not interested in sex. The truth is," she said conspiratorially, "he's right. I'm not, and never really have been that interested in sex. It's just not a big deal for me. I'm 42, and I've been married to the same man for 20 years, you know. It's not as if that whole thing is the center of the universe for me. He takes it personally; he always has. I don't blame him I guess. But I really didn't like it when I found his cache of girly magazines in the garage a few years ago. I can't believe he's interested in that smut. He said, 'What else do I have?' I said, 'Okay, do what you want, but if you are going to look at *Playboy,* then don't expect to make a stand about me not being interested in sex.'" (I didn't want to point out the circularity in this reasoning.) "I mean, is it right that a married man should have those sorts of magazines?"

"So you two have some problems around your sexual relationship," I said, ignoring the question. "We can talk about that in here if you like." She shrugged. "Or, sometimes people find it helpful to come in together to address marital and sexual issues. I want you to know that I could also arrange something with a couple's counselor for you and your husband that would be in addition to our sessions."

"Alex would never come to a place like this himself."

"Has he said that to you?"

"No, but I know he wouldn't."

"Are there any other issues in the marriage that seem important to mention?"

"Not really. That's not a really big problem, but it is persistent. Most of the time we do okay. I mean, sometimes I'm interested enough, and the problem goes away for a while."

For the remainder of the interview Dory inventoried the details of her marriage, her job, her relationship with her daughter, and the various ways she had of coping with her anxious fears. She scheduled even trivial activities into an overall plan to which she religiously adhered. She always assumed a position of control in her volunteerism and charity work. She seemed fully aware that her particular fears were irrational.

Our time was almost finished. "Is there anything else that seems important for me to understand, Dory?"

She hesitated. Clients often wait until the final few minutes of a first meeting to disclose things that they don't want to explore. Dory tried to describe a more formless aspect to her anxiety, a kind of dread that snuck up on her when she was off her guard. "It's worse at night when I'm falling asleep. You know, you're not quite asleep yet. Then this kind of clutching feeling happens."

"Show me where you feel that clutching feeling."

"It's kind of here in my tummy." She placed her hand on her solar plexus. "And it's just awful. It's almost like something's coming to get me. It seems silly, I know. But it's like something *bad* is in the room."

Our time was up. We agreed to see one another twice a week to start.

Like many psychologically unsophisticated clients, Dory imagined that I would be able to do something to relieve her of her anxieties and fears without her deep participation in the hard work of therapy. In the sessions after our first meeting, Dory shied away from my invitations to wonder what thoughts or feelings might be attached to the anxieties she described. She chose instead to concentrate on descriptions of external events and circumstances. She highly monitored and edited all of her self-expressions. Part of this process was formal and intentional. But I also had the sense that it wasn't as if she were just hiding the parts she felt but would not say. Rather, I could see that she so sanitized her self-experience to conform to a rigid inner template that parts of it were lost to her as well.

However, she did begin talking *about* all the things she disliked in her own personality, and on this topic she was eloquent. She talked about her perfectionism, her controlling habits in her interpersonal relations, her overly judgmental and critical streak. She knew that she worked too hard and wasn't good at relaxing and being spontaneous and fun. Dory also described problems in her relationships that she knew emerged from those qualities. I thought that at least she was self-aware enough to make that connection. She had read all the self-help books and then had gone on to make lists and schedule goals for implementing their suggestions. She noted the irony. Ah, at least she could poke fun at herself. She had self-diagnosed her personality disorder. There was something endearing about her dogmatic but sincere attempts, her awareness of her unawareness.

In our third session I observed, "Dory, I have the sense when we're talking that you need to keep your guard up, and that it's hard to speak to me before you measure your words, as if you might say something you don't want to say."

"What do you mean?"

"Well, your arms, for instance."

She unfolded her tightly crossed arms and shifted nervously in her seat.

"And when I ask you a question about what you think or feel, you often refer to something external that is happening in your life, have you noticed that?"

"Yes, I guess so. I guess it's just a little scary to talk to a strange man. I mean what are you going to think?"

"I see, you might say something that I would think badly about. Remember how I mentioned in our first meeting that you can say *anything* you want in here."

"I know I *can,* but what would happen?"

"What *would* happen; what is your fear?"

"Lord, I don't know, the ceiling would come crashing in!"

"It feels like something bad would happen from outside of you. I would think badly of you, and what would I do?"

"You wouldn't do anything; you would just privately think terrible things."

"Ah. Is there anything that I'm doing that seems to confirm that expectation for you . . . anything at all?"

She paused and reflected, shook her head, "No, I can't think of anything."

"Dory, I'll make a deal with you. You agree to always try to say what you are thinking and feeling in here with me, and I agree to tell you what I'm thinking and feeling if you ask me. What do you think of that?"

"I can ask you any time?" she seemed suddenly animated.

"Any time you want."

"That sounds good, except," she suddenly looked apprehensive, "that I might not like what you say." She brightened again, "But that would be better than just imagining it."

In our next sessions I could see that Dory was trying to be a "good client." She tried her best to talk freely and openly, but she seemed to be ruled by an inner directive to maintain control. Her repression seemed nonselective, and she merely skimmed over the surface of her inner life like some water bird, only occasionally dipping in and plucking out a tiny fish. It wasn't much to sustain our work together. I'm not sure why I felt so patient and interested. Maybe because I could see that she was trying her best. Perhaps it was because there was something almost elegant in the interrelatedness and impermeability of her defenses. It was like a complete pattern that makes sense.

I remembered that many years before I had arranged a perfect display of framed art on a wall in my gallery. Each size and theme of the individual pieces worked perfectly with the ones adjacent to it. But nothing sold. On a hunch I removed one of the central artworks, disrupting the symmetry of the whole. The other pieces started selling. I wondered which of Dory's defenses would need to come down first for us to be able to get access to the rest of them, and to her inner world.

By the eighth session, just as I was having a hard time staying empathic, she also began to run out of gas. I could see that it was becoming more difficult for her to manage her impression with me, preserving the conventional front. It was taking too much energy to just talk about her negative attributes without wondering what was underneath and how she shaped this self-perception. She also seemed a little more trusting of me. She began to take some chances. Cracks started to appear in the facade. Expressions started to appear on her face. Then Dory said something that seemed to express everything I had experienced with her.

"You know, you keep asking me 'what happens' when I try to talk about what I think and feel, and I just keep shutting you out because every time I want to tell you things I feel such *shame.* I mean that is the one feeling that is always there. Well, that and guilt. It's as if I'm not allowed to express feelings . . . not that they are bad by themselves, but because, I don't know, what will it lead to? I might not be able to keep a handle on the rest of it. That's when I get so nervous, and I have to get away. I have to do something to get myself together or that sense of dread just is too strong. But then I feel guilty because I know I've wasted your time and also for not doing what I need to do. But more and more I think about our talks. I can't get them out of my head, like when I'm at work. I feel like you can help me get away from this guilt and shame if I can just take a leap you know?"

I could see her core issues beginning to become enacted in her experience of our relationship. "On one hand you fear I may condemn you," I reflected, "and on the other you feel guilty for letting me down. But you also feel a sense of obligation to yourself, like you are letting yourself down for not taking this risk . . . it seems like a leap of faith. With me you might be able to open yourself up to all your thoughts and feelings without it overwhelming you, but you're not sure."

"Exactly! And somehow I know that *you* don't think I'm letting you down. It's something I do to myself. I'm just always beating the crap out of myself."

This was starting to feel like a therapeutic conversation. "Yeah, I see that. That's a hard way to live. You have to keep a tight lid on yourself all the time, but that's becoming harder and harder to do, and of course, you become more and more anxious."

"Right! And I'm afraid of what I might find if I let that go. I'm trapped!"

Dory described how every ambition she might have, every spontaneous impulse she felt, had the life sucked out of it by having to march it in front of the tribunal of her own harsh conscience. She beat herself up for everything she did and thought. She said she felt relieved that I could see and acknowledge her pervasive guilt . . . and appeared grateful that I thought it was problematic. I knew that she had wanted me to legitimatize her negative view of herself as she inventoried her faults. She was able to say that she wanted *me* to punish her for them but that this was changing as she came to trust me more.

"There's something you do that just kind of confuses me, but it also helps me."

"What's that?"

"When I talk to my girlfriends about my negative side, they all try to make me feel better and tell me I'm not really that way. But you don't try to talk me out of it. You help me to understand how I see myself, and I think, 'Well, I don't want to see myself like that anymore!' You don't try to make me feel better!"

"And that's what you wanted me to do when you came in here?"

"Yeah!"

When I acknowledged the legitimacy of her self-perceptions only, Dory began to respond. She no longer wanted me to dislike her negative qualities; she wanted my permission to dislike her punishing guilt.

More had been happening than I realized as I had been patiently listening and reflecting and trying to call out the person behind the mask. I was glad to imply to her this permission. It was a helpful little piece of transference. Clearly, she didn't realize how obvious it was that her guilt permeated her self-expression. I took her signs of relief as an indication that she might be willing to let me play a mediating role between her harsh and demanding conscience and whatever sequestered fantasies, feelings, and thoughts had been hunkering down behind the walls. I knew that when some threatening emotions are repressed all the others tend to become muted as well.

There was something about Dory, something that let me know she had been waiting a long time to fill up the hollow and empty places with something vital and alive. Though all former attempts at immediacy and engagement had been thwarted by that impermeable social conventionality, I felt a new sense of possibility that we might be able to work productively.

————

The next session began with this exchange.

"So I'm always running ragged because he gives me too much to do," she said, describing her work problems. "Everyone can see it but him. It's so unfair. I don't know what to do." She had been over this terrain in the previous session and had resisted any attempts to understand her role in the dynamic. It was time for an attempt at *second order* change.

"So, when you find yourself being treated unfairly, you're at a loss to respond. It just seems like you have to buckle under and conform to his desires."

"Right, I just can't say no."

"You can't?"

"I can't. I'm just not good at saying no to someone in authority. I've always had that problem, and I'm just too intimidated. It makes me nervous just to think of asserting myself. I've read those books. I can't do it."

"I see. Dory, I want to try a new technique I just learned about that helps people learn to say no. It's a little strange though because it relies on seeing the world from a different perspective. So what I want you to do, is just to stand up," she stood, "and go over to that wall there," she went, "and just stand on your head, using the wall for support . . . you can put your legs against the wall to brace yourself. You have to do this to get the different perspective." I was making this up as I went.

Her mouth dropped open; she looked at the wall, and shifted uncomfortably. I just sat in my chair calmly.

"You want me to stand on my head against this wall. Are you serious? But I'm wearing a dress."

"Oh, yeah. That is unfortunate. Oh well, it can't be helped."

"I don't want to do it."

"I know, it's a little weird, but, you know," I shrugged.

"I can't do it," she said laughing nervously.

"You can't? You don't know how to do a headstand? I can help you." I made a movement as if to get up out of my chair.

"No, I *can* do a headstand; I just am not going to right here, right now, especially wearing this dress."

"You're telling me you are not going to do this headstand?"

"I'm sorry, I just can't."

"You just said you could."

"Well, I can, but I won't!" she said irritably.

I smiled widely, got up from my chair and took her hand, shaking it vigorously. "Congratulations! Well done!"

"What? What?" she said mystified, "What in the world is going on?"

I became suddenly still and said, smiling, "You just said NO to a man with authority. I'm the doctor, right? I said, Dory, you have to do this headstand, and you said no, you refused! As it turns out, you do know how to say no!"

She started laughing as I explained this. It was as if she had just learned she was on *Candid Camera*. "I was not about to stand on my head," she said laughing as she shook her finger at me.

"I know, I pushed you pretty hard, but you put your foot down . . . ha, ha, you get it? . . . you put your foot down."

She rolled her eyes. "I don't know why I have such a hard time saying no to *men,* it's only with men who have power that I struggle. I mean, for a second I actually considered doing what you asked!"

Thank God she didn't, I thought, or the intervention really would have backfired. Then again, we could have used that to sort out what she experienced by complying.

"I can deal with women, those above me and below me, no problem. With men I find myself either secretly disliking them, or eager to do whatever it is they want from me. That's why I take on too much at work. But then I resent it."

"So, that seems important to explore in our sessions. At least now you realize you can say no when you *really* want to. You actually did it."

"Well, my boss doesn't ask me to stand on my head."

I gave her a surprised look.

"Yeah, on second thought, I think sometimes he does! I guess I can say no if I want to!"

———

A few sessions later, as she was talking about her husband, Dory had a wonderful slip of the tongue. When things are going along well with a client, I usually don't put too much stock in pursuing these little events. It may be something, or it may just be a neurological backfire. But I also remembered that she had amusingly once substituted "erotic" for "erratic" when describing her performance at work. With Dory, as locked up as she was, I was willing to pursue anything.

She said, "When I used to hate Alex, before we were married. . . ." She had meant to say, "date." I might have merely found it amusing and not made a point of it, but I had become increasingly aware of an undercurrent of hostility when Dory talked of Alex. Perhaps it was again time for a little interpretation.

"Dory, you just said, when you used to hate your husband."

"I meant date."

"I know you did." I smiled at her. She knew what I was after but pretended she didn't. "Dory, I wonder if you would take a second here and not say anything, just be silent and let my words guide you. Can you do that?"

"Yes, I suppose."

"Okay. I want you to clear your mind, just relax, close your eyes if you want." She closed them, and her willingness surprised me. "Now, can you tell me what comes to mind when I ask you about a time when you have been really angry at someone, anyone, at any time in your life. A time when you just thought you would burst with anger. What's the first picture or image that comes to mind?"

We waited.

"I can't get anything, nothing's coming to mind."

"Just wait. See what comes up in your imagination." We waited.

"I can't . . . I can't remember being really angry. I mean, I don't get angry . . . I just get sick! It would probably be better to get angry, I know. I mean, I get *annoyed* with Alex, and we have arguments sometimes. I get *irritated* with people all the time. Getting angry was just not something we did in my family. I guess it was *un-Christian*."

"So you get sick instead . . . wow."

"Yeah, I mean, especially if you're a girl, you know."

"So it's un-Christian . . . good Christians get sick instead of mad. What about that whole deal where Jesus went into the temple and overturned all the money tables and stuff? He seemed pretty angry."

She smiled and shook her head. "It's just not a part of how I was raised."

Big surprise, I thought. She seemed to have lost all feelings that did not fit some internal template for "acceptable."

"What other things aren't you allowed to feel besides anger?"

She knew the answer to this question, and ticked them off on her fingers: "Envy, pride, lust, revenge, selfishness; you know, all the big ones. I was raised around good people. You know, if you felt those things at all, you weren't supposed to advertise it. I once got mad at my uncle, he was a pastor, and he took a switch to my behind. I learned real quickly to not show I was mad."

"I see. Okay, let's try something else."

I had wondered if Dory might not respond better to hypnosis in our work. I had recently been to a seminar where a therapist had demonstrated a guided imagery technique for getting at emotions. With a particularly well-defended client like Dory, I thought it might be worth a shot.

"Dory, if it's okay with you, we're going to do something a little different today called a guided imagery. Are you willing to try that?"

"Sure, I guess," she said hesitantly.

"You can stop any time you want. All you have to do is listen to my voice and let the pictures form in your imagination and describe those pictures." I began the relaxation phase, which lasted about 10 minutes. Soon her chest was rising and falling evenly with her deeper breathing, and her head tilted slightly downward as she forgot about her social mask. We began the next phase by creating an imaginary lobby, or home base. Soon she was walking down a long hall with doors lining either side. Behind the doors, I told her, were rooms that contained whatever was written on the door. The names on the doors were whatever she wanted them to be, and she didn't have to feel responsible for whatever that name was; it could be anything. She responded willingly, though her voice was much slower. Her face looked so different without the characteristic tightness around the mouth and eyes. I invited her to signal me if she wanted to stop in front of any door whenever she felt like it. She nodded. I asked her what was written on the door.

"Guilt and shame." We had again explored these feelings in the last session. Dory had talked about how they came up as she tried to express herself with me, but she also had explored their origins in her early upbringing and fundamentalist religious indoctrination. But could she really let herself into that room?

"Do you want to open that door?"

"No," she said, "I've been opening that door my whole life. I'm going on. There's a door on my right that says 'disappointments and broken hearts.' I'll pass, thanks. Wow, it's weird that the names on the doors are there. There's another room on my right that says 'Jesus.' I don't think I'll open it. There's a door on my left that says 'don't you wish.' " She paused.

"Do you want to open it?"

"Yeah, I'm opening it. There are all kinds of models, male and female. They are all walking around in sexy underwear and the latest fashions, and there are photographers and flashbulbs."

"Do you want to go in and be with them?"

"No, I would be too embarrassed. They would say, 'what's that flat-chested lady doing in here. She's too old. Get her out of here.' But there's one lady . . . she's smiling at me."

"What does her smile mean?"

"Her smile means that it's okay, you can come in if you want. She's got a clipboard and she's directing the photo shoot. She seems to be in charge of it. I think maybe I'll come back here later." She was going strong without me now. "I can see a door further on that says 'Screams,' but there's another closer door, and it says 'Sad.' I'm opening it, and I see my daughter behind it. She looks angry with me like she usually does. I feel so sad because I want her to know that I really love her even though she feels she can't stand me right now. I want to tell her that."

"Go ahead and tell her."

"I love you honey. I'm sorry I wasn't the mom you wanted." Dory started to cry! Tears ran down the now sad, not anxious, face. It was the first pure emotion I had seen her express. "I don't want to stay here, it's too hard."

"Okay, close that door."

"I want to come back out into the lobby now."

"Okay, do you need to run back out, or can we walk?"

"We can *jog*."

A few moments later her eyes were open, and she was dabbing at her ruined eye makeup. "You tricked me," she said.

"How so?"

"You didn't warn me that might happen." Truth was, I didn't think it would.

Dory felt I had tricked her, but she took to this simple approach. She seemed to need a device to help her articulate what was in those many rooms of her heart. She asked to use it each time we met, and each time she went a little farther in the corridors. I started really enjoying our meetings together, and I think, despite her discomfort, that she did too. She opened doors labeled "regrets and disappointments," "things I want," and "fears." Each time she went a little farther, and each time I could see her summoning more of the sectioned-off affects she had sequestered for so long. She said after each session that she felt the emotions were both alarming and "like long lost friends." She searched deeper into her self-experience than in our former talks.

I think it helped her to close her eyes during these times. She seemed more able to dispense with the social conventions that inhibited her when we sat face-to-face looking at one another. I also think it helped her that I told her that she was not responsible for the names that appeared on the doors. This was cheating a bit, but I was willing to fudge a little to get past the censorship that had constrained her in previous sessions. She knew well enough, on another level, that she would eventually need to own and integrate what she discovered in the rooms of her inner life. So we pretended together that it was mysterious how the names appeared, and I suppose, in some ways, it was a little like conjuring.

Despite her progress, Dory didn't surprise herself in quite the same way as she did when she met her daughter on the other side of the sadness door. She had gotten wise to what could happen. On the other hand, I contrasted the risks she was taking with the iron grip of her despotic conscience's strict demands, and it felt like progress. I was giving Ms. Steitz a run for her money!

In one session Dory surprised herself and me. She had approached the "screams" door a number of times but was always too afraid to open it. This session she did. As she entered and described what was behind that door, she began to actually scream! It was not a top of the lungs scream, but for Dory it qualified as a yell! She started out angrily yelling at herself, not for being guilty but for *feeling* guilty when she knew she should not. She admonished herself for berating herself. Then she yelled at her husband for ignoring her, for always being away, for the way he held the paper and controlled the TV remote, for the way he smelled, and the way he told dumb jokes at parties. She resented his *Playboy* magazines and what she assumed was his masturbation to them. She threatened to leave him unless he made an effort at making her feel more loved. She was tired of living with him. He was a lousy lover. She said, "I'm so darned angry at you . . . No, I'm so damn angry at you . . . I'm so damned angry at you, you bastard!" And then in a quieter, venomous voice, "I hate you!"

I was a little startled by this sudden outburst and felt like I had started some kind of nuclear chain reaction. I thought her head might spin around like that possessed little girl in *The Exorcist.* Apparently she felt the same way because she suddenly wanted to run back to the "lobby." She sat shaking on the sofa, and then tears rolled down her cheeks.

"I'm sorry!" she said. "I'm so sorry."

"What are you sorry for?"

"I won't do it again."

"Dory, there's nothing to be sorry about. You were just . . ."

"Oh, God. I'm so ashamed. I wish I could take it back. I didn't really want to say all of that. I mean some of it's true. It's probably all true. You must think I'm just awful." She looked in her purse for her car keys.

"Where are you going?"

"I think I'd better leave."

"I think you'd better stay. Just sit and collect yourself."

She sat, occasionally shaking her head, as if she couldn't believe the things she had just said.

"I can't imagine what you must think of me."

I could see that she wanted for me to draw the chalk circle on the blackboard and point her to it, that it was the response she was used to and that she was expecting.

"So this is it, eh? Your real feelings come spilling out and I must want to punish you for them. Remember our deal?"

"Yeah."

"Would you like to invoke it?"

"I don't know. Maybe not."

"Okay."

She sat for a while.

"Yes, I want you to tell me what you think," she said.

"I'll tell you. I think that you have been stomping down these feelings, all your emotions, for a long time. I know you feel ashamed and guilty when you feel your real emotions. But I think these are just as much your right to have as any of your 'Christian' feelings. You were able to stumble across some more of what belongs to you here today. You've been working up to it because you know you need to. You don't need me to convince you of that. That's a good thing. Remember, you don't need to act on anything. Just because you feel and say it, that doesn't mean you have to do something right now. I'm glad this happened. It feels like we are really working now."

She seemed to ponder this. I let her sit. After a while I said, "Look," I pointed up with my finger. She looked up.

"What?"

"The ceiling hasn't fallen in." She shook her head; she wasn't buying it. "You expect me to condemn you now." She nodded her head. "So if I say I think you did well today?"

"I can't believe you."

"How so?"

"I'm not sure I'm ready to feel good about myself."

"You might need to hold onto that image of you as unworthy a little longer?"

"I guess."

"That's okay. You don't want to change too fast."

"Are you saying I *should* feel guilty?"

"No, I'm saying you might need to hold onto your guilt like an old friend for a while, just to keep your bearings."

She looked at me like I was crazy, which was fine. The session was over, and we had to stop.

———

Dory surprised me by coming to her next session, but she admitted that she had pondered canceling. In all the months we met, she never missed an appointment and was always on time, which I suppose made sense. She was still ashamed and wished that she could take it all back. Still, she was so eager to explore more deeply some of the unspoken (and spoken) religious and family rules that had contributed to many of her "unacceptable" feelings becoming invisible to her normal way of being.

But she was afraid now and didn't want to stir things up again quite so much. On the other hand, she admitted, she felt lighter, freer, during the four days since we last met. She had some energy too. But she also expected that "a lightning bolt would come down out of the sky and strike me dead."

I had been waiting to make an interpretation concerning one of her anxieties and wondered if an opportunity would arise. I knew that she might struggle with it; it might be a little premature. However, it was important to piggyback a new insight onto the emotional arousal that might make it stick. A perfect timing opportunity did arise in the conversation. Dory had again been reflecting on her anger at Alex, being fearful but not surprised at its intensity. I had realized that my former idea that she feared abandonment was wrong. I seized on her current expression of ambivalence.

"Well," I inserted into a pause, "at least perhaps you know why you worry so much about him having an accident or not coming home."

"Why?"

"Perhaps you don't want him to come home. Do you think that's possible?"

"What?" She sat staring at me. "Are you saying I *want* Alex to have an accident, to get killed?"

"Sometimes when people feel strongly one way about something, and they can't make sense of it, it's because deep down they feel exactly the opposite . . . but that's too hard to acknowledge straight on. I do wonder if your fear that Alex might have an accident might express that, on some level—that you want him to not come home."

"No! Of course not! What kind of . . . I mean I'm not so awful as that. You must really think I'm terrible. Oh God."

"Perhaps I'm wrong. It was an impression I had that I thought I would share with you to check it out. I don't see it as something awful. In fact, if it were true, it would come from your efforts to be 'good,' to not acknowledge what you often perceive as 'bad' feelings."

She sat silently.

I waited. Nothing. "Your face looks blank. I'm wondering what's going on with you."

Nothing.

"This would be a good time to practice saying what you are feeling."

"All right. I'm angry at *you!*"

I was thrilled. "Tell me how you are angry at me."

"I'm angry at you that you think I am so low that I would want my husband to have an accident so I could get rid of him!"

"It really makes you mad at me when I say that maybe you feel so worried about him because you really want to be rid of him."

"Yeah. What gives you the right to tell me that? It just makes me mad."

"You're mad. What right do I have to attribute these motivations to you? How do I get off saying that?"

"Yeah! You've got a lot of nerve." She crossed her arms and sat sullenly for a while.

"How did that feel to tell me you are pissed at me?" I said after a while.

"I'm still mad. It felt pretty good."

"Good. It seems that you feel I was really off the mark with that comment, and you were able to let me know that and I . . ."

"It's partly true," she interrupted."

"Ah. Help me see how it's true, and how it's not."

"The part that's true is that I'm so worried that Alex might have an accident . . . because I really want him to." She unconsciously put her finger over her mouth, then slowly shook her head. "If I'm honest about it, I really want him to not come home. That's awful, but it's true. But I *don't* want him to die or anything. I don't *really* want him to have an accident. I'm just so mad at him, and sometimes I think, I wish he was not around, you know? It's not like I want something to really happen to him. But sometimes I want to be free . . . free of this marriage. Oh God, I can't believe I'm saying this."

"That's important to realize. You may get worried and fear for Alex because it's the opposite of your real but forbidden feelings of anger. Because it's hard for you to own just how angry and resentful you really are in your relationship, you may sometimes, or all of the time, want to be free of it. That doesn't mean you want him to *actually* have an accident. It's the mind's way of dealing with those forbidden feelings but also of expressing them as well. Do you get what I mean?"

"Yeah, I hate to admit it. But I *completely* understand. But I still feel guilty for wishing ill on my husband . . . even just in imagination. It makes me feel so *sinful.* In my family we don't get divorced, and we don't wish our husbands were dead!"

"Well, maybe you should just allow these feelings to be there without having to do anything about them right now. As for feeling sinful, what if you thought about it this way: God created your mind to work in a certain way, and yours is working in the same way as everybody else's. I mean, sometimes people tend to protect themselves from things that are too upsetting or scary. There's nothing original or unique to

you about this. The trick is just to know yourself as well as you can.
Then, at least, you can better understand what you are experiencing and
why. You can make choices. Does that help at all?"

"A little I guess."

I could see by the shell-shocked look on her face that it didn't help
at all.

The next session Dory didn't need to use the guided imagery. She was
distressed and had things she wanted to talk about right away. I was a
little worried that now we might be going too fast, that she would over-
reach her ability to integrate the thoughts and feelings that seemed to
be bubbling up to the surface.

"Remember when you said I could talk about any dreams I had?" I
nodded. "Well I had a couple of real upsetting ones. I don't ever remember my dreams, but this week I did. In the first one, I came home from
work and I was in my bedroom getting undressed. Alex was downstairs
watching TV; I could hear it blaring the news. I opened up my closet—
it's a walk-in closet—and I was going to hang up my suit, and when I
pulled aside the hanging clothes, there was a man standing behind
them, and I screamed. But then I realized it was my boss, David. He
was standing there in his suit. He looked pretty ridiculous under my
shoe rack actually. Anyway, I said frantically, 'What are you doing
here?' I was standing there in only my underwear, and I held up the suit
so he wouldn't see me. He said, 'Waiting for you, what else?' I asked
him, 'Do we have a presentation tonight?' He laughed and said, 'No,
nothing like that.' Then he leaned out to kiss me, but he fell over Alex's
bowling balls . . . they're usually in his closet in the carrying bags; I
don't know what they were doing rolling around in my closet."

"I can't imagine," I chuckled.

She looked at me and smiled curiously.

"Is the shoe rack hanging up like that in real life?" I asked.

"No, it's on the floor. So, anyway . . ."

"Oh, I'm sorry, I thought you were finished."

"So I tell him to be quiet, we have to get him out of the house without Alex knowing. But then I can hear from the top of the stairs
that the news on the TV is talking about me! I look out the window,
and there's a camera crew, and they're reporting the story of how I'm
trying to get David, my boss, out of the house! That's the end of it. The
second dream . . ."

"You don't want to reflect on this one first?"

"No, I have to tell you the second one," she said, as if she had been containing it for long enough and had to discharge it as soon as possible. "In the second dream, I wake up in the middle of the night, and I go down the hall because a light is on. I open up Sherry's, my daughter's, door, and she's home. And then I realized that David is now in bed with *her*. I rush in and start shaking her and say, 'What are you doing, what are you doing?' David gets out of bed and starts to put on his clothes. She says, 'Get away from me; you're driving him away.' I say, 'he's not supposed to be here in the first place you little whore!' I can't believe I said that to her. Then, believe it or not, you rush in and separate us."

"What is it like for you to tell me these dreams right now?"

"I'm shaking."

"So there's a lot going on for you with these dreams if you're shaking when you tell them. It seems as if you wanted to get them out as soon as you could."

"Yes, but it's also difficult to tell them to you. That might be part of my shaking. I can't imagine what you'll think. Actually, I can imagine what you'll think, and it's not good."

"So, that old boogey man is there. You believe I will think badly of you for dreaming these dreams."

"Well, maybe more for what they imply."

"What do they imply? What comes to mind for you right now as you recall them?"

She sighed loudly, as if she had been dreading what she also wanted to do . . . deal with the dreams. But I had the impression she just wanted to get rid of the discomfort, not necessarily understand them. The dream images threatened her. That seemed like the place to begin.

"Dory, what seems most threatening to you about these dreams?"

"You're going to think I'm awful, but after I was startled that my boss was in the closet, I was also kind of thrilled by it. That kind of parallels something that's happening in real life. I mean, I get very nervous when he's around me, and I have to admit that I'm having an attraction there, you know?" I nodded. She took a deep breath and exhaled loudly. "So when he shows up in my closet, it's kind of a mixed thing. I don't want him there . . . I mean there's no question that in real life nothing is going to happen. But I do want him there too. Something's wrong with me. I can't stop thinking about him, day and night, and it makes me more and more nervous at work. We work really closely together, and I think he must be picking up on something. I worry that he can read my mind. I mean, I know he can't, but I feel like it must be so apparent. When I put on my makeup in the morning and I'm looking in the mirror, I'm thinking of him, how he'll see me. And I feel like it's so obvious when I'm around him, like everyone can pick up on it."

"Just as when he's in your closet there's a news crew broadcasting it . . . and your husband may pick up on it . . . he's watching the television."

"Yeah, exactly."

"So I wonder if your fear of someone being in the house works in the same way as your worry that Alex will have an accident and not come home. On one hand, you would like for your boss, or someone like him, to be in the house waiting for you. But, of course, you don't want that as well. Perhaps your fear that someone really is in the house is more a reaction to you not wanting to acknowledge these powerful sexual feelings and attractions. It expresses both sides of your fear. What do you think about this?"

"It feels like it's . . . I'll say accurate, because I can't say it's *right,* that sounds like I approve of it! And what about my daughter? I feel bad for calling her that name, even if it was only in a dream."

"In your dream I think maybe your daughter really stands in for a part of you that wanted to be in bed with David. But you don't feel too good about those feelings; you call the part of you that has these sexual urges a whore. One Dory is fighting with another Dory, and I come in to help sort it out. You have described Sherry as free and able to do what she wants. You are appropriating that in the dream to express another side of you."

"But that's so wrong! You must think I'm terrible."

"You expect that I will think you are terrible for having these sexual feelings?"

"Yes."

"Let's go there for a moment. Help me understand all the ways in which I will think you are evil for having these feelings."

Dory related that in her family sex, like anger and all other "unacceptable" feelings, was forbidden to acknowledge. But sex, especially, was a taboo topic. She came from a religiously conservative Christian background, and her sense was that sex was dangerous and wrong, especially in any context other than marriage. She was a virgin when she married, and her first experiences were not pleasurable. It got better over time; Alex was a kind man, and he tried to invigorate their sex life. But at some point he had given up. Now it felt perfunctory and stilted. She thought her husband "oversexed." She thought that I might punish her like she anticipated others in her life would punish her. She thought that telling me these things would "just ruin everything."

"But there's something really hard to say . . ." I nodded. "I've never really had, you know, when Alex and I go to bed together . . . I've never experienced . . ."

". . . an orgasm," I said for her.

"Right . . . except, well, recently when I think of David . . . I, well, I touch myself." Her neck flushed a scarlet red. She looked like she might bolt from the room.

"You masturbate while you fantasize about David and you had an orgasm?"

"Yes. A number of them," she said seriously.

I had to mask a smile. There was something very funny about how she said "a number of them," as if she were being precise. I had to stop myself from saying, "how many *exactly?*"

"How was that . . . it must have surprised you?"

"Amazing! I mean . . . Oh God!" It was the first truly spontaneous expression I had heard her utter in therapy. I laughed out loud with pleasure. Her eyes got wide.

"You shouldn't laugh at me! This is bad . . . I'm really bad!"

"I know," I said laughing again, "you are bad, you are so bad!"

"You stop that!" and now she laughed too.

"Okay. . . . I'm stopped." We sat for a second in silence and then both of us started laughing again, "a number of them!" I repeated, between laughs, using her voice.

"Oh! You are bad! Pastor Jenkins would not like you at all!"

"Bring him on; I'll kick his ass." Her eyes got big again, and her mouth dropped open. Then she laughed even harder.

"I stopped believing in the devil when I was little. You better hope I was right or the devil's going to get you!" she warned, wagging her finger at me, but clearly enjoying this.

"Bring him on. I'll kick his ass too!"

"Ha!" she chortled, "pride comes before a fall."

"While some take pride in *coming* at all," I rhymed spontaneously. She paused; it took a moment for her to get the off-color joke. I smiled as it dawned on her.

"Awwwhhh," she exclaimed, and her face became incredulous. "You are not embarrassed by this at all, are you?" she said, and there was a kind of freshness to her face after all the laughter. She looked 10 years younger. "Here I am thinking the ceiling's going to crash in when I tell you this, but you really don't think this is a big deal," she said appreciatively.

"Dory," I said with a care I truly felt for her then, "It's the same old thing. I think one of the reasons you are so afraid of your sexual feelings when they burst through is that you have kept them stomped down for so long. It's like your anger; the more you try to ignore it, the more powerful and dangerous it becomes for you."

"You don't think there's anything *wrong* with me? I mean, it seems so out of proportion. I'm thinking about David all the time."

"It's out of proportion because it's ignored. My guess is that David's just the medium you're using to try to get back in touch with yourself. No pun intended."

"Oh! I'm not talking to you anymore."

"Sorry. Okay, I'll quit. Maybe you need to take a long look at your marriage. Is that a place you want to invest yourself and your erotic feelings? If so, or even if not, what kind of changes do you need to make there? You've described Alex as a nice man, yet you feel angry too. He wants for you to become more sexually invested, but what do you need to change about the relationship for you to feel that you want to do that? There is nothing wrong with you having powerful sexual feelings." She looked more in one piece than I had ever seen her. Her face looked natural, composed.

"You know, in that second dream," she said calmly, "when I went in and found David with Sherry, I think I was more *jealous* than anything. It's like I told you, she is free to do with her life what she wants."

"So are you." Her head kind of ticked, as if this statement had some property that physically struck her.

"Boy, that would be a different way to live if I thought that."

"Yes, it would."

———

Our sessions slowly began to take on a new dimension. It was not as if Dory's personality became radically different; she was still bound by the same habits and style of relating to herself and the world. Dory was still a rowboat. But she had carved out a little area in her self-experience more protected from her punishing conscience, where previously forbidden feelings, fantasies, impulses, and ways of thinking could be acknowledged and find some expression.

As the sessions progressed into their sixth month, she said she began to feel better physically as well. She had less fatigue, more energy, even occasionally, a sense of vitality. She worried less about her health. She had stopped worrying about Alex having an accident, and, with coaching, was more willing to acknowledge her angry feelings to him. Much to her surprise, far from punishing her for this, Alex said that it finally felt to him as if Dory was at least partly "fighting fair." This, in turn, raised him in her estimation. When Alex admitted that he had secretly been thinking of leaving the marriage, Dory was shocked but admitted that she had been fantasizing about it too. They began talking and expressing to one another some long-held grudges and resentments. This seemed to destabilize the marriage temporarily—many sessions dealt with Dory's feelings that "things were falling apart"—but Dory and Alex seemed to regain some kind of balance that kept them going.

Although Dory gradually became willing to experiment with her angry feelings, it was more difficult for her to find and express her sexual feelings. Contrary to what I had assured her, she said, the more she tried to acknowledge what she felt, the more powerful and overwhelming her sexual feelings felt to her. She had sexual dreams and found herself having sexual thoughts about men she had just met. Having discovered her ability to orgasm, she continued to "touch" herself, but felt alternately delighted and terribly guilty about it. She could not include her husband in this discovery, she said. Things were "too up in the air." But Alex surprised her again.

Dory related that Alex had taken her out to a very expensive dinner. Alex was a miser, she said, and never spent money except on practical things. "I thought, as I looked at him across a $50 bottle of wine, where did my husband go?" she said. "I was more worried about the money than he was!"

But Alex didn't stop there. He took Dory to the Kennedy Center to see the Cirque du Soleil, something she had always wanted to do but that Alex had previously said was a waste of time and money. She began to notice in herself the first stirrings of affectionate feelings toward him.

"I'm not sure I want to give up the control," she said, in one session.

"How so, how does your control play out between you and Alex?"

"In the past he has controlled the money, and I . . . I've controlled the sex. I hate to say it like that, but I do think I use withholding sex as a way to express anger toward him. I know it gets to him, but I feel like if I actually *wanted* to have sex with him, it would be like losing something. Right now, it's more like a chore."

"So now that he has declared a kind of détente, he's spending money on you and taking you out, and you are fighting fairer, you wonder if you can do a kind of arms reduction, and bring the sexual relationship back into the marriage on a more equal basis."

"Exactly. I'm not sure . . . I'm not sure I'm ready to *love* my husband. I guess I'm not sure if I'm ready to love any man. That sounds awful, I know." These self-punitive statements and her appeals for my absolution had grown less over time, but reappeared every time Dory confronted a new area of growth where she felt unsure.

"So there's a choice you have to make. Do you want to take a risk and make yourself a little more vulnerable in this relationship, potentially improving it? Or do you want to feel a little more protected and safe, but living with things the way they are between you? Of course, there's also the choice of ending the marriage, but I just heard you say you're not sure you can love any man. Would a new man be any better for you?"

"Putting it like that, I think I'd like to take a risk . . . with Alex, but it feels really scary."

"Describe the bad thing that could happen if you took the risk."

She thought about this. "You know . . . I don't know. It's hard to name except that I might feel like I would have to let go of something. I would have to just kind of trust in something I don't understand. It's like a foreboding feeling."

"Let go of something," I repeated, focusing in on the part that I sensed held the most possibility. "Describe what you would have to let go of. You look like you're holding on pretty tightly right now!" I noticed that she was grasping the arm of the sofa tightly.

"Yeah, I know! What would I have to let go of?" she wondered aloud. "I guess if Alex and I made love and I, you know, had an orgasm with him, I would feel like . . . I don't know . . . like he has power over me or something. Like he won! Also, I don't know, if I let go . . . how far would I fall? Would it kind of take me over, you know."

"Okay, so there's a power thing there, you might lose power. But also, when you masturbate, you can kind of control how much you experience, but if you really let yourself go with another person . . . what might happen. You might fall into some bottomless well."

"Exactly. But as you say it, I don't think Alex would take advantage of me or anything. I mean he wants me to be interested and involved. I just never have."

"Dory, this may sound strange to you, but can you imagine a scenario in which you would have power and control but still be sexually invested and engaged?"

A shy look passed over her face, she said, "I actually had a thought, a fantasy, of ambushing David. You know. I would have control over everything and tell him what to do . . . you know; he would have to follow my instructions."

"Could you appropriate a part of that scenario with Alex? What if you ambushed him, told him what to do?"

"He would think I was nuts!"

I shrugged. "Have you ever taken control before or been on top?"

"No," she said shyly.

"Well, I wonder if that's one way you could have a little more control over the interaction."

"You think he would be okay with that?"

"From what you have told me he would be okay with whatever you decided you needed to revive your relationship in the bedroom. And you seem to want someone with whom you can express these powerful erotic feelings. Why not try your marriage?"

"Duh . . . I mean it kind of makes sense, doesn't it. I don't think he's very good at it though."

"So maybe you'll both have to figure out a way that makes you better at it."

"You mean I can tell him if it's bad? I could tell him he's crummy at it?" She had a smile on her face.

"Maybe you could find a way to instruct him about what works for you without it really costing him, without him having to leave his bowling balls in your closet."

"I wondered about that!" She laughed. "I wondered why you smiled when I told you that part of the dream, but I was too shy to ask."

"You can always ask in here. In any case, that's my association, not yours!"

"What about the shoes?" she asked.

"What?"

"You asked about the shoe rack in the dream; the rack was over David's head instead of on the floor. Why did you ask about that?"

"What comes to mind when you conjure up that image?" I inquired.

"I don't know . . . My shoes are over his head. They could fall on him. My heels could hit him in the head. I could knock him out with my shoes."

"As you say that I have two impressions, one is that you could put him under your heel, a control thing. The second is that you could be a knockout in those shoes!" We were having fun.

"Ah, I like that second one better," she exclaimed.

"Okay, you go with that one."

I realized that Dory and I really liked and had gotten comfortable with one another and that she trusted our relationship. She felt freer than ever to reveal herself to me; she knew I would ally myself with that part of her that accepted, not punished, her. Was her growing trust with me why she was now willing to slowly take some new risks with Alex? I thought, so much of what happens in therapy occurs way below the level of interpretations and specific interventions and builds slowly over time.

Over the next few months Dory's relationship with Alex did improve. We laughed a lot as she described how she awkwardly "ambushed" him, telling him exactly what she wanted him to do, which was essentially just to lie there and provide something rigid. He was as shocked as she had imagined, but more grateful than she anticipated. She felt comfortable controlling things and learned how to achieve an orgasm in their encounters. They went into couples' counseling with another therapist for one session a month to address the many issues that arose as they became more invested in one another. Gradually, she thought she might be willing to share a little of the initiative and control. Alex wasn't complaining.

As Dory's more severe and problematic defenses had slowly yielded to an increased ability on her part to pay attention to more of her inner world, her specific anxiety symptoms lessened. She no longer feared that someone might be in her house. Whatever anxiety she felt about Alex's travel she thought was more genuine because now she had actually missed him on occasion when he went away. She still felt a sexual attraction to her boss, David, which lessened as her relationship with Alex improved. But having learned to observe her feelings and impulses more carefully, she realized that it was not just David but *any* man with power or authority at her work who elicited in her an erotic charge. As she realized that her erotic feelings got co-opted for other power and security needs at work, these impulses lessened as well. Sexual issues moved into the background of our work together. As they did, gender politics moved forward as she explored more legitimate methods of getting influence and power with men in her professional life.

Her public speaking fears lessened. I had the impression, however, that now that she was more available to herself she also wanted something more from her other relationships. This demanded of her greater openness, flexibility, and risk. New social anxieties emerged as old ones were laid to rest. As she gained in skill, she moved the goalposts backward. It felt like a good struggle. She was now confronting the even more difficult task of changing lifelong habits and her interpersonal style. At times she felt hopeless that she would ever get past a sense that she was inherently flawed. She saw how her perfectionism and controlling style, her insistence on order and her attention to ridiculous detail, undermined her capacity to relax and be spontaneous.

Still, learning how to "let go" in these other areas, to tolerate ambiguity and uncertainty, was like trying to become someone else, she said. She pushed against her own limitations, impatient with herself as she tended to be impatient with others. My suggestions that she learn to accept some of her quirks and to just work with them with greater awareness seemed like a "cop out" to her. She could not accept, despite my repeated interpretations, that this lack of tolerance of her "faults" precisely mirrored the problem. Though she was still tough on herself, at least now, she said, it pushed her in the right direction toward greater growth more often than greater guilt.

In one session a long silence filled up the space between us. She was looking down at her lap, and finally looked up and smiled, saying nothing.

"Where were you just now?" I inquired.

"Oh, I was thinking about something that happened when I was a little kid. It's something I've always felt terrible about."

"You want to remember it aloud?"

"I guess. It was when I was about 6 or 7. My parents had sent me to live with my uncle and aunt for the summer. He was the uncle who was the pastor. My aunt, she was really strict, but I liked her. She was a few months pregnant at the time. I was so jealous of that baby. I think I got some special attention from my aunt, and I also knew I was going to get shipped back to my home with my three brothers and sisters. At my aunt's I was the only kid around. Anyway, she was going to the store, and I asked if I could go too. She said no, she was just doing a quick trip. But I snuck into the back seat of the car, and when she was going

down the road I jumped up from the back to surprise her. She was surprised . . . more than I wanted. She swerved a little and hit the edge of
the road, and that caused her to *lose control* and go in the ditch and
crunch the front of the car. I was thrown forward against the seat and
got a bloody nose." She paused, and shook her head.

"Ouch, so you got a lot more than you bargained for. Did you get in
a lot of trouble?"

"Oh yeah, but that was not the worst of it."

"It gets worse?"

"Much worse. Right after that my aunt had a miscarriage. She lost
that baby. I've always felt so awful about that."

My God! Dory caused her aunt to lose control and it caused a miscarriage? Certainly this must have been a formative event that contributed
unconscious fears of incredible damage occurring if she herself lost control or did anything impulsive. I sat with her pondering this. It fit with
Dory's personality, but I was strangely unmoved by the story. I could see
that it distressed her to talk about it, but something didn't add up. I
reminded myself that there was also that part of Dory's interpretive set
that inclined her to blame herself for anything that went wrong even if
it wasn't her fault. I decided to pursue it.

"So you feel like you caused that miscarriage." She nodded. "And
have you ever talked about this with your aunt, at the time or since?"

"No, we never discussed it. It was always something I felt too bad to
bring up."

"And how about with your family . . . was it ever mentioned or
discussed?"

"No, I think my father might have helped to fix the car, but that was
about it."

"So that's been something you've been regretting for a long time.
Huh," I mumbled, and raised my eyebrows and shrugged.

"What?" she said, in response to the gesture. "What are you thinking?"

"I'm thinking it never happened."

"What?"

"I'm thinking that it never happened."

"It happened! I remember it," she said annoyed.

"I believe you. I believe you remember something that really happened, but I just doubt that your memory of it corresponds accurately
to an actual event."

"Why do you say that?" she said petulantly.

"Because it's too good a fit between your feelings of jealously about the pregnancy, your desire for your aunt's exclusive attention. It's too good a fit because you tend to feel guilt when your 'unacceptable' feelings crop up because you think they will do damage. And how is it that nobody—nobody—ever talked about this?"

"Maybe it was just too upsetting for everyone. Maybe they just didn't want to throw it in my face!"

"Dory, when did anyone in your family show restraint about evoking shame for perceived mistakes? Sometimes our memories are accurate at describing a subjective experience of something but don't necessarily represent events themselves. You connect your disobeying your aunt and causing that accident with her miscarriage. I question that connection."

"Well, you're just wrong about it."

"Okay, I'm wrong," I shrugged. "Is your aunt still alive? Can you ask her about it?"

"I couldn't ask her . . . it would be too, I don't know . . ."

"So it's better to live wondering whether you caused her miscarriage."

"All right, I *will* ask her." Dory sulked.

I realized that when you mess around with a person's constructed narrative you really disrupt the story they tell themselves about themselves. It's about more than what happened. The meaning they make of themselves is open to question. But Dory's meanings were now open to question. She had worked hard and could challenge the old assumptions and memories. I don't know why I felt certain her memory was a screen memory standing in for an early configuration of self-experience. I hoped I was right.

———

Dory sat on the couch our next session and began, "I owe you an apology."

"No you don't. If you owed me an apology, I'd know about it."

"Well, in any case, I talked to my aunt, and she was amazed that I thought I was the cause of the miscarriage." Dory was shaking her head. "She said the accident happened just the way I remember. And she said she had a miscarriage . . . but that the miscarriage happened a whole month *before* the car crash. She couldn't believe I've been blaming myself for that. How could that happen?"

"So how do you feel about having this conversation with your aunt?"

"Relieved. And confused! It's as if I've been carrying this thing for a long time for no reason! How did you know?"

"It was a hunch. It just didn't add up. It didn't have the ring of real life to it. It did have the ring of being an expression of the guilt that you struggle with about lots of things."

"Well, now I don't have to feel guilty about that anyway."

I smiled, "One less thing."

"Yeah! Actually, I think that over this past year I learned to not be guilty about lots of things . . . but there are many more in there!"

"So it's the process of how you feel the guilt, not the things themselves, that seems important."

"Yeah, I guess that's true."

In one session Dory announced that she and Alex had decided to move to Alabama to take advantage of a job opportunity. We spent three or four pleasant sessions together reviewing that past year, reminiscing and enjoying our time, working up to goodbye.

"We should have done this more often," she observed after a silence.

"What, just hung out together chatting about stuff."

"Yeah, it was always so intense and such hard work."

"You did work hard in here didn't you? I guess that's why we have the luxury of looking back over it with satisfaction now."

"I feel like *we* worked hard. I know I'm a handful. Those first few months I didn't know if you would let me come back. Now I can talk to you about anything, and *most* times I'm not worried what you will think about it. How am I going to do that again in Alabama? I don't want to start all over again."

"I bet it'll be a lot easier for you now."

"Yeah, maybe so. I'll cross that river when I come to it."

I knew she would, and as I contemplated the metaphor, I realized that she had changed in my eyes, just as she had in her own. She looked a lot less like a rowboat, and a lot more like her Gloucester namesake. Our therapy had shown Dory how to take her nose out of the circle, and maybe, as she crossed that river, she, too, would learn to sing. Take that, Ms. Steitz!

> The water is wide, I can't cross over
> And neither have I wings to fly.
> Give me a boat that can carry two
> and both shall row, my love and I.
> —Folk song

CASE FIVE DISCUSSION
Anxiety, Defenses, and Guilt

MY FIRST IMPRESSION of Dory was that she had packed herself tightly in an armor of conformity, rigidity, and self-inhibition that prevented any freedom of movement and squelched her vital powers. The protective shield of her managed and formal presentation contained and constrained her, but it also fended off the world around her, protecting her from anything new, unpredictable, or spontaneous. As she sat erect on the sofa, her articulate but clipped way of speaking conveyed a sense of absolute control. This need for control quickly became apparent in our interactions. She seemed to want to manage our exchanges, to apply a kind of rigid protocol to the proceedings. Even when Dory wished to share with me her distress and her struggles, she did not do this spontaneously but catalogued and read them like a list of groceries.

I saw that Dory's need to manage the situation was not just in response to the uncertainty inherent in a first therapy session; it permeated every aspect of her life. How, I wondered, with this rigid formality, could she respond to the new opportunities that are born in the uncertainty and ambiguity of therapy? Could she loosen her grip, relax the muscles in her taut face, speak an immediate and authentic word? As it happened, Dory possessed a resilient spirit and a longing to break free of the constraints that subverted her vital energies.

Dory's outward expression of control and formality countered an almost continual state of inner anxiety. Dory was always on "high alert." She rarely seemed to be free of a sense that something dreadful was about to happen. The outer circumstances or problems that she identified seemed out of proportion, however, to the degree of threat that she attached to them. Dory knew this. She could sense that she imbued these external problems with far more threat than they actually contained. Her reality testing was fairly intact, but she was confused and helpless to understand or resolve her anxiety.

Dory was also quite cognizant that she was plagued with a sense of guilt that seemed out of proportion to whatever actions or transgressions she felt she committed. Like her anxiety, her guilt seemed pervasive. It settled like a layer of dust over all the rooms of her inner life. It collected in the corners like dust balls that grew to the size of tumbleweeds, and when she was particularly vulnerable, her guilt blew through the living room of her consciousness, upsetting all the furniture. Dory speculated that her troubling guilt was tied to her early relationships and rigid fundamentalist religious instruction. She had partly re-storied her religious beliefs but thought that her early instruction still held a kind of power over her that she could not completely overcome.

Though Dory sensed that her anxiety and guilt were out of proportion to the circumstances of her life (an awareness that motivated her to seek therapy), she had little awareness of how defensively her personality functioned. Why would she be motivated to have such insight? These defenses helped to protect her from the subjective threat of becoming overwhelmed and destroyed by her anxiety and guilt. They also protected her from being re-injured in other relationships. Dory's defenses were "ego-syntonic"—she had lived with them for so long— they felt like "who she was." They were pervasive in her personality. Over time her defenses had shaped and influenced her demeanor and interpersonal style in ways she could not begin to perceive. If asked about certain defensive *behaviors,* Dory might have been able to acknowledge them but would have related them to some perceived *outside* threat. Quite logically, since defenses by their nature function outside the conscious awareness of the person, she had little idea of the function, for instance, of her repression. She had little sense that the most subjectively threatening things in her life came from her own thoughts, feelings, fantasies, and impulses. By the time she came to therapy, she was in an all-out war with herself.

The Traditional Psychodynamic View: Understanding the Parts

Freud asserted that anxiety is the central problem of mental illness. Indeed, Freud's metaphor for the mind, the "structural hypothesis" of id, ego, and superego, includes a central role for anxiety as shaping the consciousness of the person. Freud related the appearance of anxiety to what he called "traumatic situations" (Brenner, 1973). A traumatic situation is one in which the person's psyche is overwhelmed by an influx of stimuli that is too much for it to either master or effectively discharge. When this happens, Freud believed anxiety develops automatically and that the person develops ways to counter such unpleasant experiences. Such traumatic situations naturally occur in early years when the child's developing ego is still forming and has difficulty containing overwhelming internal states. For instance, if the nursing infant needs its mother to respond to its hunger, but the mother is unavailable or unresponsive, a primitive, biologically based, and automatic type of anxiety emerges.

Over time, a child learns to *anticipate* or *predict* an impending traumatic situation and to react to it with anxiety *before* it becomes traumatic. Freud called this type of situation a "danger situation" and this type of warning anxiety "signal anxiety." This anticipation of danger serves to mobilize the forces available to the person to meet or avoid the crisis. For instance, now the child can anticipate the mother's absence that would give rise to a future traumatic situation. The signal anxiety motivates her to behave, act, or to do something to reduce the anxiety. For instance, the child might cling to the mother, or do something that is impossible for the mother to ignore.

Early danger situations involve the anxiety associated with the loss of important caregivers or their essential functions. But as the child grows, the danger situation more often involves the loss of the important person's love or the threat of punishment. In other words, the danger situations become increasingly subtle as the child grows and participates with others in mutually gratifying exchanges. This does not mean that anxiety in itself is problematic; indeed, "it is easy to lose sight of the fact that the role of anxiety in enabling the ego to check or inhibit instinctual wishes or impulses which seem to it to be dangerous is an essential one in normal development . . . it is a necessary part of mental life and growth" (Brenner, 1973, p. 79).

The increasing emergence of the child's sexual, aggressive, and other developmental impulses complicates the nature of the perceived potential loss or punishment as well as the potential to become overwhelmed by powerful stimuli. Now the child increasingly experiences the emergence of *internal self-states* as a potential danger situation. The child begins to react to certain thoughts and feelings in ways that neither express nor diffuse the energy contained in these states. In other words, the child begins to develop some adaptive defenses to maintain equilibrium. There is a characteristic set of danger situations in early and later life to which the person has developed characteristic responses. These danger situations (loss of love, expression of erotic urges, fear of censure or rejection, and so on) and the responses that accompany them may persist *unconsciously* to a greater or lesser extent throughout life.

To use the terms of Freud's metaphor, when the ego opposes the emergence of an id impulse, it is because that impulse will create a danger situation. Signal anxiety warns of the danger and alerts the ego to mobilize opposition to the emerging dangerous impulse. In psychoanalytic language, the ego's opposition to the impulse is called a defense, or the defensive opposition of the ego. Anna Freud (1966/1936) called these defensive operations of the ego against the id, *defense mechanisms*.

"The id says yes and the ego says no in every defensive operation (Brenner, 1973, p. 91).

It became clear to me early in our work together that Dory mobilized in her personality a number of defense mechanisms to oppose threatening internal motivations, impulses, and fantasies. I could see that she had suffered early disruptions and conflicted feelings about many of her legitimate feelings and needs and that she continued to do so as an adult.

Freud's model continues to generate controversy. New explanatory theories have supplemented or replaced much of the orthodox thinking about the forces that shape personality development. This is especially true with regard to the importance more recent theories place on social and relational forces that operate systemically in mutually influential and recursive patterns. However, the genius of Freud's seminal ideas still serves as a reference point in defining clinical observations. Most therapists affirm that anxiety plays a central role in pathology and attest to the phenomenon of defense mechanisms in psychological life. Clients marshal these defenses even in the therapeutic setting, and it is important to recognize them as they present. These defenses include the following behaviors:

Repression: The ego keeps from consciousness any unwanted or threatening id impulse (including memories, desires, wishes, or fantasies). There grows a *conflict* between id and ego at the locus of the repression (for example, Dory's conflict around many of her feelings, urges, and fantasies because they often embodied unwanted and threatening impulses).

Reaction Formation: One of a pair of ambivalent attitudes or impulses is kept unconscious by an overemphasis or exaggeration of the other (for example, Dory's fear that her husband would have an accident).

Undoing: Usually takes the form of an action that has an embedded meaning; that is, the action negates the harm the person unconsciously believes results from some wish, fantasy, or impulse (obsessive rituals, for instance).

Denial: The unconsciously motivated behavior of "not seeing" some piece of *external* reality. (Therapists-in-training often confuse repression, a squelching of *internal* impulses, with denial, a refusal to acknowledge a reality *outside* of oneself. I almost always manage to "forget" my dentist appointment.)

Isolation: This defense comes in two forms. Isolation of *affect* involves keeping threatening or unwanted feelings from being integrated with the rest of the person's affectual life. (Usually this defense mutes all the other affects to some extent.) Isolation of *thought* involves a period of brief mental blankness that keeps a thought from being integrated with preceding and following thoughts.

Projection: Attributing to another an unacceptable impulse or wish of one's own (for example, Dory's belief that her boss must be sexually attracted to her might not have any basis in the boss's behavior but in her own unacceptable attraction to him).

Turning Against the Self: This involves the expression toward the self of impulses and urges that are frustrated or too dangerous to express toward their original objects.

Regression: The person avoids anxiety by reverting to a former state of development associated with comfort and safety.

Identification/Introjection: The person fends off anxiety by "taking in" another person and identifying with their behaviors, values, goals, and so forth.

Of course the third component of Freud's structural model is the superego, which embodies internalized moral laws as well as idealized aspirations. The superego is analogous to the concept of "conscience" except that often the processes of the superego are largely unconscious. Dory's conscience or superego never gave her a break. Dory's superego was not merciful and self-affirming; rather, it was harsh and punitive, full of critical self-observation. She more often disapproved than approved of herself, even by her own strict standards of moral rectitude. She had a heavy burden of repentance imposed by her unforgiving superego.

Part of our work necessarily involved muting the voices of the internal judges that inhibited Dory's self-expression. Every time she disclosed some previously forbidden thought or feeling, Dory felt tremendous guilt at having allowed these parts of her self-experience to escape and be seen by me (and by herself). She imagined that dreadful things would occur after she had let down her guard, that lightning would come down and strike her. In other words, the disapproval of the superego becomes one of the adult's danger situations, and it manifests as guilt. Dory was eager to escape the tyranny of her over critical conscience, however, and soon began to allow my accepting and forgiving presence to exist side by side with the stern retribution of her internalized judges. She began to be able to choose between different versions of herself.

Perhaps I have never had a client who so completely fit with what psychoanalytic theory describes as the dilemma of the obsessively organized client. It was clear that Dory's repressed sexual and aggressive feelings and fantasies manifested in different compensatory and protective defenses that had shaped her personality and her relationships. Her anxiety, symptoms, and defenses were textbook. Clearly, however, the course of the therapy was anything but orthodox. Certainly I employed the method of interpretation as one intervention designed to help make her unconscious conflicts conscious. However, there were many other aspects to our relationship and work that facilitated her transformation. Insight is rarely, if ever, enough to provoke lasting change.

An Existential View: Keeping the Pieces Together

From an existentially oriented therapeutic perspective, the person and her world are a unitary and structural whole. One cannot separate the person from the larger relationships and influences in which she is embedded and still have the same phenomenon. "Self" and the "World" are always dialectically related. Self implies the world, and the world, self, and each is understandable only in terms of the other. As May states it: "World is the structure of meaningful relationships in which a person exists and in the design of which he participates. Thus, the world includes the past events that condition my existence and all the vast variety of deterministic influences that operate upon me. But it is these, *as I relate to them,* am aware of them, carry them with me, molding, inevitably forming, building them in every minute of relating. For to be aware of one's world means at the same time to be designing it" (May, Angel, & Ellenberger, 1958, p. 59).

Like the dynamic model, the existential approach to therapy also affirms the central role of anxiety in the development of client's symptoms and suffering. No less interested than psychoanalytic approaches in deep psychological exploration, these approaches nonetheless seek to preserve whole structures of experience. The emphasis is not on isolated psychological reactions and processes in themselves but on the *psychological being* or *ontology* of the person who is doing the experiencing. The effort to always contextualize the defenses, anxieties, and problems within the totality of self-experience of the person affords a different view into the same terrain of the client's inner world.

> Anxiety is not an affect among other affects such as pleasure or sadness. It is rather an ontological characteristic of man, rooted in his very existence as such. It is not a peripheral threat that I can

take or leave, for example, or a reaction which may be classified beside other reactions; it is always a threat to the foundation, the center of my existence. Anxiety is *the experience of the threat of imminent non-being.* (May et al., 1958, p. 50)

From this perspective, anxiety always involves an inner conflict between the two poles of "being" and "non-being." This does not mean that anxiety merely involves one's concern about whether one is alive or not. Each person shapes his or her being within relationships, ideas, and aspirations that have *value.* We do not experience anxiety over things or losses that we do not cherish. Anxiety occurs when some *emerging potentiality* or *possibility* faces the person, some possibility of fulfilling his or her existence. But there's a catch. The realization of such possibility and potential involves destroying present security, and this gives rise to the tendency to deny the new potentiality. Growth and change are difficult and often painful, but they are essential to preserving the vitality of life. In other words, if there were not some possibility of opening up, some potentiality striving for realization and expression, we would not experience anxiety.

Existential thinkers observe that this is why anxiety is bound up with the problem of choice and freedom to create one's own life. If the person did not have some freedom to fulfill some potentiality, he or she would not experience anxiety. Freedom is a scary business, and a person sometimes surrenders freedom in the hope of getting rid of unbearable anxiety. As Dory discovered, it sometimes feels safer to deny one's potentialities though this ultimately leads to a diminished existence. A person can surrender freedom by retreating behind a rigid wall of dogma, symptoms, or defenses. The person begins to constrain life choices, to withdraw and protect in efforts that mute anxiety but that squelch one's vital powers.

Dory certainly was reluctant to embrace her freedom to create her life as she wished. She referenced her daughter's ability to live the life she chose as if this were impossible to her. Her rigidity and personality style kept her anxiety contained but at the expense of her creative energies and zest for life. Dory was fearful of her own potentialities, imagining that they were like a runaway horse over which she would have no control. Dory's amorphous anxiety, like all formless dread, wanted to become an identifiable fear. She could not tolerate an anxiety without edges, pervasive in her being; it felt too much like annihilation.

As Dory's amorphous anxiety became translated into external fears, she had identifiable things to avoid. For instance, Dory could check her house to make sure no intruders were present (the threat can be objectified and can pass), but she could not acknowledge the anxiety attached to her "shameful" desires and potential to become more sexually fulfilled. Of course, because this and many other of her potentials were left unexpressed, Dory was assailed by a million fears from which she felt compelled to continually protect herself. In other words, her legitimate *ontological* anxiety over her unrealized potentials turned into unproductive *neurotic* anxiety as she battled her "sinful" impulses and irrational fears. When she began acknowledging her unrealized potentials, her longing to "shed her old skin" propelled her to new possibilities and transformed her neurotic feelings of shame and guilt.

From this perspective, there is a difference between being guilty, and having guilt feelings. In other words, guilt does not only arise from a violation of internalized precepts from one's parent's, religion, or society, and which are metaphorically "housed" in the superego. Like the experience of anxiety, guilt is also ontological (having to do with one's whole *being,* embedded in one's human condition). This form of ontological guilt is rooted in self-awareness. It emerges from the experience that I can see myself as someone who can choose or fail to choose. Ontological guilt emerges when a person fails to live up to her inherent potentialities, relinquishing the freedom to choose and create life in word and deed. A person rejects freedom by failing to be authentic, by conforming to outside imperatives that lock up potentialities, by denying one's own self-expression and internal urges to engage with life fully. Ontological guilt reminds a person that she is forgetting her being and merely pretending, only *seeming* to be alive and participating fully with others. Ontological guilt occurs when one has injured the order of the universe by not living up to one's human potential, or has prevented someone else from doing so.

There is a distinction, then, between neurotic guilt and ontological guilt. Neurotic guilt emerges from the person's violation of introjected moral laws and precepts that *do not find affirmation and legitimacy in the person's being* and in the authentic experience of living. These imperatives are merely encoded rules that do not fit with a person's self-experience but which none the less hold sway over thoughts, feelings, and actions, the violation of which causes guilt *feelings,* which can lead to symptoms. Ontological guilt, on the other hand, has constructive effects in the personality, alerting the person to "pay attention" to expressions of choice and freedom and indicating when a person has some obligation to repair the injured order of the inner and relational universe. Just as neurotic anxiety is the product of normal anxiety that a person has been unwilling to face, so neurotic guilt can be the result of ontological guilt to which the person has not responded with a sufficiently authentic action. In other words, it is neurotic guilt from which the therapist hopes to help liberate the client. Existential or ontological guilt, on the other hand, is the therapist's ally and points the way to the unrealized potentialities within the person.

Constructing a Theory

In my own growth as a helper I have naturally sought to find points of contact between different theories and explanatory systems of therapy. As I work with each client, his or her particular need or issue evokes in me a different response and method. Each system of describing the human condition seems to capture a piece of reality. For this reason I have a natural aversion to signing on to any single system as a faithful disciple. I guess I am a psychological heathen. However, if I have accepted a single tenet as the "truth," it is the familiar mantra that "it is the relationship that heals." I am, therefore, most inclined to theories that reflect this precept and that address themselves to how each of us forms as a person-in-relation.

Existential concepts applied to therapy capture the philosophical tone of this holistic perspective; it is a great context in which to conduct one's activities. However, the existential canon, even in psychology, lacks specific developmental models that adequately describe personality formation. Conversely, traditional psychoanalytic models have wonderful explanatory systems regarding development but are largely deterministic, drive oriented, and often insufficiently attentive to the person's relational world. Many of Freud's foundational assumptions derive from a reductionist model based on modes of inquiry in the physical sciences. These assumptions derive from investigative methods that presuppose a split between the observer and the phenomenon being observed. Traditional psychoanalytic models are essentially "one-person" psychologies that emphasize an individual model of human consciousness. Though the individual is influenced by the environment, the person is contained within his or her own "bag of skin" and develops largely in response to internal forces and processes.

A theme throughout this book is that as clinical models have evolved in response to new ideas in constructivism and systems theory, they increasingly emphasize understanding human behavior and development by emphasizing the interrelatedness of persons in complex and mutually influencing systems. The systems in which we develop as persons do not just affect us, we interact with the world of significant others and with the natural world in ways that serve to construct the very architecture of our being. This idea is resonant with the existential emphasis on preserving whole structures of experience and avoiding breaking individuals down into component parts such as drives, complexes, and so forth. These perspectives also concern themselves with the evolution of individuals *within* larger systems and, therefore, speak to the nature and course of individual development.

The Intersubjective Nature of Self-Experience

The intersubjective approach draws from psychodynamic and existential ideas and redefines essential concepts systemically into an internally coherent model. The foundational concepts are significantly inflected by the postmodern and constructivist ethos discussed previously. Put simply, intersubjectivity theory asserts that human experience always forms at the intersection of two mutually influencing subjectivities (Natterson & Friedman, 1995; Stolorow & Atwood, 1992). A person (including a therapist) can never presume to have access to an objective reality but constructs a personal reality as she participates in the subjective relational field constituted by participation with the world and others. The only "reality" that anyone can presume to have is one's own subjective world, the subjective worlds of those with whom the person participates, and the unique reality that emerges at the intersection between the two.

What happens when the intersubjective world of the child is lacking in essential relational qualities, and how does this relate to the formation of unconscious anxiety, defense, and guilt?

> When a child's experiences are consistently not responded to or are actively rejected, the child perceives that aspects of his own experience are unwelcome or damaging to the caregiver. Whole sectors of the child's experiential world must then be sacrificed (repressed) in order to preserve the needed tie. This we have suggested *is the origin of the dynamic unconscious.* (Stolorow & Atwood, 1992, p. 32)

This idea represents a radical break from the past, because it supposes that the *primary* force shaping the development of personality (and the unconscious) is in relationship. This idea is heresy to the traditional Freudian model because the origins of the dynamic unconscious are not to be found in the libidinal and instinctual urges and drives that exist solely *within* the person. Rather, the dynamic unconscious forms out of the *emotionally laden interpersonal processes* that characterize the child's interactions within a particular intersubjective context. The origin of the unconscious is not the drives but dissociated and repressed emotional states and frustrated developmental longings. The dynamic unconscious forms because the child cannot keep certain self-experiences available and integrated and at the same time preserve needed connections with others. Faced with the choice of being faithful to one's own developmental integrity or the perception that one's self-experience could damage needed relationships, the child will almost always section off the offending (but legitimate) thoughts, feelings, or fantasies. This shift to characterizing the unconscious as a product of relational processes has far-reaching implications.

The first implication is that the repression boundary between conscious and unconscious life is fluid and shifting, a product of relational processes. The boundary between conscious and unconscious self-experience depends on the changing responsiveness of others to different aspects of the person's experience. In other words, if certain parts of self-experience went underground because they created disruptions in important relationships, those aspects of self-experience would likely become more available if they were welcomed or celebrated in other relationships. The strength of the repressive barrier depends on the person's assessment of how likely it is that he or she will be hurt if the person allows the reemergence of the forbidden thoughts or feelings.

Different intersubjective contexts, then, evoke different configurations of self-expression and experience. This is one of the reasons clients repeatedly observe that they know themselves better in the context of their safe relationship with the therapist. As described in many of the cases in this book, the resistance of the client can be seen to fluctuate depending on the degree of receptivity and attunement of the therapist to the client's inner world. The key idea is that a person's unconscious forms when important, affectively loaded aspects of self-experience are sectioned off from normal functioning. These important self-experiences are repressed because their expression upsets important relationships and threatens needed ties. Later, perhaps as an adult in therapy, when the person encounters an empathic intersubjective context where these disowned affects are safe to express, the repressive barrier is weakened.

This weakening occurs as a result of the process *between* client and therapist in the mutually influencing system. The sectioned-off aspects of self-experience are then available for reintegration within the whole of the person and the person's relationships with others.

The notion of a fluid boundary forming within an intersubjective system is quite different from the traditional notion of repression as a fixed *intrapsychic* barrier. The degree to which clients have access to all the aspects of their inner world is partly dependent on the accurate and facilitating empathy of the therapist. Empathy and insight-oriented interventions such as interpretations are, therefore, two sides of the same coin. They are modes of understanding and validating the client's inner world and, in the economy of participation, the currency of the unconscious realm.

Another implication of locating the development of the unconscious in relational processes pertains to the experience of conflict and anxiety. Conflict takes form when primary affect states of the child cannot be integrated into the whole of self-experience because these affects failed to evoke the attuned responsiveness from primary caregivers. These sectioned-off and unintegrated affect states become the source of inner conflict because they threaten not only the person's psychological organization but the stability of essential relationships. Thus, affect dissociating defenses are activated that show up in the therapy relationship as resistance. Once again, it is in the defensive dissociation of affect states provoked by early derailments of affect integration that the origins of what has traditionally been called the "dynamic unconscious" can be found (Stolorow & Atwood, 1992).

Thus, a defense substitutes for a process that originally happened with other persons (Teyber, 2000). The person's generic conflicts form over time into inflexible interpersonal habits and strategies that themselves become problematic and injurious. An experience of oneself in relationship begins to form that structuralizes these negative and frustrating patterns and lowers the sense of self-efficacy and esteem. This developing personality structure might include an unstable self-image, pathogenic or self-defeating beliefs, and fragmented and unmodulated affect states that engender confusion and conflict. Because the person moves from failure to failure, the individual's relational skills do not improve or change with new, more productive interpersonal exchanges. Some of Dory's defenses became characterological, such as her obsessive-compulsive personality style. Other defenses were rooted in more transient psychological states (such as her reaction formation about fearing that her husband would be injured). Though these defenses helped Dory to cope, they also interfered with her ability to be fulfilled and actualized in her life.

Thus, the manifestation of defense mechanisms indicates that the person may be fending off a flood of stimuli from repressed impulses or urges (the Freudian view) but also that sensitive and sequestered affect states are being hidden and protected from retraumatization. The person wants and needs to express these inner potentialities but holds them back in fear, vainly attempting to satisfy and address them through secondary transformations that fail to sustain or nurture the person at his or her core. The promise of the therapist is that the sectioned-off affects and longings can find expression and become resolved through participation in the facilitating empathy of the therapeutic alliance, an alliance that will "stand in" for those important other relationships in which the injuries were first sustained. It is a hopeful offer to the client, but he or she nonetheless suspects some possibility of reinjury by the therapist. The *sustained* empathy of the therapist, however, convinces the client that a safe environment exists for the expression of long-frustrated developmental needs. As these needs do finally emerge in response to the therapist's validating attunement, the client's vigilance grows for any sign that this attunement will fail or be withdrawn in response to the client's hidden and sequestered longings becoming apparent. This defensive walling off of central affect states, which attempts to protect the person against reinjury, also translates into the necessity for disguise when such states are represented in dreams (Stolorow & Atwood, 1992).

Clients specific defenses typically manifest in three characteristic ways (Teyber, 2000). First, client's block their own needs *intrapsychically* and respond to themselves in the same hurtful ways that others have responded to them (for instance, Dory's perfectionism, self-criticism, sexual inhibition, and controlling rigidity).

Dory's defenses quite obviously stood in for processes that happened with significant others in her life. For instance, she was repeatedly punished for expressing un-Christian feelings and behaviors such as anger. Sexual feelings were so forbidden that she did not begin to dare putting them into words or actions. She had absorbed the sense that any "unseemly" feeling of jealousy or even a sense of independence or pride was not to be allowed. Dory once observed that her mother had told her repeatedly that anyone "who truly loves Jesus" would never be sad because Jesus had suffered more on the cross! Because her environment was not resonant to her emotional developmental needs, and because Dory was interpersonally fearful for having "inappropriate" feelings, she soon learned to punish herself without these significant others being around. She learned to block or dissociate her feelings and needs long after she moved from home and the consequences of having her feelings emerge were no longer relevant. Now she responded to herself the way that others had in the past: She was "sinful," "shameful," and deserving of retribution. She gave extraordinary power to these introjected others. Her conscience stood in for an angry God.

Clients also defend against anxiety and block the expression of needs by *reenacting* in current relationships the same conflict that was originally experienced in earlier formative relationship. Dory's sexually controlling, passive-aggressive relationship with her husband, and her shutting down, at first, of any ability to self-reflect and become available in the relationship are manifestations of this.

The third way clients block the experience and expression of the conflicted needs is by eliciting the same unsatisfying response from others in current relationships that they received in their childhood. Dory's expectation and certainty that I could not help but revile and reject her once she began to reveal herself to me was an expression of this type of defense. But her defenses also pointed to the location of her injuries, a thread leading us through the chambers of the labyrinth.

At the same time that clients are trying to block their needs through their defenses, they are simultaneously trying to get these hidden longings met in an indirect way. They look to the therapist to somehow see past the protective shell and into the delicate parts of their longing for connection and understanding. Showing me the direct way to those longings was difficult for Dory. Indeed, she had trouble acknowledging them herself. Therapists are inclined to view the unconscious wishes and impulses of the client as problematic. But Dory showed me that her unconscious processes were preserving something vitally important to her. As her trust in the therapeutic relationship revived in her the hope that she could find again what she had long ago lost, she allowed the signs to appear that would guide us both.

✗ ℟

Oh Mother, Where Art Thou?

Broken down shacks, engine parts
Could tell a lie but my heart would know
Listen to the dogs barkin' in the yard
Car wheels on a gravel road

Child in the back seat, four or five years
Lookin' out the window
Little bit of dirt mixed with tears
Car wheels on a gravel road.

—Lucinda Williams

The Shenandoah Valley of Virginia is one of the most beautiful places in the country. Bordered on the east by the Blue Ridge Mountains, and sheltered on the west by the Allegheny range, the valley stretches between them, long and narrow, for 250 miles from Winchester to Roanoke. If you stand at the top of one of these ridges, you can panoramically view the well-kept farms and fields laid out like a giant patchwork quilt and hear the sounds of lowing cattle grazing across the bucolic countryside. All along the valley the rolling pastures contrast with the small cities, towns, and hamlets that make the whole so picturesque.

The culture of this region is rich and varied. The legacy of the early German, English, Irish, and Scots settlers lives on underneath the veneer of pop culture in the religion, music, and art, enabling the region to retain its cultural character. Larger towns like Charlottesville and Harrisonburg have universities that provide a contrast to the agrarian origins of the culture and economy. The turn of the century homes in the old sections of these towns gradually give way to the newer suburban neighborhoods with their split-level and ranch houses. Beyond the city limits a few old estate farms with large Victorian, Federal, or Georgian style homes and huge bank barns intermingle with more modest clapboard-sided farmhouses and fields. These rolling fields of cropland and pasture undulate over the landscape for miles to the foot of the forested mountains. There, small communities nestle in the hollows and hills, and some are tucked away even further in the backwoods of the mountains.

In these outer regions small houses and mobile homes, unpredictably ramshackle or prim, are scattered about, stringing along the imperative of utility wires and roads. In some of these out of the way places dwell the remnants of the mountain culture of the Blue Ridge. Years earlier, a young woman had fled the poverty and insularity of one of these backwoods communities to come over the mountains to try to make a new life for herself. Now she sat in my waiting room waiting for our first meeting to begin.

Darleen had heard through a nurse friend that I taught in James Madison University's graduate programs and that I was conducting research on eating disorders. As I greeted her in the waiting room of my private practice, I introduced myself briefly, and she acknowledged me with a demur nod. She seemed self-possessed, even sophisticated in her appearance and gait. Darleen took a seat on the couch, crossed her legs, and looked around the office. She noticed a cushion propped next to her, placed it on her lap, and folded her hands on it. I settled into my chair and asked, "Well, Darleen, what brings you here to meet with me today?"

She was stylishly and meticulously dressed in a blue business suit. Her brown hair, cropped neatly at the shoulder, framed her oval face and perfectly proportioned features. "She is quite beautiful," I realized, as I noticed her clear blue eyes floating in a complexion like alabaster.

"I heard that you are good at workin' with people who have eatin' disorders, and I reckon I've had bulimia since I was about 21."

Whoa! I had to stop myself from blurting. Darleen spoke with an accent that twanged like a banjo string. Definitely not from the middle valley, too distinctive . . . but her vowels were not drawn like a deep-south accent. West Virginia for sure.

"How old are you now, Darleen?"

"Thirty-four."

"So you've been living with this for quite some time."

"Yeah, a pretty long time. I was in a treatment program for 10 days. It was the kind where you go and stay at the hospital and spend all day workin' in groups and doing art stuff and hearin' about nutrition. That was about two years ago. I went because my daughter was so worried about me. She's always watchin' me to make sure I'm not going to throw up. If I'm too long in the bathroom, she bangs on the door and says, 'Mamma, what're you doing in there.'" Darleen cocked her head as if her ear were pressed to an imaginary door and mimicked her daughter's attentive listening, "Mamma, you better not be throwin' up in there." She smiled shyly. "It's embarrassin'."

I usually find this particular regional accent jarring, but as I listened, I had to stop myself from smiling with pleasure at the melodious and unique sound of Darleen's voice. The lilting inflections gave it a musical quality; she said "yeah" almost as if it were a two-syllable word: Yeayuh.

"So it's upsetting for her if you're too long in the bathroom, and you try to hide it from her."

"Yeah, I try to hide it from everybody . . . my boyfriend, my daughter, everybody at work."

"Do you have to throw up a lot?"

"Maybe twice a day; sometimes only once if I can stop myself. I can't hardly eat nothin' without wanting to go the bathroom and get it back out."

"You mentioned your time at the treatment program. How did that work for you? Has there been a time when you felt able to control it, when you could stop yourself?"

"When I first got out of that program I did pretty well for a little while . . . a few weeks maybe. But then I just kind of slid back into it again. They put me on an antidepressant, Prozac, and that helped some, but I started gainin' weight from that so I quit, and now I'm on one where you don't gain no weight."

"Darleen, how do you feel about your weight, about how you look right now?" I asked, aware as I looked at her that she possessed a figure that was full in bust and hips, slim at the waist, and well proportioned to her 5 foot 9 inch frame. She was very attractive, certainly not overweight.

"I think I look like a fat cow," she said, the sudden tone of disgust emphasizing the statement.

"It feels to you like you are really overweight. How much would you need to lose to feel good about the way you look?"

"About 20 pounds; that would put me down to about 105."

Just as I thought she would, Darleen set an impossible ideal for her body type and height. Most women would have been more than content with a shape and appearance like Darleen's. Like many of the "if only

I . . ." statements people create for themselves that mark an elusive future "happiness," Darleen leaned out to embrace some fantasy version of herself, a version that bore little resemblance to her present possibilities and represented much more than the ability to get into a smaller dress. I knew already that part of our work would need to focus on exploring what those fantasy constructions stood in for. What longings, conflicts, frailties, or imperatives were secretly deposited in this persistent but frustrated drive to thinness? Now, however, I needed to know just how Darleen's bulimia played out in her day-to-day life.

"Darleen, help me understand how this bulimia happens in your life . . . some of the things you think and do that seem most important for me to know about."

"Okay. I guess I just can't stand the feeling of food in my stomach, especially if I eat anything but salads. It just don't feel right. When I do eat somethin', I got to get it back out, and I sneak off to the bathroom. But then I get hungry, and I eat again, and it starts all over."

"You said it doesn't feel right when you have food in your stomach . . . can you say more about that?"

"It just don't feel right . . . like I feel bad about it. I think about how it's makin' me fat."

"So the feeling of it being bad is not that it makes you sick to your stomach . . . a physical feeling, but more of an emotional feeling of 'bad.' "

"Oh yeah, it's feelin' bad about myself . . . like I've just done *somethin' wrong* that's gonna put on 5 pounds. But sometimes I just lose it, lose control. And it's like someone else takes over, and I find myself eatin' everything in sight, and I can't stop myself. It's like I'm watchin' myself and I say, 'What are you doin'?' but I just do it anyway. But later I feel bad again, and I have to throw it all up."

"How much later . . . till you throw it all up?"

"It depends, maybe 20 minutes . . . maybe half an hour."

"But when you're doing it . . . it feels good?"

"For a little while. It's almost like I get kind of high, but after it feels bad pretty quick. I imagine all those calories going straight to my thighs and my butt, and I have to get rid of it."

"How does it feel when you purge?"

"It's weird . . . the purgin' part feels good," she admitted shyly. I guess cause I'm gettin' it out."

"It's after you throw up that you feel bad again. If you had to name a feeling for 'bad,' which isn't really a feeling . . ."

"Right."

"What would you name it?"

"I don't know; it's just bad. I feel bad about myself . . . like I messed up . . . like I'm ashamed of myself. Mostly after it's done I feel kind of numb. You know, like I can't feel nothin'. That's why I can't figure why I can't stop it."

"Ashamed and numbed out are some of the first things that come to mind about it when it's all done."

"Yeah, like I'm no good or somethin'."

Darleen contemplated this statement for a few moments, then diverted the conversation. She spoke at length and in great detail about her habits of eating. I realized that she would be happy to use our time obsessively talking about food, its preparation, calories, when she ate, her preferences, her binging and purging. I knew that past a certain point this sort of discussion would be unproductive and could potentially "eat up" all of our time together. I gently steered her back to talking about herself. Her bulimic profile seemed textbook. It was time in this first interview to shift gears.

"Darleen, I'm very interested in your difficulties with bulimia, and I want to talk more about how you might use therapy to address that, but let's back up for a bit. I'd also be very interested to hear more about you . . . about your story. Tell me a little about yourself."

Darleen explained that she had grown up on a little hardscrabble farm in the hinterlands, just over the mountains in West Virginia near the Virginia–West Virginia border. Her family lived in poverty, and when she was 17, she dropped out of high school, left the farm, and eloped with her boyfriend. As she continued telling me stories about her origins, I realized that Darleen had a wonderfully colorful way of relating her life, and her narrative was spiced with regional expressions that accentuated the effect. She was a good storyteller, and her melodious voice made her accent and syntax charming, creating pictures and scenes in my imagination.

"I saw Gary's old pickup truck tearin' down the long dirt road to the house, kickin' up this big rooster tail trail of dust behind him. I was sittin' on the porch with my daddy, and Gary skidded up, and this big cloud of dust went back over the truck and I couldn't hardly see it, and when it cleared, Gary was leanin' over the front seat and callin' out the passenger side window, 'C'mon girl . . . let's go get married!' So I ran off the porch and hopped in the truck, and off we went like thunder."

I could picture Darleen fixing up the ramshackle little house she and Gary had rented and imagined her as she described going from door to door trying to sell mail order merchandise and Mary Kay cosmetics to her poor neighbors. "I wanted that pink Cadillac like livin' . . . but I never even came close."

Not only did Darleen not get her pink Cadillac, but things had not gone the way she planned. At 19 she was divorced and living alone with her 1-year-old child. Gary "was a good for nothing drunk," he "screwed around with just about everybody" and eventually "ditched her" for another girl. But he came back, and when he did, he expected her to "take up with him" again. She had had enough. But it wasn't easy to get away from Gary.

He turned out to be "more of a problem than I could possibly have imagined." As she said this, she looked distracted and sad. She muttered, "He messed me up for livin' with anybody else. I don't think I could ever marry Eddie."

"Eddie?"

"Oh, my boyfriend now. He's a good man, and he wants to get married, but I told him never again."

She resumed her story, and I made a mental note to follow up later on her first marriage. Eventually she had moved over the mountains to Harrisonburg, "to get away." She got a clerical job that enabled her to get off welfare (she was embarrassed to admit she had been on welfare) and provided her enough to scrape by. Darleen was proud, though, and in her mid-20s she managed to finish her high school education through an adult degree program.

As she talked, I could see that her ability to work hard combined with her natural intelligence had enabled her to steadily acquire better positions. By the age of 32, she had taken a few courses at the local community college and had risen in position in a small company where she worked in the human resources department. She wanted to quit renting her apartment and buy a little house out in the countryside for her and her daughter. Now she was worried that her bulimia would jeopardize her job. Two of her friends at work knew of her eating disorder. They had warned her that her bosses had noticed her absences from her desk when she went to the bathroom to purge (or to contemplate purging, which happened even more than the actual vomiting).

"One of the worst parts about it is this lump I got in my throat. I feel it every time I swallow, right about here," she pointed.

"Is it there all of the time?"

"Almost all the time . . . more if I'm upset."

I surmised that her frequent vomiting might have caused erosion of her esophagus, a not uncommon symptom, especially because I had the sense that she was probably hiding the truth when she reported that she purged two times a day. I felt certain it was more.

We agreed to meet twice a week to start. She was to follow through on a medical consult to examine her throat as well as a consult with a nutritionist to construct a meal plan. Like many bulimics, she had been counting calories for everything she ate, but Darleen possessed little real understanding of proper nutrition. Her stern discipline would give way to uncontrolled bouts of eating and then follow with compensatory behavior such as purging and exercising. Her three hours a day at the gym took up most of her leisure time, and she felt guilty, she said, about not spending more time with her daughter.

"Darleen, as you describe these events to me, can you recall what was happening in your life at the time you first started to think a lot about eating and first started purging?"

She sat silently for a while reflecting. "Yeah," she paused, "it was when my mamma passed away," she said in a suddenly meek and child-like voice, radically different from her normal strong and musical voice.

"I can see from the change in your face and your voice that recalling that touches some very strong feelings right now."

"It's hard to talk about without cryin'. I visit her grave a few times every week. I can talk to her there, and I know she can hear me and can see me," she continued in the meek voice.

"You were very close, the two of you."

"Very, very close," she continued in the childlike voice. "She went away suddenly. I was in the hospital with her. I held her hand. The doctors had to pull me away screamin'." She paused briefly, and then said, "I went to her grave and started diggin' it up with my hands. I think I was losing it."

"That's quite a thing to do. As you talk about it now, even after all these years, you look very despondent."

"She was my best friend." She raised her left hand and looked at her nails briefly. There was something in the gesture that seemed to require comment.

"You looked at your hand just now."

"Oh," she folded her hands on the pillow again, and looked up. I cocked my head as if to invite her to say something about it.

"My nails are all tore up."

"Ah," I responded. I was not interested in her nails. I thought I would like to explore more about her early reaction to her mother's death. But then I had a disquieting thought: "Is your work tough on your hands?" I was fishing, not wanting to voice my suspicion.

"No," she said meekly, and I saw a blush spread across her face and neck.

"When you said that you went to your mother's grave and were upset and dug with your hands . . . was that soon after she was buried?"

"Last week," she said quietly, averting her gaze toward her feet.

I was thrilled by our first meeting. Darleen was interesting, easy going, and pleasant. She seemed motivated and receptive to building a therapeutic alliance. Her flair for describing her life absorbed me in her story, and the one and a half hour meeting flew by and had extended to two hours. I gleaned from her narrative so far that she had fled her old life, remade herself, and cultivated a new persona, creating something for herself that was different from anyone else she knew.

She had also disclosed a lot about herself. There seemed to be a temporal and emotional connection between the death of her mother (and her persistent grief) and her bulimic symptoms. She had tried to dig her mother back out of her grave using her bare hands! My many associations with this powerful image created a vivid picture in my imagination. For me it possessed a sense of pathos deeply reflective of the kind of folk myth or song born from the culture from which she fled. I noticed that Darleen hadn't referred to her mother's "death," describing it euphemistically as "passing" and "going away."

Then there was that accent! "What a stitch!" (Darleen had used the expression.) That voice, so incongruous with her sophisticated and stylish appearance. And what about that other voice . . . the disconnected, meek, childlike voice that sometimes emerged when she talked about her mother's death? It seemed to speak for another area of her self . . . to imply to me a lack of integration as she tried to access different aspects of her thoughts and feelings. Her background fascinated me too. Multicultural therapy, I realized, is about more than ethnicity and race. Darleen came from roots that extended deep into the Appalachian slopes of her ancestors. Her family had lived on their farm at the foot of the mountain for generations. She had inherited a culture, a set of expectations and values very different from the clients I was used to seeing.

My experience treating bulimia argued that the emphasis these clients placed on body image, when they measured themselves against the pervasive cultural ideal of thinness, was a secondary transformation of more fundamental conflicts. This is especially true in cases like Darleen's—she already possessed a body that was as near to this cultural ideal as her body structure would permit. How had her inner energies become diverted into this particular symptom?

By the time Darleen and I next met, I had a plan for how to approach her therapy. She had expressed most interest in immediately addressing her bulimic symptoms. Her idea of therapy was that she had a problem that she wanted fixed. She had little notion of therapy as a mode of exploration into the other realms of her experience. Therefore, I thought that a cognitive behavioral, solution-focused approach would satisfy her desire for quick concrete progress. Research underscored the utility of this method for treating bulimia, and she had responded positively to her inpatient treatment where this model was employed. But she knew no way of consolidating her gains, and when she exited the program, had backslid. Since part of therapy involves uncovering a client's particular ways of thinking, interpreting, and making sense out of life events, I wanted to know what cognitive and behavioral configurations represented Darleen's drive toward an ideal body. Like so many women with eating disorders, had she instilled the messages implied by the glossy ads that if she could just achieve the body she held in her imagination that ideal acceptance, love, happiness, sex, respect, and self-esteem would be hers forever? As part of this approach, monthly meetings with a nutritionist would help Darleen take specific steps to regulate her diet.

However, I also hoped to eventually invite Darleen into a more thorough exploration of her rich inner world and see if she warmed up to the process of discovery. There was just too much good stuff in here to ignore: the death of her mother and her continuing grief, the creation of a new persona to go with her new life, the allusion to something keeping her from ever getting married again. Darleen had no notion of therapy as a means of growth, actualization, and self-cultivation; she thought of me as a medical doctor and her reporting to me of her life circumstances as a kind of diagnostic exercise that I required to help her. She did not realize that therapy had already begun.

———

By our next meeting Darleen had consulted the nutritionist. She expressed excitement about implementing her new meal plan and felt supported by having a structured approach to her eating. She was going to keep track of her meals and keep a food diary to ensure that her nutrition was adequate. We talked about what the implementation of this new structure would mean to her.

"Darleen, I'm a little concerned about how the nutritionist framed this with you. These are good goals, but there seems to be no acknowledgment that your binging and purging is not going to disappear overnight. It might be a slow steady process of changing."

"We didn't talk about that much. I got to get aholt of this thing though. I need to quit or it's gonna get me fired or somethin'. I can't live no more with this, so I got to do it now."

"Yeah, and I admire your enthusiasm for changing it, and I believe that will happen. Let me ask you though, are you intending to completely quit all binging and purging right away?"

"I'd like to. If I stick to this plan, I think I can lick it . . . I can try. I've got everything written out now, and I can plan meals for a whole week at a time."

"Yes you can try . . . and that's the important thing. Let me ask you, what will it mean if you do real well for a bit and then find yourself out of control, like you described it, and binging and purging?"

"I reckon it will mean I'm messin' up."

"That's the part that concerns me. Maybe it doesn't have to mean that."

"What else is it then? I'm either messin' it up or not."

"Maybe not. Maybe success could mean that you're making some progress toward your goal . . . not that you have to do it all at once, but a little over time." She looked a little disappointed. "I don't mean to squelch your enthusiasm, or imply that you won't succeed. I'm just thinking that you've relied on this bulimic stuff for a long, long time, and maybe at first it would be good to have some goals that mean reducing rather than eliminating your bulimic episodes."

"What do you mean rely on it? I hate havin' this stuff going on. It's not like I like havin' to throw up all the time. I'm kind of hoping I can just give it up. Rita said that if I follow this diet I might lose a little weight 'cause I won't be eatin' much sugar or fat."

"What I mean by rely on is that binging and purging is doing something for you. It's important to you somehow. We might need to wonder how it's important as you give it up."

"It ain't doing nothin' for me except wrecking my life. If I can lose some weight on this new diet, I think I can quit."

"Okay, we'll see how it goes. Maybe you can go cold turkey."

By our third appointment, Darleen had consulted with her doctor about her throat, and he had conducted a complete physical, including blood work. He found only very minor irritation in her esophagus, her blood work appeared normal, and she seemed fit in every way. Darleen was relieved at this report, though mystified that the exam had not revealed what she perceived as a physical obstruction in her throat. By our third session, she also let me know that our talking together had affected her deeply.

"What about our meeting seemed to affect you most?"

"I don't know . . . I started thinkin' what you meant by my bulimia doing somethin' for me. I had to binge and purge a bunch this week, and I felt real bad about it. But I can't figure it out. And just talking about all these things made me think about them a lot: that time with Gary, thoughts of where I grew up, all that stuff about me changin' to get where I am today. I never talk to anyone about that stuff."

"Or even your grief about your mother's passing," I offered, but she ignored this invitation.

"I guess I've been thinkin' about the way you asked me how much would I have to lose to be happy . . . to put it like that. I was askin' myself, is that what I really think . . . and I thought, yes! It's so stupid, but I do think that if I lose that weight I'll be happy, and knowin' it's stupid doesn't change the way I feel about it. I hate my fat cow body."

"So it's one thing to know in your head that losing 20 pounds won't really make your life perfect, but knowing that doesn't make you any happier about the way you appear when you look at yourself in the mirror."

"Yeah, exactly! I can't hardly stand in front of the mirror. I hate it."

"All you can see is how fat you appear to yourself . . . and I imagine that when other people tell you that you look great, that you've got a great figure, those compliments just bounce off of you, and you think they're wrong."

"It don't matter how many times I hear it, it don't make no difference. Eddie tells me I look great. My daughter tells me too . . . everybody does."

"Well, I guess hearing it from me too won't make any difference then. So one thing we know for sure is that no amount of persuasion is going to talk you out of seeing yourself as fat and unattractive."

"I reckon not." She laughed that I put it so bluntly.

"Then let's accept your view of that. You, Darleen, are a real heifer," she put her face in her hands and laughed harder. "Oh, my God!"

"I mean, we're talking about a real Bessy here."

"I get the point!" she put her hand down from her face and looked at me directly, eyes wide, but enjoying that something in this conversation was different from any other she had had about the topic.

"So help me understand why being as *huge* as you are is wrecking your life, and how things will change when you transform into Barbie."

And so it began with both an acceptance of, but also a challenge to, the ways that Darleen saw herself. In the following seven or eight meetings two main interpersonal processes emerged as our relationship unfolded. On one hand, Darleen had trouble dropping her conventional and charming social demeanor, her "false face." She was not used to the idea of therapy as a relationship unlike any other where the normal rules of social engagement do not apply. Like most clients, I could see she wanted very much for me to like her, and she was working hard to keep me engaged and approving. On the other hand, Darleen was bright, and she quickly picked up on the spirit of the enterprise. She was able to look inward and describe to me what she saw. She began to give voice to all the private ideas and fantasies about her body that she had created over the years that had never been articulated all at once, but that survived as half expressed, vague wishes. This seemed to be one area where she could drop her front and be genuine and disclosing.

"You know a guy, when he sees a real attractive slim girl, and he's checkin' her out . . . you know that he is really thinkin' that he wants her. Those kind of girls, they got it made because that's what everybody wants, you know. I mean it's just the way it is. They're the ones who get what they want."

"In other words, those are the girls who are happy and fulfilled. If you can be like those real slim waiflike women, then you'll be happy and fulfilled too . . . and whatever guy you're with will not check out the other girls, and what . . . it will ensure that he will never cheat on you?"

"Exactly," she said, but less assuredly after my reflecting her assumptions back to her, "he won't cheat on you 'cause you got what he wants anyway."

"Oh, I see. So losing that weight also gets you perfect assurance of fidelity in relationships with men . . . like an insurance policy. You don't have to worry anymore about your man being unfaithful."

"Yeah, I reckon," she laughed.

"You laughed when you agreed with me."

"Well, when you say it, it sounds funny. But I guess that's what I think. I do think that if I get my size I won't have no guy cheatin' on me. I guess that's kind of simple, isn't it?"

"Do you have any concerns about Eddie cheating on you?"

"No, he says he's happy with me and the way I look." I raised both my hands in a "go figure" kind of gesture. She smiled.

"I guess I kind of worry about a guy cheatin' because of Gary and just, you know, how guys are." I raised my eyebrows, challenging the generalization. "Not all guys I reckon. I mean, I trust Eddie, I do."

"So losing weight will not make any difference to whether Eddie is going to be faithful or not?"

"I reckon not. He says he likes me the way I am. I just expect bad things to happen, you know, even when there's nothin' wrong with a guy."

"I'm confused . . . I'm sorry, I'm a little dense today," I said, intentionally misunderstanding her, "you say that you have nothing to fear from Eddie, he likes you the way you are, and you feel he's a faithful guy, but also that if you lose more weight, that what you already have will be possible. I don't get it."

"Well, Eddie's not like other guys. You know, he ain't the best catch in the world."

"Do you mean that if you had a better guy than Eddie, that he might not accept you the way Eddie does unless you lost weight?"

"Yeah, 'cause he would have higher standards. But as I say it I think, he wouldn't be a better guy if that's all that matters to him."

"Have you ever heard of Groucho Marx?"

"No."

"He was a comedian. He once said that he wouldn't want to belong to any club that would have him as a member."

Darleen laughed. "I know what he meant. I never did think I was good enough for any guy that would have me."

"And if a guy would have you, like Eddie, that must mean he's not so desirable."

"Oh my God . . . poor Eddie!" This time I laughed.

"But if you lost 20 pounds, you'd be good enough for any of them wouldn't you?"

"I reckon I ought to get a date with Groucho."

———

As the sessions progressed, we discussed specific triggers to her binging and purging episodes and created behavioral alternatives that would help her bring these episodes under control when she felt ready to implement them. (I had learned well from my work with Chloe that one does not try to take symptoms away from a client . . . even when the client is as motivated to give them up as Darleen appeared to be.)

Bringing her fantasies out into the light of day, giving words to these thoughts and wishes, made them sound very different to Darleen than when she kept them to herself. She was amazed, she related around the eighth or ninth session, to see how increasingly "ridiculous" some of her ideas about herself now appeared.

"Is your embarrassment that I may be judging you for having these thoughts?" I asked.

"No, I don't feel like you're makin' fun of me. It's just that I've never talked about it before. Stuff I think looks different to me after I say it to you."

"Something about giving it words makes it sound different to you."

"Yeah, I guess. I see how it don't make no sense. Sometimes when I say somethin', and it don't seem like it's important, and then I see this little smile on your face as you're looking at me, and I know it's something you see that I don't."

"And that alerts you that . . . hold it . . . I need to look at that because he's seeing something differently from the way I see it."

"Yeah, and then I can kind of see it too, different, and I leave here with my head all messed up."

"How messed up?"

"Real messed up."

"I mean, in what way do you feel your head is messed up?"

"Just confused, you know, and like I don't know what I'm doin', and I think about this stuff all week."

"You don't know what you're doing. And from the way you said it, that feeling of confusion doesn't sound pleasant."

"No, it ain't no fun, but I guess it's good."

"How so?"

"'Cause I just look at what I'm doin' instead of just doin' it. I find myself wondering about the kind of stuff that you wonder about when we talk in here. It's different. When you ask me, 'What will your ideal body get you?' I think of all kinds of things."

"Tell me some more of them."

"Well, I'd feel better about myself in lots of ways. I mean I hate it when people ask me where I went to school 'cause I got my GED and it's embarrassin' when everybody else went to college. And you know, Eddie's a good guy. He has a good heart, and he helps me a lot, but he ain't that great to look at," she said shyly. "I know that's not the most important thing."

"But you assume it's the most important thing when others evaluate you?"

"I reckon I do . . . because I'm a woman. You know, if I looked real good, I might be a part of that group and get invited to the good parties and stuff."

In this new fantasy circle of friends, people threw parties where they sipped drinks, said witty and intelligent things, and wore expensive clothes and drove expensive cars. Darleen imagined that Trent, the regional manager of her company, her boss's boss, belonged to this world. He would occasionally breeze into town in his BMW, full of stories of travel to Europe and boat charters in the Caribbean. It was the "world of Ralph Lauren" like she had seen in commercials where ideal beauty and money seemed to give one access to all the things that were the opposite of the life she had fled, and which she kept hidden from everyone in her new life. It struck me that this fantasy world represented the opposite of shame.

"So you fantasize that you could belong to this club where all the beautiful people hang out together."

"And that would be really good, but I'd be afraid that they'd find out."

"Find out what . . . that you are an imposter?"

"Yeah, that I'm really, you know, white trash."

"You think of yourself as 'white trash?'"

"They would think of me like that."

As the weeks progressed, Darleen began to realize that losing weight might make her look more like an ideal purveyed by the ads, but no amount of weight loss could change the way she felt about the "invisible body" inside the one standing on the scale. She had, of course, been unable to instantly give up her bulimia. She had "messed up," and she realized that therapy was going to be a longer and more difficult project than she had optimistically believed. Underneath her slowly crumbling facade, a mild depression started to emerge in her demeanor and expression. She seemed to trust me enough to show it to me, and it seemed like a good opportunity to take our work to a deeper level.

In one session she talked about her feeling of being an "outsider."

"I just think they don't really see me the way I am . . . and that's a good thing."

"Ah, they don't see you the way you really are," I repeated for emphasis. "I wonder, can you help me see the way you really are and imagine that showing me could be a good thing?"

"What do you mean?"

"I mean, most of our talks involve thoughts and feelings that are somewhat related to your goal of dealing with bulimia. But what if we widened our scope a little. If others can't see what you see about yourself, could you talk to me about what you are hiding from them, about how you really see yourself? Could you share with me what you feel and think that you normally don't show to anyone . . . anyone at all?"

She hesitated. She had worked hard these past few months to give words to the beliefs and private meanings that underscored her feelings about her body. She had also begun exploring configurations of self-experience that had gone unexamined in her transformation from backwoods farm girl to rising junior executive. But I realized that this was a woman who had also worked hard for years to cultivate a persona designed to elicit praise, approval, acceptance . . . to present herself well, and she was not about to completely drop it all for me. I knew she had not anticipated this sort of interaction as part of the deal when she started therapy. She started telling a story.

"I don't know why I have to keep doin' the same crazy stuff. When I was little, my daddy said that I was real pretty, so I don't remember feeling this way about my body."

She had told me this before, and I had been interested, but it was clearly a diversionary tactic. "Darleen," I interrupted, "when I invited you just now to help me see you the way you see yourself, it seemed to imply that we could take our work to a deeper level than we have been so far. How do you feel about that?"

"I don't know. I already told you more than I have told anyone." She paused and changed tacks. "Yeah . . . it's fine. I mean whatever we need to do to get rid of this. I just hate livin' this way."

I heard what Darleen said, and she appeared sincere. But I also had the impression that she would say or do anything she thought I wanted to hear. I had a fantasy that behind those words stood a great forest and on the edge of it, nailed to the trees, were signs that warned: No hunting, fishing . . . trespassers will be . . . ? I wasn't sure what would happen to trespassers, but I didn't want to be one. I wanted Darleen to invite me onto her land.

"How's that going for you . . . in our meetings, I mean, sharing with me more than you have ever told anyone?"

"Good . . . really good. I look forward to bein' here every time. I always think about stuff after I leave. I'm not binging near as much, maybe two or three times a week, but I'm still purging after meals almost the same as before, maybe a little less. I just can't stand to have the feeling of food in my stomach. I've been going to the nutritionist and that's working out well. I'm learning a lot," she smiled at me. There it was again. I suddenly had the impression that she offered these observations to me to convince me she was being a "good client," and more, that I was being a "good therapist."

In fact, looking at that charming smile I realized that Darleen had been one of the most cooperative clients I had ever seen. She had made herself interesting, had followed through on all suggestions. Here she was, smiling at me sweetly . . . so cooperatively. "Ha!" I realized, on some level she knows she is a good-looking woman because she's using her charming smile on me right now. I had the thought, she's trying to keep me in the parlor having tea when I want to throw open the other doors in the house where the rooms aren't so tidy. Yes, she was charming me the way I imagined she had cultivated the ability to charm everyone, and in that she was recapitulating in our relationship what she did elsewhere. I would have to explore that with her.

After the session I wondered about my own part in this interpersonal process. What kept me holding my cup of tea and smiling back? Had I chosen to collude with Darleen by sticking with material that she let me know was not too distressing? Were we talking "about" things rather than creating a riskier sense of immediacy and "being in" them with her? No, I would have been bored if that were too often the case, and I wasn't bored.

Okay, I braced myself to ask: countertransference? I liked her a lot. I found her attractive, charming; I enjoyed her stories (but, I thought, they always put her in an appealing role). I felt effective and important to her, and that was nice, perhaps a little too nice. I was more encouraging with her than with most of my clients. Why was that? She seemed to elicit an especially strong supportive impulse in me . . . too supportive, and I had been feeling a kind of protective paternal instinct. Was she working me, and was I colluding with her from some need of my own? Damn!

I realized that she was not the only one who wanted very much to be liked. She was somehow communicating a message to me that said, "Whatever you do, don't hurt me . . . like and approve of me, and I will like and approve of you." It was a pretty good deal, and it felt nice to me. But I knew that the therapist has to shake things up, risk the client's displeasure, participate in conversations about things that cause distress or pain. What interpersonal process was keeping me from knowing that while we sat together? It also raised the issue, how much should I allow her to set the comfort level, and how much should I perturb the process to create a climate of productive change?

I reviewed what we had achieved so far in four months of twice weekly therapy. Her bulimic behavior had moderated a little. One thing I certainly knew was that Darleen had a new and different sense that her "fatness" was not an external fact but had everything to do with the way she interpreted that image in the mirror. Though she still saw herself reflected as fat, she also had come to realize that this interpretation was connected to a larger self-perception that reached into all facets of her life. The process of examining her latent assumptions had also disrupted her notion that a change in her appearance would alter her idea of herself or fundamentally change her interpersonal world. She was also developing a greater capacity of "reflective self-awareness." Our conversations taught her to pay attention to her own thoughts, feelings, and action in a way she had never done before. Though she wanted me to see her approval-eliciting false face, she had also revealed herself in our sessions, and together we had created a therapeutic alliance.

But there was a shadow there too. The pleasant mutual gratification that existed somewhere in the background of our relationship had not yet derailed the productivity of our work, but it would eventually if it continued. Why had we not explored the unresolved grief I had seen in her for the death of her mother as well as that first marriage that "ruined her?" What more powerful indicator did I need than that image of her digging in the dirt of her mother's grave with her bare hands. I realized that early on I had brought up these issues in our sessions and that she had expertly diverted me from them, and I had colluded with her by letting them go.

Empathy, I reminded myself, is not merely an attitude of emotional resonance with the client, being sensitive to and mirroring displayed affect. Rather, empathy is an investigative stance that also requires participation with aspects of the client's inner world that she could not yet articulate or display, even if these thoughts and feelings might be unwelcome or painful to her. Being empathic with Darleen might mean I would upset and distress her and even cause her pain even though something about her elicited in me a desire to avoid this.

After all, her bulimia had been altered to some extent, but she was purging at least once a day she said, and clearly this still played an important role in her functioning. Darleen had tried to implement some of the concrete behavioral alternatives we had discussed, and sometimes they worked for overcoming her "extra" bulimic sessions, the ones she could manage to give up through an effort of will. She tried going out to places that did not contain strong triggers for her. She called a friend, journaled about her feelings, went to a support group, but often she found herself in front of the refrigerator, and shortly after, hanging over the toilet bowl. I knew these behaviors must still be powerfully connected to the self-experience for which they substituted.

We both knew it was time for a change. I sensed that she didn't want it and that I did. Now, here she sat with that pillow in her lap, smiling this message to me like a seductive invitation that some part of me wanted to accept, "You're a great therapist, I'm a great client. Let's not have any unpleasantness." Darleen had been paying for our second session per week out of pocket and the agreed upon time to move to one session a week had arrived.

"I tried to do some journalin', but I had five episodes this week . . . only two at work though. Saturday and Sunday I didn't have none."

"Two days in a row."

"I was with Eddie all weekend. There was a couple of times I really wanted to, but I just couldn't get away without him noticing. That was hard."

"Maybe that's good enough for now," I offered.

"What do you mean?" she asked, with a sudden sense of heightened attentiveness.

"I mean that part of our work has been about reducing your binging and purging because it threatened to interfere with your work. Now you're back to the point that you were when you left that clinic, and things seem okay at work now. You only purged twice at work."

"I do feel pretty good about cuttin' it down."

"You should feel good about it, but I get the sense that to give it up more than you have would be a really hard thing to do." She looked at me questioningly, and I had the sense that she was weighing whether or not to be straightforward in her response.

"To tell you the truth," she said hesitantly, "I can't imagine it. It's hard now." A pause, and then disqualifying this message, "but I ain't about to give up on tryin'."

"Okay, it seems like to further reduce it would be really hard, but to not try would kind of feel like giving up. But the binging and purging is not so disruptive as it was when you came in."

"Not nearly!"

"Okay, and things seemed to have stabilized at work. Darleen, I think it's time for us to explore why you *shouldn't* give up any more of the binging and purging."

"Say what?"

"I think, now that it's not totally disrupting your life, it's time for your bulimia to talk to us and tell us what it is and what it wants. Let's talk to the part of you that *wants* to binge and purge. The part that defies your attempts to control her."

I expected Darleen to be entirely mystified by my referring to her bulimia as a separate entity and to protest my entirely sincere observation that we not try to antagonize this part of her further. I offered this intervention not merely as a paradoxical confabulator but as an invitation to relieve herself from the repetitive cycle of trying and failing without further understanding the function of her symptoms. Clearly, an examination of the cognitions and behaviors she felt able to access, even in the context of a supportive relationship, was not going to completely suffice in her situation. She really had made progress, but it was time for a leap forward, and I knew that this meant addressing the other issues she had been avoiding. I had invited her to "show herself," and I knew she was holding out on me. I expected Darleen to be mystified, but she surprised me.

"It's so weird to hear you say that."

"Say what?"

"That my bulimia needs to talk and tell what it wants . . . it's so *weird.*"

"Tell me how it seems weird to you."

"Because, even though I don't like it, that's how I've always thought of it . . . like it's somethin' apart from me . . . like it's something separate but a part of me. I don't know how to explain it," she said frustrated but also excited.

"Keep trying."

"It's like you know how when you're a kid and . . . ," she hesitated.

"Go on, I hear you."

"It's stupid . . . ." I raised a finger and cocked my head. This was a signal that had evolved between us. "Okay, I know, nothin' you say in therapy is stupid. Okay, like when you're a kid and you have an imaginary friend . . . God! (Pronounced "Gaawd!" Her accent became more pronounced as she got more animated.) I can't believe I'm sayin' this . . . it's kind of like that."

"That bulimia is like your imaginary friend," I interrupted (I was getting excited too). She shook her head, no. Now I was confused. I tried again.

"That your bulimia is like an invisible real friend," she nodded her head, yes.

"That it's like my *best friend*," she said in that little girl voice. We sat together silently for a moment and took this in. She broke the silence with her normal voice. "Isn't that crazy? To say that your eatin' disorder is your best friend!"

I had only heard her use that term once before, and it struck me then as well . . . she had described her mother as having been her best friend. No, she had described her mother as her best friend in the *present tense*. She was clearly not putting these two statements together.

"Well, I guess no one wants to just give up their best friend," I offered.

She shook her head, and said, reverting to the little girl's voice, "but I don't know what it's trying to tell me."

"You sounded like a little girl when you said that just now, what are you feeling?"

"Helpless. I don't know what my bulimia is tryin' to tell me."

"Helpless . . . can you say a little more about that feeling of helplessness."

She fended this invitation off by merely shrugging. Then, "I just can't feel nothin' about it. I don't know what it's tryin' to tell me."

When we next met, I was excited to further explore this idea of speaking to that other part of Darleen's self-experience, the invisible bulimic best friend. I knew this was the part of her that had no intention of giving up her eating disorder and that spoke with that little girl's voice. But as she sat in the session, it became clear that Darleen had no intention of dropping her guard again. She had her pleasant demeanor on and was talking about her disappointment in having binged and purged.

". . . and it feels like I ain't gettin' nowhere. I was at the gym too. At least I have Eddie and my daughter comin' with me now."

"I thought after last session that you might give yourself a break from trying so hard to control her."

"My daughter? She wants to come to the gym."

"I don't mean your daughter." She looked confused, and then comprehending.

There was a long pause, and then she said quietly, "I was just talkin'. You shouldn't put so much into everything I say. I thought about what I said later, and it's true, but it don't mean nothin'."

"Well, maybe not, but it seems kind of like you are giving up on your best friend pretty easily after all she's done for you."

"What do you mean? My bulimia hadn't done nothin' for me except mess things up."

"I don't know, that sounds like pretty shabby treatment to me. I have the impression that the part of you that wants to binge and purge has taken pretty good care of you and has no intention of quitting, and that we ought to pay attention because it's saying to you . . . this far and no further. She's given up as much of her ground as she's willing to at this point. I think we ought to listen to that."

"And you think that's okay?" she said suspiciously. "This far and no further."

"I do think it's okay."

"Nobody's going to believe this, I swear."

"What?"

"That my head doctor wants me to stay bulimic."

I shrugged. "I'm not saying that. I'm just saying that this part of you had worked very hard to help you, and perhaps we have not appreciated her as much in our talks as we should have."

Darleen turned a long searching gaze on my face. I wanted her to see I was sincere, that I wasn't playing games. This was no therapist trick. I wanted her to bring all of her self into our conversations.

"You're serious aren't you?"

"I am."

"Jesus, Mary, and Joseph. Well, I reckon I thought when I left here that you were foolin' with me. It's strange though," she paused, and looked suddenly sad. "When you said let's listen to what she has to say, I felt excited, but then I didn't know what she had to say at all."

"You look disappointed."

"I am. It's like this part of me that is so . . . I don't know . . . *there* . . . but I don't know how to say it."

Okay, I thought, now we're onto it, and even though she can't seem to get to it herself, I'm going to risk a firm shove. "Well, I guess we'll just have to figure out what language it speaks. Darleen, when you just said that your eating disorder is your best friend, I was reminded that you used that expression another time . . . the first time we met."

"When I said my mother is my best friend?"

"Yeah."

"What are you getting at?" she said suspiciously, the first edge of defensiveness I had seen in her.

"I'm remembering that you said that you started binging and purging around the time your mother died."

"Yeah, about that time," she said resignedly. "There was a lot of stuff happenin' then."

"I've had the impression you have wanted to avoid talking about your grief, even though the first time we met you told me that you had been digging at your mother's grave with your bare hands."

She put her face in her hands. "Oh, don't mention it. It was so stupid, I must have been crazy that night," she caught herself and unconsciously peeked guiltily out between her fingers to see if I was doing my "nothing is stupid in therapy" gesture. I saw her out of the corner of my eye and felt an inner smile, but I wasn't going to dilute the power of this conversation with levity.

"Can you speak of how you experience that now?"

"You mean when my mamma had her heart attack?"

"Yeah, or how that happens in your life right now. It sounds like it's alive for you in the present."

"I don't know if I can."

"You didn't come to therapy to talk about that, did you?"

"No, but I kind of understand now why you can't just take away my problems," she said, reflectively.

"That would have been nice, huh?"

"I don't know . . . maybe not. It's just that I get real upset if I think about some things, but I see that it's all kind of stuck together too. I see that what's going on with me kind of comes out in other ways with my eating and all. I just don't know if I can do it."

"I know it's upsetting. But I think you're right; it's all connected. It's important to our work to look at some of these important things in your life you have mentioned. My guess is that it's part of what this other part of you wants to say to us." She sat in silence for a bit, occasionally looking up sadly at my attentive face. Her chest expanded and fell in a deep sigh.

"Well, one thing was awful about mamma's heart attack," she began, "I didn't expect it. I was stayin' at the house because Gary was huntin' for me, and I was scared." (Darleen's phrasing was almost always meaningful and intentional. I made a note to return later to her fear of Gary "hunting" for her.) "I came in and found mamma on the kitchen floor, barely breathin'. Daddy was off somewhere on a job. Mamma looked up at me like she wanted me to help her, and I could see she was afraid and confused, and all I could do was run for help 'cause she didn't have no phone. So I got in the truck and went to the next house and called the ambulance, but they didn't come for a long time. I guess they was lost and couldn't find the place. I finally tried to drag mamma out across the yard and into the truck, you know, like this." She demonstrated putting her arms under her mother's shoulders. I nodded. "I felt sick to my stomach seeing her head floppin' around on her neck as I dragged her out. It looked like the head of a deer on the back of a pickup truck . . . you know, all stretched out. I had her half in the pickup when the ambulance finally came, and they took her to the hospital. I stayed by her side all night long, and I held her hand, but in the mornin' she was gone." Tears were welling in her eyes, and she tried to force them back.

"Darleen," I said gently, "you can cry in here."

"I know." A pause. "They had to drag me out of that hospital room. I wouldn't let them take her. Daddy had to hold me when they wheeled her out and I was screamin'. I couldn't bear to think of her in the ground. I still can't think about it." Then the tears did start rolling down her cheeks. "After the funeral I couldn't leave her. I went there every day. I slept on top of her grave a few nights 'cause I just couldn't stand to leave, thinkin' of her there all alone. I think I was crazy. My dad used to come and find me there and take me home." She was quietly weeping, and I sat with her silently in her grief. After a while she said, "I go there a few times a week and talk to her, and I know she can hear me and see me."

"You feel as if she's watching you."

"Lookin' over me like an angel."

She was backing away from this overpowering grief. It was enough for this session.

Over the next few sessions Darleen spoke of the devastating loss she felt when her mother died. Picking up on my repeatedly referring to her mother's "death," Darleen slowly began to use the same term and to dispense with her euphemisms. I felt she almost needed permission to use this language and that this alone represented a move forward in her grieving process. But more than this, it represented a step toward differentiation. As she spoke I realized that Darleen and her mother had never become psychologically separated. They had lived together emotionally fused into a kind of "I am we" identity, a mutually dependent and protective alliance against all the harsh circumstances of their lives.

Her mother was her "best friend," not in the way that mothers and daughters share a facilitating "self-building" intimacy that helps the daughter to become a separate but connected person. No, she and her mother were best friends with each being the "other half" of the other, and this had helped to insulate them both from being vulnerable, alone, unprotected.

"Me and mamma, we was always together doin' stuff. She loved me. We worked in the garden and around the house. She didn't like me to be away too long. Partly that was because sometimes when daddy would come home he' be all drunk and falling down. But he was an angry kind of drunk. I've seen all kinds of drunks growing up, sad drunks, pitiful or happy drunks, but daddy was an angry drunk. Sometimes he'd come home and mamma and him would start to fightin', and he would beat her . . . not real, real bad. He never did break her bones or nothin'. But she would be all bruised up. I would sometimes yell at him to quit, and sometimes that stopped him 'cause he didn't like me to see them fightin' . . . he never laid a hand on me."

"So you helped to protect your mother from him. He seemed to listen to you some. How did that feel, to have more power with your father than your mother had, and to feel that it was your job to have to protect her?"

"Terrible, 'cause I didn't have enough power to stop it entirely. He felt bad about me cryin' when I would see them fight. After their fights I would go lie down with mamma in her bed and she'd be cryin' and say she was going to leave him, but she never did. She didn't have no place to go to. Mamma and me slept in the same bed up until the time I married Gary. We was that close. I miss her so much . . . like a piece of me is missin', like a big giant piece of me is missin'."

"Like a piece of you is missing," I repeated for emphasis. "I guess you don't have to look too far to understand how you're trying to fill up that missing piece," I interpreted.

She looked up at me, paused, "I know it . . . it sounds strange, but it makes sense," and then, in that meek little girl voice, "'cause I just don't know what I'm going to do without her."

"So there's a part of what 'she,' your bulimic best friend, is trying to say to us. You really feel lost without your mother, even after all this time, and something about your bulimia expresses this, and at the same time, helps you to not completely realize or accept it."

Darleen looked up at me suddenly, tears welled in her eyes, and it looked as if a wave of recognition swept over her as she contemplated these words.

"Help me understand, Darleen, what it has meant to you to have your mother die? Let's talk about this piece of you that's missing."

"It's the part that I can see her face, and I know I'm going to be all right because she's takin' care of me and got her arms all around me and lovin' me. We talked about everything. We didn't have no secrets from each other. She said I was her darlin', and I knew I was even more special than my two brothers . . . you know they was closer to my daddy. My mamma said me and her would always be best friends, and I know she didn't know she was goin' to go because she wouldn't have left me. She said she wouldn't have no reason to live if it weren't for me. I don't understand why God would take her then. She looked so scared as she was dying on the floor, and I couldn't do nothin' about it."

"You could sometimes protect her from your dad, but you couldn't do anything to protect you both from her death." She shook her head.

"Nope, I couldn't do nothin'."

"Darleen, you're weeping."

"I know it. I never cry, and here I am sobbing like a fool."

"Maybe these tears are also expressing something of what that other part of you wants to tell us."

"I know it," she said, her face in a mask of grief.

Over the course of the next few sessions, Darleen continued to explore the dimensions of her own grief and loss. For the first time she spoke of her feelings of helplessness that she could not prevent the abuse by her father. She even admitted that she felt that the family violence and her "best friend" relationship with her mother might have held her back from "growing up normal." She revealed the "terrible guilt" she felt at having "run off" with Gary. She knew that she wanted to get away but that it left her mother vulnerable and alone with her father.

"Darleen, you said that you felt guilty running off with Gary because it left your mother alone with your dad. Then you mentioned that she had her heart attack. As you were talking, I had the sense you were implying a connection between those two events."

"I know," she said in the meek voice, "I've always known that if I didn't go that she wouldn't have died."

"You feel that your leaving caused your mother to die. Tell me, how would your staying have prevented it?"

"I don't know. I guess I would have been there to help protect her. Maybe she was heartbroke I left."

"Darleen, I can see you really feel a lot of sadness and guilt about this, and I'm not trying to talk you out of those feelings, but didn't you say to me that you were going to see her every day, just like when you were living at home?"

"Yeah. It don't make no sense does it?"

"What does it feel like if I ask you if your mother could have died because it was just her time and that it doesn't have anything to do with you leaving home?"

"She did used to say that 'God chooses the time and the place and God has his reasons that nobody can't know.'"

"Yeah, that maybe there are things beyond your control. Darleen, you're weeping again."

"Dern it! I don't know why I have to always end up cryin' in here."

I felt now that I understood another dimension of Darleen's bulimia. When her mother died, it was as if she had had a piece of her self ripped out of her. She was not only bereft, she had also lost what was essentially a part of her inner architecture and structure. This part had to do with being able to comfort herself, support herself emotionally, provide her with a feeling of connection to another. Neither she nor her mother knew how to feel okay without the other being physically present. Apparently she had not been able to internalize an intact mother's care-giving functions enough so that as she grew up she could essentially "carry her mother with her" and access inner resources in times of stress or trouble. In a climate of abuse, their relationship had been so actively and palpably dependent that she had not traveled far enough away from her mother psychologically to make this transformation into a more autonomous and independent person. Further, her mother's death had left her with an overpowering sense of vulnerability. No wonder she spoke of her mother "watching her," of her "conversations" with her at her grave site, of "knowing that she's my guardian angel." These were Darleen's ways of trying to summon up the spirits of her own inner capabilities to keep her safe and intact.

But this didn't always work for her. She had created an external, concrete way of ensuring that she did not have to incorporate the loss of her

mother. Just as she had partly transformed her existential crisis of
mother loss and her own ultimate separateness into the external problem
of her bulimia, she had also kept herself from fully acknowledging her
mother's death by her graveside vigils. She could convince herself that
they still had "conversations" and that she was protected by her mother
like an angel. But when these comforting notions failed her and the full
force of the finality of death broke through in her consciousness, that
was when she found herself in an altered state ("I must have been crazy
that night") frantically digging in the dirt of her mother's grave with
her bare hands in a desperate attempt to stave off accepting this finality.

How then, exactly, did Darleen's bulimia "fill in" for the experiences
she was attempting to access? I resolved to explore the details of what
she did and felt when she engaged in her bulimic episodes to see how
they provided something that she so desperately needed. I looked forward to our next sessions with anticipation to see what Darleen could
tell me of her conjurations, for I now saw that deep in her hidden
rooms, away from the parlor where she had tried to entertain me, she
was practicing to raise the dead.

But the sparkly things of life have a way of attracting our attention
away from these glances into the inner world. Magpies all, we each
sometimes look to the external things of life to ease our suffering and
mute the voice that whispers into our ear that we will pass this way but
once. Darleen appeared at her next session breathless with excitement to
relate to me that Trent, the golden boy, the "Ralph Lauren's world" representative, had asked her out on a date. Trent, whom all of the women
at work thought was "hot" but also a "user." Trent, who Darleen had
once described as "way out of my league." Eddie had quickly faded into
the recesses of her imagination. I lamely questioned whether Trent was
allowed to date employees. I resented him already.

I noted the reemergence of my countertranference with surprise. Was
I jealous, I checked in with myself? No, I sincerely didn't think so, at
least not sexually. Well, maybe a little sexually, I admitted. I had occasionally caught myself not fully paying attention as I admired the
beauty of Darleen's face. And true, the appearance of Trent had evoked a
little of the jilted boyfriend feeling in me. What the hell was that? I
took stock. I was in the final stages of a divorce in a 17-year marriage.
Could it be that I was taking from my meetings with clients some gratification—being needed, admired, relied upon, appreciated—that I was

currently lacking in my personal life? Was Darleen's turning her attention elsewhere making me feel less important when I was feeling a need to feel valued and special? That felt accurate. All right, so I was a little jealous, but I was going to be aware of it and had it under control. The main thing, I told myself, was that Trent was wresting her attention away from our hard won gains in therapy. Darleen would put on her best persona, her falsest face, to win Trent's approval and affection. This would happen just as she was really dropping those masks with me. The best I could hope for was the opportunity to Monday morning quarterback as the whole thing played itself out.

Was I being too pessimistic, jaded? Could I not let Darleen enjoy this sexual conquest that communicated to her that she was "in Trent's league"? She had spoken of him before, and I had always had the impression that he was shallow, self-involved, and arrogant, but I didn't know him. Maybe he was a great guy and his interest in Darleen was more than just exploitation. I looked at Darleen's glowing face, her shapely legs, and I doubted it. In addition to mild jealousy, Trent's arrival on the scene had also suddenly revived some paternal, protective countertransference. I felt like telling her to be in by 12. Surprised, I marveled at my own processes. Somehow this unsophisticated, seemingly helpless backwoods country beauty had evoked a kind of erotic attraction/damsel in distress reaction from me. I had to laugh at myself, the incongruity between my own self-image and the feelings I was having in response to her shifting attention. Somehow the awareness helped it to dissipate.

Each week she came in to report on what new adventures she and Trent were having. They went in his BMW out to the Shenandoah Valley vineyards for wine tasting. They went to nice restaurants and the movies. This week they spent the weekend at the famous and luxurious hotel at Hot Springs, Virginia. They had ridden horses and gotten massages. They had, of course, become lovers. I hated that guy.

Darleen spent most of her sessions talking about these events. I listened with attention, commenting on only what she gave me—basic reflecting and active listening. I knew that if I questioned a single illusion, rained on her parade with only a slight sprinkle, Eddie and I might as well be sitting at a bar together commiserating about a woman we once knew. She would disappear from therapy as fast as falling in love.

Darleen's romance with Trent took up all the space in her life and in our sessions. She wanted to talk of little else. There were a few times when something Trent said or did gave her anxiety, but she always offered the most generous interpretation of his actions. Coworkers warned her that Trent liked to date "the good looking ones," but not to get too attached because he never stuck with any of them. Darleen ignored them because she thought they were just jealous. Sometimes she felt an inclination to talk about an "issue" or "problem," but I sensed that she did this dutifully, that she didn't know how else to make sense of our sessions. It was almost as if she were asking me to bear witness to a miracle, the fulfillment of all of her hopes. I made a few feeble attempts to encourage her to reflect on why she felt this relationship was "it."

I once observed that when she talked of Trent it was often not about the man himself but about the exciting things they did together. What was Trent like as a *person* I wanted to know? She dutifully provided an inventory of his many virtues, with the exception that he tended to drink too much and was inclined to say things about "Blacks and foreigners" that she found objectionable. But she had grown up around that sort of thing, and she let him know that he was incorrigible. I just held onto the string and waited for the kite to come back to earth. I felt that we had lost the brief opportunity to take her therapy to the deeper level that we had approached. What had I to offer her that could compare to the delight of falling in love? The prospect of self-examination, painful growth, and awareness? "Come dear, let me lead you to the mouth of this cave . . . go on in . . . I'm right here with you." Then she disappeared from therapy.

It didn't happen all at once. At first she couldn't make a session because of illness. Then she and Trent went out of town. Then she came to a session. She began to express doubts about her ability to afford further therapy. She thought she could manage on her own now. Trent had told her about his sister. She was in therapy, but it didn't help her, so she had gone to a weekend retreat at "EST" and had loved it. Trent didn't believe in therapy. She would be in touch if she needed to schedule an appointment.

A month went by with no word from Darleen. The hour we had met was a hole in my schedule, an empty space in the orthogonal grid of my week that had not yet been filled with a new appointment. I realized that I missed her. Then one day I saw that my secretary had her written in on my schedule. Darleen followed me from the waiting room, went through the door, took her seat on the couch, and looked around.

"Where is it?" she inquired with a look of mild distress on her face.

"Where is what?" I asked.

"My pillow, I got to have my pillow."

"Oh," I said with a laugh. I went to the closet and took out the richly covered Victorian style couch cushion, fringed with tassels. I had forgotten that Darleen ritually placed this cushion on her lap or by her legs and held or absently stroked it for much of our sessions together. I had put it away thinking that it looked a little out of place in this contemporary office. Though I must have seen her take it up many times, I had not realized that it was so important to her sense of place and safety.

"I love this pillow," she said stroking the rich velour fabric. It reminds me of those big fancy antique sofas." She put it on her lap, and looked up. "It's good to see you."

"It's good to see you too."

"I guess you thought I was hightailin' it out of here."

"I wondered."

"I reckon I wondered too."

"You thought of not coming back?"

"Yeah."

"Yeayuh," I mirrored her accent smiling.

"You think my accent's a hoot, you should hear my daddy."

"So what made you avoid coming for our talks?"

"Our talks! Well, where I come from people don't talk like what happens in here. I don't know. I was so happy with goin' out with Trent, and we were talking about sad stuff in here. After leaving here I just couldn't stop thinkin' about all the stuff we talked about, and it was makin' me crazy. I don't know, I reckon I just needed a break. I was so happy going out with Trent," she repeated, but sadly this time.

"That seemed to be going really well for you."

"Then all hell broke loose."

"Oh."

"He seemed like such a good guy, but he was screwin' around the whole time. He turned out to be a jerk like most of the guys I get messed up with. I thought this would be different. She described the long scenario of how she had discovered that Trent was also dating another employee in a different town.

"Would being thinner have kept Trent from cheating on you I wonder?"

"You don't . . . even I know by now he would have been a jerk. I guess I'm no better than he is though."

"What do you mean?

"Remember when I said I was going to break up with Eddie? I never did it. I never told Eddie I was going out with Trent."

"Oh."

"That's awful, isn't it?"

"I wonder why you decided not to tell Eddie?"

"I don't know. I told Eddie I just needed some time alone. I guess I knew somehow that Trent was too good to be true, but it felt good to have him want to go out with me. I guess I was keeping Eddie on the line."

"A fall back position when Trent didn't work out."

"Yeah . . . and I . . . I don't know. I didn't know what Eddie would do. Maybe he would go crazy and kill me."

"Darleen, it really surprises me to hear you say that. You have always talked of Eddie as if he is a gentle, affectionate guy. Has he ever shown you a violent side?'

"No, he wouldn't hurt a fly. I know he would be real upset though."

"I'm sure he would be . . . but do you think he would hurt you though?

"I don't know . . . you never know."

"Darleen, I'm curious about this expectation. I wonder if seeing your dad beat your mom gives you a kind of extra fear about the kinds of bad things that might happen if you displease Eddie?" This seemed self-evident to me, almost so obvious as to be patronizing, and I was surprised when she silently shook her head, no. I was about to launch into an explanation about the powerful effect of early modeling, but the devastated look that emerged on her face stopped me, and I kept my mouth shut.

She said in that little girl voice, "The reason I came back is because you told me that I always show people what they wanted to see." I nodded. "And how you said I could tell you about myself like I don't with anyone" . . . more nodding . . . "I'm afraid of it . . . I been listenin' to that other part of me, but it's harder to do it alone. I been listenin' hard, but I'm afraid to tell you everything because you'll see what I really am." A long silence.

"Darleen," I said gently, "I don't know what it is that you want to tell me that you think might cause me to be disgusted by you, and that you think will make me stop liking you. All I can say is that nothing you could tell me will cause me to reject or punish you. I will like you regardless of anything you reveal about yourself to me."

"You say that now."

We were out of time in the session. Darleen asked if we could meet at our regular time again.

At our next session, we sat in silence for a long time. I did not want to pursue her around these "secrets"; she would have to take the lead if she wanted to go further. She did.

"When I married Gary, we were going to live next to my mamma and daddy's place, but after we were married, Gary didn't want to anymore."

I thought, Gary had no idea that Darleen was not about to leave her mother.

"So we moved to the other side of the county. At first it was okay, and he was nice to me. Soon I found out he was screwin' around. When I found it out, I put it in his face and said that I could do the same thing. I just wanted to get in his face, you know?" I nodded. "He beat me up so bad I was unconscious. I woke up on the floor, and he was gone. But he came back, he always came back, and over time it got worse and worse. I went home a few times, but he always came and fetched me. At first I used to fight back with him, but then he would get even worse, and once he hit me with a shovel and broke my jaw."

"Jesus, Darleen. What you were going through sounds terrible."

"It was bad. But it got worse."

I shook my head. "It's hard to see how it could get worse."

"Yeah, but it did. He started in not lettin' me leave the house to visit my folks. He said my mamma was always against him, and when I tried to go anyway, he beat me up so bad with his fists the next thing I knew I was wakin' up in the hospital. He got arrested for that one. When I was there, they took some x-rays of my face, and the doctor said the bones in my face was all criss-crossed with little lines from old fractures from all the times he hit me."

I looked at Darleen's beautiful face and imagined that underneath the fair complexion her facial bones bore the fractures that recorded the history of her hard life, of her poverty and abuse. And more, they traced the fractures in the structure of her invisible self, the self she loathed and kept hidden away from the view of any who might want to know her.

"I had a few months to think about it while he was in jail. I went home, but I knew he would come after me again, and he did. He came walking up the porch and told me to get in the truck."

"I told him to get the hell off the property. I swear I said it just like that. I had a restraining order against him. He was not supposed to come anywhere near me. But he wouldn't leave."

"Jesus, what did you do?"

"I shot him."

"You shot him?" I said incredulously. I felt like the story was starting to sound like something out of *Deliverance.*

"I actually didn't *mean* to shoot him. I meant to fire at his feet, but it must have ricocheted up and got him in the ankle."

"That must have surprised him."

"Yeah, I should have shot him in the head," she said bitterly. "He left me alone after that because he got arrested again for violating the restraining order. I didn't get in no trouble at all. But now he's back."

"He's back! Now?"

"After 16 years. He wants visitation rights with Brenda."

"He just reappeared on the scene out of nowhere?"

"Yeah, well, not out of nowhere. I used to see him around once every six months maybe. It was awful. I'd get panic attacks and have to get away from wherever I was. They made him pay child support through the court, so I never had to see him or talk to him. Of course he mostly didn't pay. But now I have to go to court to fight his petition to see Brenda."

"It's as if your old life that you have worked so hard to leave behind you has suddenly intruded on the new life you have created."

She nodded, resignedly, "Exactly. How am I going to face him in court? I have a panic attack every time I think about it. Eddie is wonderin' what in the world is wrong with me. Now, not only do I throw up, I seem scared to go anywhere."

"You mean Eddie doesn't know about any of this past life?" She shook her head. "He comes from a good family. I don't think they would understand."

"I think maybe you underestimate him. So this is another way . . ."

She interrupted me, "that I've hidden from everyone, even the ones who are right around me. You see what I mean?"

"About what?"

"About really being white trash."

"No, I don't see that," I said.

"You still think I'm worth seeing in here?"

"Jesus, Darleen, of course I do."

Our sessions became still richer. She had opened up the door from the parlor and let me in to more of the rooms, some of which were haunted by the ghosts of her past, some of which she was afraid to enter in the present. Over the next four or five months, Darleen became more open, not only about the life she had left behind but about her life in the present. I also noted that as Darleen and I became more and more "real" to each other, my countertransference attraction and my feelings of wanting to protect her receded. She increasingly dropped her false face and allowed me into her inner world of thoughts, fantasies, and feelings. We worked together exploring the multigenerational legacy of abuse that she had experienced and witnessed and identified the ways that it influenced her view of herself and her relationships.

She decided to become more open with Eddie, and contrary to her expectation, he and his family were sympathetic to her. She was so grateful, that Eddie seemed to rise in stature in Darleen's imagination. She didn't imagine any man could accept her past. We also rehearsed how she would cope with having to confront Gary once again.

After prevailing in the hearing, she said she realized that Gary was "nothing but a burned out drunk," and that he no longer loomed so large as a menacing presence in her imagination. More than ever, though, she grieved the death of her mother, and I was astonished that her grief never seemed to lessen in its intensity. It seemed to have a life of its own, just as did her persistent bulimic symptoms. Although her bulimia took up much less space in her life and she rarely binged, she continued to purge after normal meals three or four times a week. I wondered that she seemed to need less to "take something in" than to "get something out." Her weight remained stable.

"What is your bulimia trying to tell us?" had become a frequent inquiry every time her symptoms got worse. And Darleen got much better about making connections between what she was experiencing just before her uncontrollable purging episodes. It was connected to so many things, she said; she had so many ways of feeling bad about herself that it took a lot of attention to sort it all through. Darleen had long since observed that she tended to "switch" when she wanted to purge, "like it's another me that takes over." Like most persons with bulimia, she felt better after purging: freer, more in control, less upset. I wanted her to access the feelings that she somehow got in touch with when she made this switch into an altered state. I was certain that that little girl's voice I had often heard was connected to whatever resided on the other side of that partition.

Darleen had never been willing to acknowledge the importance of her description of both bulimia and her mother as her "best friend."

"Darleen, when you 'switch' and you feel yourself compelled to purge . . . for that moment, don't you feel your bulimia is really taking care of you, that it is really the thing that helps you survive?"

"In that moment I feel that it's the only thing keeping me from feeling like total shit."

Darleen had never before used anything resembling profanity in our meetings. "So it takes care of you, it helps you."

"Yeah, it makes me feel good about myself for that moment . . . but it switches back so fast, and then I feel even worse about myself than I did before."

"But for that brief moment you feel comforted."

"Completely."

We had been over this terrain many times before, but this time I took a new tack. I had the sense that there was something about Darleen's mother "watching over" her that connected her to those states that she accessed when she binged and purged.

"And when you talk to your mother at her grave site, don't you kind of feel the same way—looked over, taken care of, like she's with you and can see you?"

"She's watchin' over me and helpin' me, and I know she hears me."

"There's something about your purging that you feel bad about afterward. I wonder, is it the same as when you visit with your mother, or are you ambivalent? I mean, do you feel mixed about visiting her grave, or is that something that only makes you feel good?" I was grasping here, but I had an intuition that grieving at her mother's grave put Darleen in touch with the same self-experiences she accessed when she purged. That her grief, if not her purging, might be more willing to reveal the part of her that lived on the other side, the part that spoke in that little girl's voice.

"It's funny you should say that because I feel good as long as I'm there where she's buried. I fix up the flowers and make sure her grave is real pretty. But after I leave I feel kind of bad."

"You feel bad. Help me understand what 'bad' means."

"Right, I knew you were going to ask me that . . . bad is not a feelin'. I feel kind of like I'm lettin' her down, and I feel sad and like I wish I could do something more for her."

I had an impulse, "Or that she could do something more for you."

"What do you mean?"

"To tell you the truth, Darleen, I don't know what I mean. I have the sense that you want to carry something away from your visits with your mother, but that it doesn't stick. Yes, you go and tend her grave, and keep it pretty, and it looks like it's all about honoring and missing her, but aren't you really looking to get something back from her? Perhaps your grieving for her is partly about grieving for yourself. You can't let her go because you need something from her, and you kind of get it when you visit her grave, but it goes away real fast. It's almost as if she's holding out on you. Maybe that's why you need to go there so often. We have asked often, what is your bulimia trying to tell you, and we've understood a lot about that. If you had to ask your dead mother, what is she trying to tell you, what would she say? How do these long years of mourning work for you, keep you from releasing yourself, keep you stuck where you are?

It was way too much. Darleen looked shaken. Her face looked ashen and flat. I had been so caught up in the flow of my ideas and words that I had not attended to how she was receiving them.

She merely replied, "I don't know. I'll have to think about that."

"You look a little shaken. What's happening with you right now?"

"Nothin' really."

"Come on, Darleen, something's happening; try to identify what's going on with you right now."

"Nothin', I told you!" she said, suddenly angry. "Just quit it!" Over the past few months Darleen had rarely become annoyed or impatient with me as I prodded. It was the first expression of anger I had ever seen from her.

"Thank God."

"What?"

"I was worried that you were missing your angry bone. I'm so glad to see that you can get angry with me."

"I'm not angry."

"You look pretty angry to me."

"Well, you will go on talkin'!"

"Yes, and I made you angry."

"Congratulations!"

"Wow, sarcastic too . . . all in one day!"

"You asked for it," she muttered. Then, shaking her head, she disavowed it as quickly as it had emerged. "I'm sorry," she said.

"No, don't be; I'm glad to see you can get angry." We sat silently for a bit. My intervention had not gone like I wanted, but at least something good could come from it. I liked Darleen's flash of emotion. It was immediate and real, even though she thought she needed to apologize. "Our time is almost up. Is there anything more you want to talk about?" She shook her head. "I just want you to know," I said, "that I feel like you showed a new part of yourself to me today. I think it says a lot that you were able to be real about how you felt about me pushing you."

"So, we should meet at our normal time?" she said as she rose from the couch and headed for the door. The implication of her question was that she had misbehaved and that I might not want to see her.

"Of course, I am not here to punish you for having your feelings."

She said, almost under her breath, "I do that myself."

"That's right," I agreed, "you do."

The following session she sat on the couch, put the pillow in her lap, and said straight out, "I'm mad at you." Great! She was practicing with these feelings in a safe environment.

"Okay, I hear that you're mad at me. Help me understand what I said or did that got you mad."

"You messed up my whole week. I couldn't stop thinkin' about what you said, and the more I thought about it, the madder I got. I went to see my mother and I was upset. I didn't feel good about what we talked about in here." She was back to describing her mother as if she were alive.

"Something changed about when you went to your mother's grave. It didn't feel the same."

"Yeah."

"And it seems like something we talked about messed that up, like it got taken away from you, and you're mad about that."

"Yeah, you made it sound like I visit my mother because I'm selfish . . . like I take good care of her because I'm really doin' it for myself."

"So, when I said that your visits had to do with needing something for yourself, you hear that as selfishness."

"I reckon, and you just kind of said it, you know, like it or not."

"You mean that last week I pushed you around a little, and you didn't like that. You don't like anyone pushing you around."

"Yeah! You're supposed to help me, not upset me even more. I wanted to purge just to make you mad, but that just seemed stupid. And purgin' didn't feel the same either."

I didn't know what exact intervention I had made, but I liked it a lot!

"I thought a lot about what you said. I couldn't get it out of my head."

"Which part? I recall saying a lot."

"You know, if I asked my mother what she wants to tell me."

"Ah, that part seemed to bug you this week. Were you able to answer that for yourself . . . what she would want to tell you?"

"I asked her. She answered it for me when I went to visit her. I mean, not like I heard her real voice or nothing, but like I heard her in my mind." I nodded. "She would tell me that it's okay, that she loves me," and then more quietly, "even though I messed up real bad."

"She loves you, even though you've made some mistakes in your life, it's okay . . . that everyone makes mistakes." Darleen shook her head no.

"Not that I've made some like mistakes that everybody makes, but that I messed up real bad, but that she loves me . . . you know . . . in spite of that."

"It seems like you have particular mistakes in mind that you think are out of the ordinary." She nodded. "Do you want to share with me what you mean by saying you messed up real bad?" She shook her head.

"I've never told anyone."

"Even your mother?" She shook her head. "I lied to you when I told you we talked about everything. There was one thing I never did tell her."

"But now that your mother is dead, now that she's watching over you . . . she knows about you messing up real bad." She nodded. "She can see what has happened in your past that you didn't tell her in life, and these are things you did that she would find abhorrent," she looked confused, "abhorrent . . . like really terrible and distasteful." She nodded. "But she forgives you . . . she says it's okay."

"No, it's not okay. She says she loves me anyway."

"Ah, okay. She loves you anyway. Do you want to share with me what your mother forgives you for?"

"Never . . . I never told nobody. Why would I tell you if I didn't tell her?" There was the anger again.

"You think that I will not like you anymore. That I will be so disgusted that I will see you differently . . . that, unlike your mother, I could never love or accept you for who you are."

"You got it."

We sat together silently for a little while. Silence is always good to let things settle in. Silence is also a good setup for when the therapist wants to punctuate an intervention. I did what I rarely do in therapy . . . adopted an oracular tone. I didn't know if it would have any effect at all, but it was an intuition that seemed right for Darleen, especially because she talked to the dead and was generally superstitious.

"Darleen, look at me." She raised her downcast eyes and gazed into mine. "Some day," I prognosticated, "even though I will never ask, you will want to tell me. It may be tomorrow, it may be next year, it may be 10 years from now. You will want to reveal to someone living what you think prevents you from being worthy of love. Do you know what will happen when you do that?" She sat stone still. "I will accept you just the same. I will still like and care for you. I will still be here to help you when you need me." I paused to let this sink in. Then, "Do you think, Darleen, after all this time together, that you have hidden yourself from me, that I do not see you? I see you."

"I never will."

I didn't care whether she told me or not. I just wanted her to carry away with her the statement that I would not reject her, and this prediction, I hoped, would help her to remember that, as if it were a piece of unfinished business between us.

———

During the following two months, Darleen's bulimic symptoms reduced a little further. She was purging two to three times a week, usually only after lunch. She seemed to be using her purging to regulate her caloric intake, and she described these incidences as less imperative than in the past. There was little of the "switching" experience that had characterized her bouts before. It was almost as if she was devoted to old habits. Importantly, the feeling of something being stuck in her throat had slowly faded, until eventually she noticed that it was gone entirely. She found herself relying more on her workouts at the gym to get the effect that her binging and purging had provided. Though she worked out five times a week for two hours each day, this seemed like an acceptable transformation.

One session, Darleen let me know that she had had enough of therapy. We had been seeing each other for 10 months. She was exhausted, she said, with this continual self-examination. She needed a break. She was sick of herself, sick of her bulimia being a focus in her life. In fact she was bored with her bulimia. She was tired of having to wonder about the *meaning* of things; she just wanted to live without working so hard at it.

I was happy for her. I recalled our first meetings: her animated talk of food and its preparation and how her binging and purging was at the center of her life. How she seemed like a pretty manikin with her false face smiling out of the display of her fake persona. Darleen and I had become slowly real to one another, and she had explored her life in ways that she never imagined were possible with another person. It was time to part ways. She let me know how much our relationship meant to her and that it had changed her life in more ways than she could name. I let her know that I cared for her deeply too, and that I was proud of the courage she had shown on this adventure we had taken together.

"I got more than I bargained for, didn't I?" she teased.

"You bargained for a lot; you just didn't know it when you started."

"I reckon."

We met three more sessions to work up to the parting and to review all that we had accomplished. She felt good about the gains and hopeful about continuing to make progress. It was a cheerful goodbye.

Seven months went by. Then one morning I noticed Darleen's name on my schedule for the week. We greeted each other warmly in the waiting room and made our familiar trek down the hall to the office where she took her customary seat.

"You put my pillow out didn't you," she said, as she placed it in her lap and began fondling the fringe.

"Yes I did."

We made small talk for about 20 minutes, catching up on all the things that had happened since our last meeting. She had gotten promoted and was looking at buying a little house in the country. She described her potential new home to me along with all the improvements she intended to make. As the hour advanced, I was a little concerned we would not have enough time left to address whatever it was that brought her in after all this time. But she knew the drill; she could get down to business when she wanted to. She paused, "Well, Eddie wants to get married. That's why I wanted to talk to you. I don't know what I should do."

"Ah. You knew that was coming eventually, and hasn't he asked you before?"

"Yeayuh," I smiled openly at the two syllables, "but now he's real persistent. He's fed up with my sayin' 'maybe down the road.' He's sayin' it's now or never."

"I guess that brings up all kinds of feelings for you. You swore you'd never do it again after Gary. But Eddie's a very different man, isn't he?"

"He's very different. I don't know how he's put up with me all this time. He's a good man. I don't know if I love him; I guess I do.

He's comfortable, you know?" I nodded, "and he's a good dad to my daughter."

"When you envision living in your little house all together, how does that picture look to you?"

"It looks real good. I wish I could make it happen sooner, but I don't know if I can."

"I'm not sure what you mean. It seems like Eddie's eager; you seem to want it. You seem to already know what you want to do."

"There's a problem."

"Oh?"

"Remember that thing I told you that I would never tell you, and you said I would, and I said I never would, and you said someday you will?" I smiled at her convoluted delivery.

"Of course, I remember."

"Well, I can't marry Eddie because of it."

"Sure you can."

"What?"

"It's in the past; you and Eddie live in the present. He loves you, Darleen, and you want to marry him. Do you want the past to control whether you can choose good things for yourself now?"

"But I can't marry him without tellin' him."

"That part's a decision you'll have to make."

"You mean maybe I shouldn't tell?"

"I don't know whether you should tell or not. And if I knew your secret, I still wouldn't know if you should tell it to Eddie or not."

"You're not being much help here," she said frustrated.

"Sorry." A long pause. "Darleen, you knew when you came in here that I wouldn't give you advice. That I would say, 'Choose and take responsibility for the choice . . . create your life.'"

"Yeah, I know." We sat together for a long time. She heaved a big sigh, and began, "After Gary beat me real bad that time and he went to jail, I was in a rough way. I had no money, and I was living back at mom and dad's house. I was a mess." She paused, then resumed in a very quiet voice, "There was this man . . . I'd known him since I was a kid, and he always tried to get me to, you know, do stuff." I nodded. "He kept being real nice, and he was always saying 'come by my place' and stuff . . . and one day . . . well, I did go there." She stopped, and sat silently.

"You went to his place; he wanted you to go there and have sex with him."

She nodded, "for money," she revealed, barely audible. She gazed blankly into the pillow on her lap, gently stroking the soft texture with her long fingers.

"Ah, I see . . . go on."

"I did it. I wouldn't, you know, lie down for him, but I did other stuff . . . you know while he was sittin' in a chair." She stopped again.

"Do you mean that you performed oral sex on him?" She nodded.

"And I let him touch me while I did that." She looked up briefly at me to check my reaction. I held her gaze and gently encouraged her to continue. "He paid me a lot of money."

"I see." A long pause. "That's the thing that is too terrible to tell . . . the thing that your mother forgives you for, that she knows about since she can see you, but she loves you anyway." She nodded.

"You said I would want to tell you, and you were right, because how can I marry Eddie if I'm really a whore?" She put her hands in her face and sobbed.

"Darleen, do you really think that makes you a whore?"

"You don't understand. I did it more than once with him; I did it whenever I was broke, and I couldn't work as much as I wanted because of my daughter needin' me to take care of her. I did it a bunch of times that year, and then I got out of there. It's where I got the money to get out and move over the mountain."

"So some good came out of it, even though you feel ashamed when you think of it." This seemed to give her pause.

"Yeah, I guess some good came of it, but how can it be good when it comes from somethin' so bad? I could never *feel* good about it, even though I thought then that I had to get me some money any way I could. I can't think about what I did without feelin' sick about it."

"Where do you feel sick about it?"

"Right here," she said laying her hand on her stomach.

I smiled, and looked at her curiously.

"What?" She looked at her hand resting on her stomach. "Jesus, Mary, and Joseph."

"Darleen, we have been too far together for me to mess around with being subtle. We have talked about how your eating disorder connects you to feelings you used to get to through your mother."

"Yeah."

"And we've talked about the push-pull kind of feeling you have about it, you know, where it kind of helps you feel better but also makes you feel bad."

"Yeah."

"I wonder, you tell me if this feels right."

"I know what you are going to say."

"You do?"

"Yeah. Maybe part of my wanting to throw up is because of how bad I feel about doing sex on him. I thought about it when I was thinkin' of comin' in here."

"That's a lot better than me saying it. And how did that thought feel to you?"

"It felt like it was just there, you know, I thought that could be a part of it. I did feel a little relieved, like maybe a bit of this is just something I don't have to do anymore. I guess I felt good about just wonderin' about it . . . like you always say about puttin' it together."

"You said maybe it's something you don't have to do anymore, and I got that you thought that maybe the past could be the past. You could leave it behind you; it doesn't have to control your life."

"Except one thing: How can I marry Eddie if he don't know he's marrying a whore? That's going too far . . . not to tell him? That's why I need you to tell me what to do. I know I'm supposed to choose for myself, but this is different. You're a man, would you want to know?"

"I want to tell you something important." She looked up through tearful eyes. "I have heard what you have said . . . you have told me this thing that you have never told anyone in the world . . . and just like I told you I would, I still care for you just the same," a pause, "I still respect you," a pause, "I still think you are a special person, worthy of love from all the people who are important to you . . . Eddie, your mother, your daughter . . . me. Darleen, see that I am not saying this to the fake you. You have let me see you completely now, and I am here."

She looked up with a grateful expression and began sobbing louder, heaving occasionally as if she were vomiting out the accumulated grief of the long history of her suffering. I sat silently with her for a long time. She alternated between periods of silence and sobbing, some sighs so great that I felt tears beginning to well in my eyes. I allowed her to see this when she occasionally looked up at my face. Eventually, she sat quietly.

"Thank you," she said. I nodded. "I guess I know what to do."

"What's that?"

"I know I can't live keeping this inside me. If Eddie can't live with it, then he can't live with me. I don't want to keep lyin' . . . I been lyin' my whole life. I have to go," she said, getting up. "I'm late for work." She didn't realize that she was still holding the pillow. "Oh," she said, handing it to me.

I handed it back to her, "Here, keep it . . . so you can remember our talks." She paused considering, "No, I think I'd like it better if I knew it was here in case I need to come back. You won't give it to no one else?"

"No, I won't. It will be here."

She stood in front of me and paused, then shyly reached her arms around me and embraced me. I held her for a few moments, and then she again said, "Thank you," and left.

———

CASE SIX DISCUSSION
Interpersonal Origins of Self-Experience

MY WORK WITH Darleen illustrated for me some of the things that can go wrong when fundamental elements are missing in the important relationships in which each of us becomes a person. Darleen's bulimia was about much more than wanting her body to more closely resemble the models on the cover of *Vogue*. Her bulimia appeared as the most overt manifestation of what was fundamentally a *disorder of self*. That is, the profound disruptions in her primary relationships had subverted her legitimate developmental needs. Metaphorically, just as the bones in her facial structure were traced with the history of her trauma, and just as she was "wandering lost" without her mother there to support her, the "structure" of her inner life became disintegrated and fractured, and important areas of self-experience were lost or cut off from the rest of her awareness. It was these lost parts of herself and her longing for connection with others that Darleen attempted to recover in her bulimic episodes.

Early in our work together it became apparent to me that Darleen's sense of her own existence was perforated and fragile. She often felt vulnerable and unable to draw on her own strengths to respond to the challenges of her life. How could she become a whole person in an environment that was so hostile to growth? I saw that the interpersonal world of her childhood provided little opportunity to develop a sense of herself as capable and autonomous. Though she eventually made a break and fled a world antagonistic to her emerging autonomy, she continued to be plagued by the conflicts and fears she carried with her over the mountain. Darleen learned early on that getting close to others can be painful and dangerous. How, I wondered, had Darleen managed to stay as intact as she did in the face of such difficulty, loss, and trauma?

Heinz Kohut (1984) argues that every child needs three essential experiences with early caregivers to develop an intact and cohesive sense of self. The first is a sense of *belonging* with others, being part of a family or community. The second is the necessity in the vulnerable years of childhood of *idealizing* caregivers, a sense that the child's caregivers have the power and ability to handle any situation to keep the child safe. The third experience all children require to develop an integrated and cohesive sense of self is reasonably accurate *mirroring.*

Mirroring describes the essential development of emotional resonance between the child and caregivers. The idea is that when the parent can accurately perceive and reflect to the child the child's own inner processes and emotional states, this engagement creates an essential shared psychological space where the separate subjective worlds of parent and child intersect. Through accurate mirroring, the child experiences her own inner world connecting with the world of others in a shared reality. This fundamental sense of connectedness is the most essential element of the growing self. Through accurate mirroring, the child learns to name and articulate feelings and to develop a wide range of emotional possibilities.

Caregivers need to be accurately attuned to the child's inner needs and feelings and to use language that accurately reflects this inner world. When the parent is accurately attuned, the child has the opportunity to gradually develop the ability to be aware of and express inner states without the parent's immediate help or physical presence. It is important that caregivers not *impose* their own "narcissistic" needs and demands on the child or seek gratification from the child in such a way as to usurp the child's own legitimate striving and self-experience. With particularly good mirroring and repeated relational events, the child can develop enormous range and subtlety of emotional expression. The child learns to contain and mediate even very strong affect states. Kohut uses the term *selfobject* to describe how a child appropriates and internalizes into self-architecture these "functions" of the caregiver. He calls this a process of "transmuting internalization." These internalized functions (selfobjects) gained from attuned caregivers become the foundational building blocks for the integrated architecture of self.

When accurate mirroring is profoundly absent, however, the child fails to develop a sense of connectedness to others and the environment. Rather than share a reality with important others, the child feels its own inner states are in opposition to the needs and requirements of the world around her. The child might then repress or split off emerging emotional states because they appear antagonistic to needed caregivers. Whole areas of inner life can become lost or sectioned off from the child's core sense of self.

This "disowning" happens because the child cannot risk alienating essential others by remaining faithful to her own self-experience. Forced to make a choice between retaining the integrity of inner life or appeasing needed others, the child tends to sacrifice this tentatively held experience of self and internalize a reality imposed from without. The child cannot risk needed ties to others by "sticking to her guns." For instance, if a child's emerging states of autonomy, anger, sexuality, or any other legitimate self-expression are experienced by the caregiver as threatening, the caregiver may be unresponsive, failing to mirror or even squelching the emerging self-state in the child. The child quickly learns that certain self-states are unwelcome or even dangerous and eventually disowns the developmental task so as not to disrupt the connection with important others. Without the mediating help of the caregiver to articulate and express legitimate needs, these affects and longings go "into hiding" even to the child as they are sectioned off from the core self. When these legitimate longings threaten to emerge, the child experiences great anxiety even many years after leaving home. Clearly, the imposition this accommodation represents can cause a lifetime of inner conflict as the person's own legitimate needs and self-experience come into opposition with the *now internalized* demands of others. Without adequate mirroring, the child fails to fully develop the internal functions that help to integrate and regulate affect states, so the child later has difficulty drawing on her own ability to self-soothe and obtain comfort in the absence of caregiver. The acquisition of adequate selfobjects through the process of transmuting internalization in relationship with others has failed. It is as if holes develop in the fabric of the self. These deficits in self-esteem and self-cohesion prevent a sustained sense of worth and well-being.

In summary, when caregivers do not respond to or actively squelch the child's affect, or if caregivers communicate antagonism to the child's emerging developmental longings or self-experience, then the child disowns, sections off, or rejects these states, creating a lack of integration in the self. Because these inner states represent legitimate developmental longings and strivings, they do not just go away into oblivion. It might be more accurate to say that they "hide away," awaiting a more receptive environment, awaiting the conditions that should have existed when these yearnings first sought expression as appropriate developmental challenges. When the distress these conflicts create eventually brings the person into the consulting room, the empathy of the therapist is often the longed for receptivity that the person craves, and these hidden and sectioned-off realms of self begin to emerge in response to the therapist's accurate mirroring. When the therapist responds with acceptance instead of rejection and punishment to configurations of self that the client deems shameful or unacceptable, this provides a new relational event, potentially creating a new "self-structure" that serves as a healing alternative to old perceptions and patterns.

Kohut's model of self-in-relation is useful for understanding how each of us may have areas of inner life that are more, or less, integrated with the rest of our personalities. Kohut, like Carl Rogers, encouraged a therapist attitude of sustained empathic inquiry to create the environment where client's developmental conflicts and injuries can reemerge and become fully expressed in the therapy. The idea of recovering something that the client has lost is an especially important idea with regard to bulimia. Clinicians have become increasingly aware that the splitting off of aspects of self in bulimic clients is profound enough that it involves the process of dissociation (Everill & Waller, 1995; Sands, 1989). These dissociate aspects of bulimia have the potential to inhibit an unfolding therapeutic dialogue because important pieces of the client's self-experience are prevented from emerging in the relationship with the therapist.

Dissociation, an alteration in the normal functioning of the person's continuity of experience, is a break in the thread that ties cognitive and emotional processes together (American Psychiatric Association, 2000). Each of us sometimes experiences dissociation, such as when driving a car on the highway and suddenly realizing we have arrived at the exit with little recollection of the past 30 miles. Talking to one's in-laws on the telephone provokes dissociative phenomena in some people. Faculty meetings are particularly good at provoking normal dissociation. At the other end of the continuum from these normal dissociative events are fugue states, where a person finds him- or herself in a strange city with no recollection of how he or she came to be there. The level of dissociation in bulimia is usually between these two extremes.

The dissociative process in bulimia tends to manifest along two dimensions. Recent studies (Grave, Rigamonti, Todisco, & Oliosi, 1996; McManus, 1995; Swirsky & Mitchell, 1996) have found that the binge-purge cycle itself is accompanied by a dissociative alteration from the client's normal self-experience. Darleen, like many bulimics, described this experience to me by using metaphors such as "something switches" just before the binging episode. She described "being out of control" and said it was "like I'm watching myself from outside, and can't stop myself," that it was "as if someone else takes over." One client described to me that "it's like a monster bursts out, and I think, where did that come from?" Darleen described a typical scenario in which "I could be doing fine, but some little thing can happen, and suddenly I'm binging like crazy, like I've lost it. But it makes sense to me as I'm doing it; it feels good. Then it changes. I feel like a cow, and I have to get rid of it. It suddenly feels bad. Then when I purge that feels good, but then I feel bad again for doing it all. After a while I got so used to it, it just became a habit, and I can't quit." These statements are familiar to therapists who work with clients with eating disorders of all kinds.

The second dimension of dissociation is what I have come to think of as the development of the "nuclear needs bulimic self." This bulimic self is an aspect of the person's identity that is a separate region of self-experience not *normally* present to the person. This region exists on the other side of a metaphorical partition in the self. Kohut termed this sort of division in the self the "vertical split." Sometime the person, often through some maladaptive behavior, can access the "content" on the other side of the vertical split, and emotions, thoughts, and needs become expressed that are different from the client's normal self-experience. These are often the fundamental unmet nuclear or essential primary needs, which are driving the bulimic behavior and have been prevented from becoming realized in more productive ways in relationship with others.

Though these important affectively charged configurations have become dissociatively partitioned from the person's normal process, they are important to the person. In fact, the bulimic episode is the "maladaptive" behavior that really represents both an address to and an expression of these frustrated nuclear needs, needs that cohere into configurations that are hidden from view, even to the client.

In other words, the nuclear needs, bulimic self keeps hidden and preserved all the lost and forgotten strivings, the precious and essential feelings and needs of the person that never found mirroring in the form of receptive and validating responses in relationships with others. All these longings live behind a door that is shut and locked tight. The bulimic's binging and purging becomes the key to open that door for a brief moment to access the parts of self normally shut off from view.

I often had the impression that Darleen wanted me to stay in the "parlor" and away from opening any of these doors. She had good reason. I might, as had others in her life, abuse, punish, or reject her if she brought these needs into our relationship. Over time, in a climate of empathy, Darleen came to trust me, her secret longings for connection emerged, and she allowed herself to be "seen" more fully. For her, this meant disclosing to me her darkest secrets that she had never revealed to anyone. For her, these secrets contained the "truth," that behind her approval-winning demeanor she was really worthless, repugnant, and unlovable. When I still accepted her despite my knowledge of her past, when she saw that the strength and warmth of our relationship did not suffer, she felt recognized and validated in a new way. She began to look to relationships outside of her "safe" one with me, and less to food, for essential connection and gratification. Darleen did not know that I saw her revelation of these secrets as incidental to what the disclosure actually meant—the gradual dismantling of Darleen's false face, which had served to protect her from real immediacy, authenticity, encounter, and love. Our relationship "stood in" for all her relationships in the past and gave her a kind of second chance to speak to the lost and forgotten aspects of herself. Darleen may not have been able to name completely with words what her bulimia was saying, but she enacted it as she became able to reveal herself and receive my regard for her.

Using Kohut's (1984) three essentials that children need to thrive, we can construct a developmental pathway for Darleen's "self" disorder and her symptoms of bulimia. It might go something like this.

Mirroring

Darleen's early caregivers were challenged in their ability to provide her with an empathically responsive environment. Accurate mirroring that would have contributed to her own affect integration was profoundly absent. Darleen described growing up in a climate of impoverishment both economically and relationally. Her father was often absent, and when he was around was often drunk or verbally and physically abusive to her mother. Because her father was affectionate to Darleen, she felt ambivalent about her relationship to him. She wanted his affection but felt that she could not trust him, and she normally kept a safe and fearful distance.

Though her mother was very affectionate ("my best friend") and sustained Darleen in these early years, her own years of abuse caused her to rely on Darleen to support her emotionally. This narcissistic use of the child by the parent sometimes feels good to the child, especially since Darleen and her mother felt they were holding onto one another in a hostile world (they slept in the same bed until Darleen left home). But this reliance on the daughter to keep the mother soothed and intact, and the "merger" that comes from it, always has detrimental effects for the daughter's developmental longings for growth and autonomy. As a narcissistic extension of her mother, Darleen could not refuse to gratify her mother's needs, especially in the climate of abuse. Darleen learned early on to take care of her mother, her only sure support. She did this even if it meant attenuating her own emotional expression and needs to soothe her mother's distress. Darleen once mentioned to me that her mother often said that she would have "no reason to live" if it weren't for her daughter's love and affection. Darleen was ambivalent about this relationship with her mother, but not as consciously as with her father.

Darleen must have gotten some inner strength from somewhere because she eventually managed to act on her impulses toward change. She felt the constraint of this mutual dependence with her mother and eventually made a break for it—she ran away with Gary. But both sides of her ambivalence were strong. Her guilt at having abandoned her mother kept her close by, and she chose (perhaps as penance?) a husband who recapitulated her mother's situation of abuse. Her marriage to Gary, however, was disastrous to any self-efficacy she might have acquired from her growing up years. The violence she suffered seemed to confirm that she must never assert any of her legitimate impulses or needs but must hide her face and keep her longings sequestered away and hidden from view. But everyone has their ultimate limits, and Darleen finally reasserted hers, shotgun in hand, in a first step toward autonomy and change.

She had tried to differentiate from her mother but feared that this would hurt her mother and sever the connection that, by now, was vital to Darleen's own sense of psychological cohesion. After her mother's death, Darleen's compulsive eating was an attempt to replace her mother and the self-regulating functions she had provided. These were the affect containing and regulating functions, which her merger with her mother had prevented her from internalizing—any remnant of which Gary had beaten out of her. But the conflict between meeting the needs of her mother and listening to the call of her own developmental strivings was still very much alive in Darleen's eating disorder. Her eating disorder both connected her to her mother (both her eating disorder and her mother were her best friend) and differentiated her from her as well. Binging was merging, purging was differentiating; both connected her with feelings and impulses on the other side of the vertical split.

Idealizing

Darleen also did not have the opportunity to properly idealize her care-givers. Rather than being a source of safety, she perceived her father as unpredictable and dangerous. However, Darleen highly idealized her mother, even into adulthood. But it became apparent that this fragile construction ("she's an angel, watching over me") often fell apart and could not sustain her. Under normal circumstances, even the child with good idealization of competent caregivers must realize that her parents are not omnipotent and all powerful. Usually this disappointment happens gradually, enabling the daughter to internalize the mother's self-regulating functions through the process of transmuting internalization. However, when this growth process happens too suddenly, traumatic disillusionment too profound for the child to handle leads to a disavowal of the idealizing needs and the emergence of feelings of insecurity and vulnerability (Kohut, 1984).

In Darleen's case, her mother's repeated abuse, her inability to change the situation, and her profound helplessness and dependency on Darleen caused Darleen both to be traumatically disillusioned and to hold onto her mother even tighter for survival. This is a particularly dual loss. Rather than internalize what few self-regulating functions her mother could offer, she instead merged with her to prevent the psychic catastrophe of feeling overwhelmed and "falling apart." Unfortunately, as in most cases where menacing abuse hovers in the family atmosphere, what becomes incorporated into the self are feelings of unworthiness, shame, and self-hatred.

Belonging

When Darleen "fell in love" with Trent, she longed to belong to the world in which Trent moved. She identified feelings of worthiness, esteem, respect, and acceptance with the society and the material things Trent seemed to possess and that seemed to make life effortless and happy. I was later glad that Trent burst on the scene, because nothing I could have said could have pierced that illusion of material happiness and belonging better than exposure of the hollowness of Trent's perfect image. Darleen longed to fit in and to escape the "white trash" community in her head to which she identified herself as belonging. Each of us wants to internalize a sense that we belong to a group that is good, trustworthy, and self-endorsing and that provides a collective sense of sustaining affiliation. After Trent, Eddie looked more desirable to Darleen. She began to realize that his "being a good man" might outweigh his being "not much to look at." It was not until Darleen began to value herself apart from her emphasis on her external qualities that she allowed herself to become more emotionally intimate with Eddie. In at least three places in her life, Darleen allowed herself to risk letting people become more important to her than food: with Eddie, with her daughter, and with me.

In the absence of these core conditions of mirroring, idealizing, and belonging, the child is vulnerable to a host of self-states to which he or she must respond. Feelings of depression or emotional instability, emptiness and hollowness, or unworthiness and despair require some response to prevent being overwhelming. In the case of eating disorders, as the capacity for self-esteem and cohesion diminish, especially in times of stress, the person develops a system of compensation whereby people are replaced with eating in an attempt to provide the missing relational experiences and the sustaining internal functions deriving from them. Of course, a host of other factors such as cultural ideals of female beauty, attitudes toward weight, and family attitudes toward body image and food impinge on the particular constellation of noxious influences.

The nuclear needs, bulimic self is under full construction as food becomes a powerful and symbolic substitute for soothing, comfort, and connection with an empathic caregiver. The early needs become increasingly split off from the rest of the person's normal functioning and are organized around these partially successful efforts at self-care. Food is increasingly called upon to provide nurturance that can only be supplied in a caring, responsive relationship (Sands, 1989). Over time, the individual invests less energy in the developmental task of learning how to have intimate connections with others and more toward fending off bouts of loneliness, depression, and fragmentation.

The nuclear needs, bulimic self is further elaborated by the bulimic's compromised ability to successfully meet new developmental hurdles such as adjusting to a changing body image, integrating sexual feelings and behavior, and becoming more autonomous. And food works! Darleen described that she felt "high," or sometimes "numbed out," and free of pain during some binge-purge episodes.

In fact, in any disorder in which symptoms substitute for frustrated legitimate self-experience on the other side of a vertical split, the symptoms representative of that hidden area of self are paradoxical. On one hand, the *bulimic behavior is a defense against* the pain associated with the relational origins of all those lost and forgotten needs waiting for the right climate to reemerge. In other words, the dissociative aspects of the bulimic episode protect the individual from overwhelming affect, anxiety, and conflict. On the other hand, the *bulimia expresses and meets the needs,* briefly, of soothing and nurturance and provides a sense of cohesion to self-experience. No wonder then that Darleen secretly cherished her bulimia as her "best friend" when it was so important to her sense of continuity and identity and met important relational needs she felt incapable of getting with people.

My relationship with Darleen made me aware of treatment issues that I have since seen manifested in almost every bulimic client with whom I have worked. Darleen entered therapy with the expressed goal of getting rid of her bulimia. She presented her bulimic behavior in negative terms and described her distress and high motivation to overcome her disabling compulsion. She revealed to me her unhappiness with her body and her low self-esteem because of it and insisted that this was the primary reason for her bulimia. She articulated the self-destructive, even masochistic, nature of her behavior, and she sincerely appealed to me to help her.

It may be an error, however, for the counselor to instantly adopt these goals and ally and collude with the client's socially desirable self. This is the client's normal presentation: part of the client's self that is perfectionistic, conforming, eager to please, and eager to adopt the attitudes and views she believes will win the therapist's goodwill. It is also the part of the client's self-experience that sincerely disapproves of her own bulimic behavior. The client expects that the counselor will agree. Often, the client is right; this is the presentation the therapist wants to see. It is certainly the presentation I wanted to see in Darleen, so I referred her to a nutritionist, connected her with an educational group at the hospital, got her a medical referral, and began discussing adaptive strategies. And Darleen followed through. She was, apparently, very open to treatment.

Darleen liked to talk "about" her eating problem, and over time, some good things did happen. For instance, Darleen began to understand how her bulimic behaviors were especially strong in times of upset and stress. There is an old therapeutic maxim about not taking a problematic behavior away without providing a more adaptive one to replace it. Darleen accepted that she could use journaling, talking with Eddie, girls' nights out, and other activities to express and diminish painful feelings. Taking advantage of "teachable moments," I also helped Darleen understand how media images and impersonal cultural standards shaped her perception of her body. This was all great except for one thing—her bulimic behavior continued almost at the same level of intensity.

One reason the bulimic behavior continued is because Darleen hid the part that needed and, in fact, *celebrated* being bulimic. Bulimia was something she did well, and she was proud that she had been able to meet some of her needs through it. Darleen's description of her bulimia as her "best friend" spoke to how important a function her bulimia played in helping her stay "glued together." Darleen put on her false face and showed me what she thought I wanted to see. It all looked good to me until I grew suspicious and realized that her smiling face was telling me, "Keep looking here! This is a pleasant place to gaze." But, of course, it is the nuclear needs, bulimic self that the therapist needs to contact for any healing to occur: the unintegrated part of the client's self that is on the other side of the vertical split.

The first thing a therapist can do to "welcome" the nuclear needs bulimic self into the relationship involves a change in the therapist's approach. The therapist often does not realize that he or she has unwittingly been communicating that this bulimic self is unwelcome and that any behaviors associated with it must be overcome as soon as possible. The therapist desires to ally with the socially appropriate initial presentation of the client, and the client seeks approval from the therapist. As with Darleen, this collusion crowds out any communications from the client about how the bulimia serves her well and has important adaptive functions that are essential to her. The client fears not only that the therapist will not accept the dissociated bulimic self but that it will be taken away from her if therapy is successful. Thus, the bulimic self tends to disappear in the therapy setting, not only to the therapist but to the client as well.

It is not enough to invite the bulimic self to become revealed. The therapist must *respect* the bulimic self for preserving essential parts of the client's experience from insult and usurpation by others. Since the emergence of the bulimic self will reveal needs, feelings, and perceptions that are very different from the client's ordinary self-experience, the therapist must provide the longed-for accurate mirroring that enables the client to begin to reintegrate these dissociated aspects of self.

A change in therapist language is sometimes useful for accessing the hidden bulimic self. For instance, instead of discussing Darleen's bulimic behaviors (something very comfortable for her to talk about and that achieved little), I directed an invitation to "the part of you that wants to binge and purge." I also responded to her oblique references to her bulimic self, the one that used that little girl voice, by saying, "tell me about her . . . tell me about that person that wants to binge and purge, and who defies your attempts to control her." Although this might at first appear to encourage the client to see herself as separate personalities, or promote fragmentation, in fact, the client experiences it as so empathic and perceptive that it promotes integration and expression of what had been forbidden and sequestered sectors of self-experience.

The therapist may even need to resort to *defending* or taking the side of the bulimic self against the socially conforming "normal" self. Once I got past the pleasant collusion between Darleen and I that served to avoid more difficult issues, I heard her disparaging remarks about her bulimia quite differently. I began to feel a pull to ally with the opposite side of her experience, observing that "you give pretty shabby treatment to the part of you that needs to binge and purge." When I began defending the very part of her that she was secretly defending against me, it upset the balance and began to diffuse any struggle she felt about defending this valued part of herself. I went on to observe that "this part of you has worked very hard to help you, and perhaps she is not as appreciated as she might be," which communicated to Darleen that I accepted and valued what she kept hidden from all others. It was then that I began to wonder what "she" (her bulimic self) might have to say. This approach usually elicits a strong emotional response from the client because the therapist communicates regard for the whole of the client's self-experience, not just the aspects that suit the therapist's goals of symptom reduction. Though initially the therapist's invitation to reveal the valued bulimic self is met with suspicion, with repeated expression of regard the client begins to risk exposure, and this becomes the critical turning point in therapy.

After Darleen and I had worked together for a short while, I found it necessary to take the focus off of her bulimic symptoms and her efforts to change them. I introduced the paradoxical message that "I'm not sure it's a good idea to give up anymore of your bulimic behaviors right now. They have been very important to you and have helped you in the past. Let's hear from the part of you that you keep hidden, the part that does not want to let go of the binging and purging." This language almost always comes as a big shock to the client. To the client's normal observing self, it does not make sense. She cannot believe that the therapist does not want to reject this part of her. From her bulimic self, however, this communication is experienced as highly empathic and confirming and relieving of shame and guilt.

The result of this change in therapist approach is almost always a shy and tentative emergence of the client's hidden needs, fears, interpersonal traumas, and developmental arrests. Once these become constellated in the therapy relationship, they may be transformed and reintegrated, helping to restore the person to wholeness.

✄ ✄

As I Walked Out in the Streets of Laredo

As I walked out in the streets of Laredo,
As I walked out in Laredo one day,
I spied a poor cowboy all wrapped in white linen,
All wrapped in white linen and as cold as the clay

Come sit down beside me and hear my sad story
Then play the dead march as you carry me along
Take me to the green valley and lay the sod o're me
For I'm a young cowboy and I know I done wrong

It was once in the saddle I used to go dashing
It was once in the saddle I used to go gay
'twas first to the drinking and then to card playing,
then on to those flashgirls, now I'm dying today

—American folk song based on the Irish/Appalachian
ballad, *The Unfortunate Rake*

A m I putting you to sleep here?" he said with a mixture of mild dis-belief and annoyance.

My head checked the beginning of its slow drift downward, my half-closed lids opened again, and I saw him looking straight at my face. I had never begun to nod off in a session before. When I meet with clients, I sit face to face with them, my chair at a slight angle to the couch. It's pretty hard not to stay awake. I felt suddenly guilty, felt an apology rising from my suddenly constricted chest to my lips. I had not slept well the previous night. My father had just been admitted to the hospital the evening before in the midst of a heart attack, and I hadn't come to this meeting with the clarity and attention that therapy demands and clients deserve. The remorseful apology was almost into words when I paused and remembered who was sitting before me.

Tim, a White, 44-year-old professional, had come to therapy two months before at the university clinic I directed. He complained of long-standing anxiety, dysthymia, and chronic problems in his relationship with his wife of 18 years. He and his wife had two children, both of whom were in their early teens. Tim had already missed two of his appointments, with no advanced notice, and he was 10 minutes late to all of the sessions he did make. Though the clinic's fees were on a sliding scale to accommodate those in the community with lower incomes, Tim asked after his third session to have his fee waived entirely. He said he was financially strapped because he was suddenly "between jobs" in the computing field. The fob on his key ring had a BMW logo.

I tried to explore with Tim what his ambivalent behavior might reflect about how he felt about coming to therapy. He insisted that his lateness meant nothing and that the fee waiver was related only to his current job status. I acceded to his request to drop the fee. I thought we could always revisit the issue if he wished to continue after we completed the agreed upon sessions. I speculated that Tim's presenting concern of "feeling trapped" in his marriage and his line of work might be an interesting training case for my students to observe on videotape. So far I was wrong.

During the six sessions we had met, Tim seemed to be unable to make any real use of therapy. He did not appear to be interested in himself, tended to be trivial in his expression, and intellectualized in his presentation. He seemed cynical about almost everything. He sat formally, his long ectomorphic frame erect in his chair, lanky legs crossed, hands folded in his lap, and he spoke precisely of everything and nothing at all. His short brown hair and meticulously clipped goatee framed a face that expressed little of his inner world of thoughts and feelings. Tim talked in the sessions, but it was as if he were merely lining up facts like numbers on a ledger. The facts of his life did not tally into some meaningful sum, and he made no connections among these supposedly relevant pieces of information. He seemed intent on being inaccessible.

My attempts to engage him in some sincere and meaningful way met with passive-aggressive diversion, stonewalling, and feigned misunderstanding about my intentions to understand him in depth. This could have allowed us to examine the interpersonal processes themselves as a starting point. But my efforts to encourage him to reflect on the process between us in the session met with diversion and a concrete inventory of his complaints. He was depressed, he said. His wife didn't understand him. He was unhappy at work, he couldn't get a break, his mother-in-law nagged him. It wasn't that any of these topics were irrelevant; what was missing was Tim's refusal to do anything other than merely trace the outlines of his problems. He was painting by numbers the picture of his life, and he was using only primary colors.

Tim refuted any attempt on my part to explore how *I* might be eliciting what I saw as his defensive and resistant demeanor. I concluded privately that Tim seemed to have little self-reflective awareness or capacity for therapy. He just seemed to want to gripe unproductively . . . for free. I believed that there was someone in there, and I had been patiently waiting for him to make an appearance in his own time. But I was also aware that this was our seventh session and that we had only one session left together. It was now or never. His statement hung in the air like an accusation:

"Am I putting you to sleep?"

I looked at him directly. "Yes," I replied. "I think you are."

"What?" he replied, incredulously.

"Yes," I said again, "I am having a really hard time paying attention to you. Not just today. I admit that today I am overly tired from too little sleep, and that's not fair to you . . . I apologize. But in most our meetings I find myself having a really hard time staying with you."

"Isn't that your job?" he said resentfully. He shifted from his crossed-legs reclining posture and sat more upright in the chair, his hands now off his lap and on the arms of the chair. Ah. I had his attention now!

"Yeah, it is, and usually I can do it pretty well. But in our sessions I have wondered if *you* are truly interested in what you are saying. I'm confused because on the one hand you are here and on the other you seem not that invested in really making use of our time together. That makes it difficult for me to stay interested in you and in what's happening here. In our talks I feel shut out to what's really important to you."

He crossed his arms again and the familiar cynical smile formed on his lips. "I thought you guys were supposed to tell me what my problem is. I told you I've been depressed and anxious."

"Yes, you have told me *about* the fact that you are depressed and anxious, but I have very little feel for what it's like to be inside your experience. You seem protective of that. When I've had trouble understanding how what you are telling me is important to you I have asked, 'Is this what you want to be talking about . . . how you want to spend our time together?' You've seemed to not want to change it, so I left it alone. But as I have also said in previous sessions, it seems like you are only touch-ing the surface of your experiences."

"I don't know why I bother coming in here," he said dispassionately, like a statement of fact.

"I think that's a great question to ask yourself. Why bother coming in here?"

"Clearly you don't give a damn if I come or not since you use it as an opportunity to catch up on your sleep." There was only a mild tone of sarcasm in his statement, but did it imply that it might matter to him whether I cared or not if he came?

"I wouldn't say that. I do give a damn, or I wouldn't be here," I said sincerely. "I think that you must give a damn too, or *you* wouldn't come. I just think that maybe you are playing it safe with me, not taking a risk in bringing to our conversation what is really meaningful to you, and I don't know why that is. You must have a good reason for it, and I've often won-dered if your sense of sarcasm doesn't mask some very sensitive areas. My guess is that it does. But it's like I said, when I have tried to inquire more in depth about you, I often feel brushed off. Then when I try to explore that, it seems to me that you discount my speculation. I wonder if you fear I might not understand or that I might reject you, both of which are often concerns of someone coming into therapy for the first time."

"Those are not concerns that I have."

"What concerns do you have?"

"I don't have any concerns. It wouldn't break my heart if you didn't 'understand me,'" he said, unfolding his long arms to make quotation marks in the air with his fingers.

"Right."

"What do you want me to say?" he said.

"I can't tell you what to say other than what you think is important to talk about."

We sat there looking at one another. His face betrayed nothing. He had regained that composure that was impervious to any intervention. I didn't know if what I was doing was therapeutic or not, but it felt like we were deadlocked. At least for a brief moment there had finally been some energy in the room. After a silence I said, "I'm aware that our time is almost up. Is there anything you want to say before we end?"

He shrugged, and shook his head sullenly.

"Okay, then. See you next week for our final session," I said.

He rose from the couch, took his jacket, and passed by me while I held the door. He left without a word. Given his inconsistency before and the events of the session, I didn't expect to see him again.

At the appointed time of our session, however, Tim appeared in the waiting room . . . five minutes early.

"I thought since this was our last session I might as well be on time," he offered as we sat down.

There was something different in the tone; was this an acknowledgment of sorts? An offering?

"It's the first time I've been here early, I know."

"Better late than never . . . no pun intended."

"So," he said after a brief pause, "you really told me what you thought of me last week." It was the first time he had commented directly on something that had happened between us.

"Yeah, I did. I felt a little bad about it later." He cocked his head surprised. I could see that it struck him that he would take up my attention outside of the session. It was true. The memory our exchange had bothered me during the week, and I had admitted to myself that my "spontaneous" expression was not only a confrontation designed to disrupt a repetitive pattern but also an expression of my frustration and embarrassment. How, I wondered, had it helped the client?

"I thought about it too," he said. Now I was the one surprised. "I'm not sure why I haven't been able to talk about things in here. I could see that you would listen to me no matter what. When you asked me if I was talking about what I wanted, I knew that you saw that I was just talking crap. It was almost a relief."

"That I confronted you?"

"No . . . well, maybe that too, but that you could see that there was more to me than what I've been saying in here. I was glad that you realized that . . . even though I gave you no reason to." He said formally.

"I could sense that there must be more to you than you have been willing to show?"

"Yes. I don't know why I do that." He shifted uncomfortably in his chair, as if even this admission was difficult for him.

"Maybe that's something we can wonder about together today."

"I suppose," and then, apparently realizing that this noncommittal expression represented the very issue we had been discussing, he said, "I mean, yeah, that would be good."

There had been other times in therapy when I felt my blunders had led to good things. I had the sense that this might be one of them. Where was the characteristic cynicism? Tim's formality seemed defensive, but at

least he allowed some interchange. Had I somehow earned his respect
with my bluntness?

"Does that happen in all of your relationships . . . that you keep
yourself so well hidden?" I thought, "let's see if he really wants to come
out and play."

"I suppose I do. I mean, Yes. I don't often trust people. I guess you
know that. I think that you just saying what a jerk you think I am
somehow made you seem a little more real. You say I've been shallow,
but you've been hiding behind this therapist persona." That was a brief
disclosure, I thought, and now he was going on the offensive.

"I don't remember saying you were a jerk, but how do you mean I've
been hiding behind this therapist persona?"

"I mean, come on," he said dismissively, "you come across as this nice
guy who's going to listen to all my crap and pretend that you want to
know what I'm really about. Nobody's that way. You do it because it's
your profession. You're trained to do it; it's not real. It can't be. I mean,
I'm a stranger to you. Why would what I say really matter to you? People just aren't like that." The smug expression had returned to his face.

"So I must be faking any real interest in you."

"You don't even know me; why would you care?"

"Ah . . . and yet you're here, seeking me out. Two things seem to be
happening at once. You don't believe I could actually care as a person
about your concerns, that I'm only here in a technical, professional
capacity. But you also seem to be saying that you want me to see past
your surface . . . to really see you . . . to realize that there's more to you
than you are showing, and that it could matter to me, and to you. Somehow my confronting you made me seem a little more real to you, like
you might be able to trust this."

"Maybe," he dissimulated. Then he again made an effort to be more
definitive. I could see that he had to make an effort to commit to any
expression at all. "I guess I was relieved to see you getting frustrated,
like a normal person. I thought, 'Ha, I knew nobody was that nice!'"

"Me getting frustrated meant to you that I was not just hiding
behind some professional 'nice guy' role. It gave you something you
needed to push against. You saw me as an ordinary person." (I also
thought he was just glad to "get to me.")

"Yeah, and somehow I felt like I might finally be able to get somewhere, like you wouldn't put up with my crap." The content and delivery of this statement seemed to convey two different messages, a
double-bind. The content seemed to indicate that he thought he
might find a way to make some progress, but the feeling I got from

his face and tone as he said it felt like a criticism of me that I hadn't enabled him to "get somewhere." I realized that Tim was an artist at being passive-aggressive.

"I see. You might be able to get somewhere if I were to respond more directly. That's the third time you've mentioned me putting up with your 'crap.' It seems like there's something ugly here that you don't feel too good about." There was a long silence. Did I see his neck flush? Hmm, what was that?

"I just meant my giving you a hard time."

"So what now? What do you want to do in our final session?"

"I want to talk about continuing, if you will. I'll pay the full fee. I've got some good job leads, so it won't be a problem."

I paused, taking in this unexpected turn of events. I was quite aware that I had contemplated Tim's termination with a sense of relief. Did he really want to continue? I could hardly believe it. I felt reluctant to commit to a further course. But another, more compassionate voice was reasoning that for the first time Tim seemed to be making an effort to engage, at least in this limited way. Shouldn't I acknowledge that? I decided to do a little more assessing before I made a decision.

"If I agreed to continue, how would you use our time together? What are you hoping to get out of it?"

"I don't know. I don't know how it works, and I'm not sure I even believe in it."

"That's not a promising start."

"Right. I guess not. I do know, though, that I've been holding back saying things that I thought I might want to talk about."

"That sounds more like it. Let's talk about those things before we decide if we are going to continue."

I felt a little uncomfortable making our continued relationship conditional on Tim's acquiescing to my requirements for therapy. Wouldn't this likely be a recapitulation of past relationships in which he was required to give up something in order to maintain needed ties, the cure by compliance? On the other hand, was I really asking him to give up anything other than his recalcitrance? Further, did we really even have a relationship with which I could bargain? It felt like a fair tactic, even though I knew that his resistance must have been covering for some very sensitive spots. At least it conveyed that if he could be available to me good things could happen. Tim nodded; he seemed to accept this "test" of whether or not our time could be spent productively.

"Okay." He paused, took a breath, and began. "I guess I thought this week about telling you something that I've only thought about discussing with my real doctor. I mean . . . you know . . . ," he stumbled. His neck began to flush again. I regarded his loss of composure as a good sign. I waved off his rising apology, thinking that even when he was trying to relate he couldn't help being passive-aggressive. But then he revealed more about himself in five minutes than he had in the previous seven sessions.

"For a long time I've had relationships . . . well, not relationships, but sexual encounters . . . not in my marriage," he explained tentatively, "with men." He stopped, as if he expected me to react in some way. His body posture, his long torso, looked taut as a bowstring.

"Please continue," I invited after a brief silence.

"Of course Maria doesn't have any idea about it. She would never accept it. She would probably rally the kids against me. I can't imagine what she'd do. Well, maybe I do imagine it sometimes. The whole thing would come apart if she knew about it. I'd lose everything." His impassive face betrayed little of his concern for these dire consequences of discovery. "I never do it, you know, around here. I always do it when I'm out of town, which I am frequently for my work." He seemed to search my face, looking for a reaction. "That's it." Silence.

"It seems like this was an important and, judging by your reluctance to talk about it previously, a difficult thing for you to tell me. What part seems most charged for you?"

"What do you mean?"

"I mean, what part strikes you as most troublesome or in need of exploration. Is it that you have been leading a secret life . . ."

". . . for 12 years," he interrupted.

"Okay, for 12 years, or is it that your sexual feelings or behavior trouble you, or your concern with discovery?"

"My biggest fear is that I will lose everything if she finds out. I mean she'd get lawyers that wouldn't stop till she had my balls in a jar on the shelf."

"So this is not something that you feel you could *ever* discuss with her."

"Absolutely not," he said, unconsciously grasping his chin and resting a finger across his mouth. It was the most definitive thing he had said yet. His eyes moved from my face to the carpet and back again.

"You look almost furtive as you tell me this right now. What has it been like for you leading this secret life?"

He paused, looked down at his lap, and said reflectively, "It's like I live two separate lives in two separate worlds. Neither world contacts the other; I make sure they don't. You might not believe it, but I care for my wife, and I love my kids. I want to protect them. I don't want to upset everything we've got."

Tim explained that early in his marriage he was alarmed to discover that his sexual relationship with his wife did little to combat his powerful homosexual attractions. He had married, he said, because it looked like the kind of life he wanted: he desired a family, a wife, Little League for the kids, upward mobility and all that went along with that. He and his wife had been affectionate, if not passionate, toward one another. They had a "decent sex life," he said. He had hoped that marriage and the achievement of this domestic life would mute the disturbing homosexual inclinations he had felt for years but upon which he had never acted. But after a couple of years of marriage he discovered how easy it was while traveling for him to meet men in gay bars, in bath houses, and in public parks. "Wherever I go I can find that whole other world."

After he began his homosexual infidelities, he reported, his relationship with his wife actually improved for a time. He felt less persecuted by his own guilty conscience: he had strayed, yes, but he convinced himself that he had not hurt anyone. His sexual inclinations, though now realized, had not destroyed everything, as he had imagined. His family would survive his sexuality now that he had an "outlet." It wasn't, he told himself, as if he had strayed with another woman. This betrayal didn't really count. He could protect his more important world, the one with his family, by keeping part of himself partitioned. He felt justified in his deceit because his activities never impinged on his "normal" sphere of activity. This was the narrative that Tim had constructed to reconcile the various and conflicting dimensions of his experience.

I listened carefully. Despite my attitude of receptivity, I felt as if Tim were explaining his case to a jury; as if he were trying to convince me that he was justified in the choices and life he created. I was not going to judge him; his sexual and personal struggles seemed quite similar to those that many clients faced. They were valid and legitimate. However, I did not accept that he was being honest with himself about his choices and behavior. His rationalizations were flimsy and transparent, designed to enable him to avoid responsibility. Tim conveniently claimed he wanted to protect the welfare of his wife and children. But at whose expense, I wondered, had his current reconciliation of impulses come? Without access to complete information, had his wife had the opportunity to create the life *she* desired?

I tried to imagine her. Was she really an unknowing innocent? Or was she, as in many cases of infidelity, somehow complicit . . . willing to "not see" to protect her own stake in something valued? Could she really not know or sense anything about her husband's other self and life? How was he not opaque or unknown to her? What kept her in the marriage, I wondered, was her life with Tim gratifying to her? It all seemed quite similar to cases I had encountered of heterosexual infidelity, except that Tim was disguising not just the encounters themselves but a whole region of his sexuality.

As Tim talked, I realized that there was another important issue involving a heightened risk of sexually transmitted disease. It became apparent that he had engaged in "well over" a hundred brief sexual encounters with strangers. Only occasionally did he meet the same partner more than once, and even then by chance. This hypersexuality, the compulsive drivenness without any pretense of relationship, would certainly need exploration. I wondered, listening to him, did his argument that he wanted to "protect" his family also mean that he practiced safe sex during all of these liaisons?

These speculations were relevant, but I could only directly intervene in the ways that I felt Tim was lying to himself, not to Maria. Privately, however, I felt a sense of heightened obligation to represent the interests, at least in principle, of his wife. Therapy is never a value-free activity. As a therapist, I often feel that I stand in for the larger community of shared meanings and values, calling the client away from alienation and back to participation. The values that I, or any therapist, embody in therapy cannot merely express an individual and privately treasured morality. The client cannot be coerced into adopting a set of values artificially imposed by the therapist. Whatever values the client adopts must emerge from the new possibilities evoked and revealed by the unfolding relational process between therapist and client as the latter's potentialities are evoked and brought to realization. Yet the process of therapy rests on some core values and principles of human interaction that the therapist hopes the client will engage and come to value in his or her relations with others. If Tim and I could establish an open and honest communication, a sense of respect and regard, and a heightened value of self-understanding and knowledge, I hoped he might begin to import those values in his relations with others in his life. I felt secure that my desire to promote those values was not merely countertransferential in the sense of Tim's disclosures activating my own unconscious material. In fact, as a student working a yearlong practicum at an AIDS response clinic, I had worked in depth with clients struggling with precisely the sorts of issues with which Tim now struggled. I knew the terrain. I also recognized the degree of denial that Tim demonstrated by avoiding talking about the risks of his encounters and by lying to everyone about his secret identity.

I knew that to immediately and directly challenge Tim's rationalizations and self-serving interpretations would instantly put us at odds and evoke his resistance. I remembered a colleague's description of the "judo metaphor" for therapy: In judo, when the opponent attacks, one does not face him head on (as in boxing), opposing force with greater force. Rather, when attacked, the judo expert steps aside and uses the opponent's own momentum to gain an advantage.

Creative misunderstanding is one way the therapist can "step aside." Creative misunderstanding encourages the client to give voice to feelings and thoughts that are underneath the client's "stated" or accessible position. The therapist may sense that the client would reject the sentiments if they came from the therapist's observation. However, if the client can be induced to articulate that which the therapist does not seem at first to understand but which resides (perhaps not fully formed) within the client, the client's own production can be credited with the insight and expansion of awareness. In other words, just "telling" the client is rarely effective.

What I wanted to evoke in Tim was acknowledgment of the subtext of his narrative, the part that was just as real and important to him but that he was less willing to articulate to me. Tim finished his explanation and looked intently at me, wondering whether he had convinced me that he had made the only choices available to him . . . looking for a ruling. I refused to pass judgment.

"So," he said breaking the silence that followed his appeal, "you can see how it's pretty complex. *There's not much I can change* under the circumstances." He seemed to be watching me closely.

"Yeah. You seem to have it pretty much figured out. I can tell you've really struggled with it," I observed, stepping aside, not arguing with his assertion that he couldn't change anything.

"What do you mean?" This was not the response he expected. He seemed truly confused. He shifted in his chair uncomfortably.

"Well, the way you describe it, it seems like you feel that these are the only choices that can work, that you've arrived at the best resolution possible, and that this works pretty well for you."

"Yeah, you can see how it's a tough situation."

"You said that. You really want me to get how it's an impossible situation to resolve, and you feel like your hands are tied. Yet you also seem to have arrived at something that you find is an acceptable compromise; even though it's hard in other ways, it also works for you."

"Yeah. That's right. Well, mostly right I guess."

"Oh. What do you mean?"

"It's the only way, but it takes a toll in other areas."

"It takes a toll," I repeated. "Do you mean that there's some part of this to which you are not reconciled or content? I got from what you said that you feel this is the best that is possible for you and your family, that there's not much you could, or would want to, change," I said, testing the water.

"It's tough . . . you know, to have a whole other part that you have to keep hidden. That takes its toll, so sometimes I wish things could somehow change."

Ah, great!

He paused reflectively. "Most of the time," he continued. "I don't even think about it when I'm here, in town. But sometimes I have a sense of panic about it. I think, this can't keep going, and I get kind of depressed about it and say I'm going to quit going out, you know, when I travel, but I always end up doing it anyway." Tim let an expression of tired misery form on his face.

"That's quite different, isn't it? There's a struggle there, another part of you that is not content at all with the need for deception. You try to tell yourself not to go out anymore, but something happens to undermine that intention. I suspect there's a sense of being compelled."

"Exactly. It's like I can't help it; like I don't have any control over it, and I'm walking down that street and I know where I'm going, and I know what's going to happen when I get there." He was becoming agitated, and repeatedly pressed his fingers into the hollow of his knee. "You said that I 'created' this scenario, but I don't feel like I created anything here. I feel like I almost don't have a say in how it happens."

"I get that. There's a feeling of not being able to stop yourself, even though you really want to, so you keep it all a secret because it seems very dangerous to other things you value."

"Exactly, that's exactly it. I value this other part too."

"Is there any part of your secret life, any part of how you relate to it, where you do feel you have a say . . . or can make a choice?"

"No."

"So that's a problem."

"What?"

"I'm surprised that you ask. It's a problem if you feel that you are trapped and also that you don't have any choices here, even if they are difficult or even seemingly impossible choices. When you describe it, it seems as if your life merely happens to you. Nobody wants to feel that they have lost the power to respond to their own life."

"I can't change who I am," he said suddenly defensive. He folded his arms over his chest.

"Ah, it feels to you like changing 'who you are,' not just 'how you are,' your choices in life. What would you say if I said that I can imagine many choices that a person might have that would address the panic and depression you say you feel when you worry that the secret world might invade your ordinary sphere."

"Like what?"

"It doesn't matter what I imagine the particular choices might be. I imagine that you wouldn't like the choices anyway. Choosing anything new would disrupt things, and I hear that, despite the ambivalence, you want things to stay the same. I'm just saying that you seem to have forgotten that you can choose."

"I don't want things to stay the same." He was inching closer to owning this position.

"Oh, okay, that's something new that I'd like to hear more about. As I listened to you, it seemed that the thing you most worry about is a fear that your two separate lives will collide," he nodded, "but that each life is important and valuable to you. But then you said that you don't want things to stay the same. How do you want them to be different?"

"I don't know. The only thing I can think of that I could do is that I could tell Maria. But that would collapse the two worlds into each other, and one would explode." The long arms unfurled and spread expansively to indicate that it would be a big explosion.

"So that's one choice."

"Not really."

"Sure it is. You don't like the implications, but it's a choice. Let me ask you a question. If you fell asleep tonight and a miracle happened that resolved all of these problems, but when you woke, you didn't know that this miracle had occurred, how would you notice that things were different?"

"Okay," he said skeptically. A long pause. I thought, he's not going to go for this . . . it sounded too contrived, but he played along. "I guess the first thing I would notice is that Maria would be cheerful and affectionate."

"Okay, there'd be a difference in her feeling toward you. Say more about that," I encouraged.

"I don't know . . . we seem to be guarded around one another as the years go on. I mean, we still talk and make love, but it's kind of perfunctory and stilted. I'm not sure how she thinks and feels about things. I've even wondered, though this would be totally unlike her, if *she's* having an affair." ("That could be a big hunk of projection," I thought.) "She would be smiling. We wouldn't have this underlying sense of anger."

"She would be less guarded, more open and affectionate."

"Yeah." He paused, "But to tell you the truth, I feel kind of bad saying that."

"Can you describe what 'bad' is?"

"Bad? I don't know, *guilt,* I guess."

"Guilt." Now we were closer to the core. I knew that Tim's guilt would contain a host of neurotic configurations, but right now I wanted to emphasize the legitimate aspects of his guilt, which I was relieved to see surfacing. "Because you keep all these secrets from her?"

"Yeah. I guess if I woke up and things were right, Maria would also somehow know about my gay side and it would be okay with her. I wouldn't have to lie to her because she would have found out about it. I guess in this miracle world she wouldn't have to find out; I could talk about it, and she wouldn't care. She would accept it. She would think it's just who I am."

I was pleased. This felt like real movement. "As I listen to you," I reflected, "what strikes me most is that you seem to value what you most lack right now . . . a sense of openness and sharing with Maria. It's as if you would recover something that's valuable to you. But you fear you would lose the very thing that's important to you if you let her see this other secret side of you. That really is a dilemma, and I can see why you feel stuck. Let me ask you something else, how would *you* be different after you woke up and the miracle had occurred, all these issues we're talking about are solved?"

"I would be happy. I guess I wouldn't be so pissed off all the time, and I'm not sure why that is. I wouldn't have to lie anymore and could have my life the way I want it without apologizing or feeling like I have to feel guilty for it. I would be able to say 'to hell with what people think.' I would also not be ashamed to be my parents' son. They're both dead now, but they were both very strong, good people. They wouldn't think much of my bisexuality or how I'm screwing up my life." A look of sadness passed over Tim's face, and I realized that this was the first true and *unadulterated* emotion I had seen reflected in his features.

"You looked very sad just then . . . it really struck me when you said 'ashamed to be my parents' son.'"

"They wouldn't understand my screwing things up," he said dejectedly.

"This 'screwing up' your life sounds very different from how you were telling me your story and describing your choices a few moments ago."

"Unless I say it's all okay . . . I don't know . . . I might have to do something about it. So I don't know where to go from here. I guess if I woke up and things were different, I would know what to do. I don't even know who I am anymore. It's no wonder Maria is lost to me; I'm lost to myself." We sat together in the silence.

"Maybe that's the beginning of knowing something new," I ventured, wanting to reframe the sense of finality in his statement.

"Maybe," he said. Then, "Yeah, I think it could be." I could see that Tim was working on his tendency to equivocate.

"I'm guessing that I'm the first person to whom you have disclosed all of this."

"I've never told anyone," he said, with a downcast gaze.

"I'm glad you were willing to share yourself with me today. It seems like we were really able to talk about important and meaningful things, and I know that you took a risk in doing that. So how does that feel right now . . . to have revealed yourself to me . . . to be seen, honestly showing me who you are?"

"It feels . . . I don't know," he said, looking up, "new. Disorienting."

"Do you feel any sense of relief at having shared this with another person . . . less alone in it?"

He shrugged, "I guess. But I'm still stuck in the same situation. Nothing's really changed."

Man, this was tough going, but at least the giant boulder of his resistance had budged a little. I felt resonant with Tim's struggle now that he was willing to participate with me. I agreed to meet with Tim for another eight sessions. I knew that our therapy would likely extend beyond this period, but I calculated that with a guarded client like Tim artificially limiting the number might provoke a sense of urgency to get the most out of each session. I didn't want him backsliding. He agreed to pay the full fee.

At the next session, however, I was disappointed to see that Tim appeared to close off again. There was little of the sense of possibility that briefly infused our previous meeting. I let 20 minutes of the session go by listening to trivia, and then I brought my impressions into the immediate process.

"Tim, it seems like we're back to talking about less important things in a kind of distant fashion. We had an important session last week, and you really disclosed a lot about yourself. Sometimes when clients in therapy do that they feel a need to quickly withdraw to protect themselves from so much exposure. I'm wondering whether you might not be feeling that now?"

He tilted his head obliquely toward the corner of the room and said, "I almost didn't come today. I thought, I don't want to come back here and get even more anxious and depressed."

"Our discussion made you feel more anxious and depressed this week?"

"Hell yes," he said emphatically, "I had dreams about it too. I thought I shouldn't have told you anything. Now you've got the upper hand, and there's nothing I can do about it." He narrowed his eyes and looked back at me, gauging my reaction. His suspiciousness seemed to be growing into paranoia with the vulnerability inherent in self-disclosure.

"I've got the 'upper hand,'" I said gently. "I might do something to you, harm or punish you, now that I know about your secret life?"

"Yeah. I hate that feeling that you have all the power now, and I'm just this little confessing client who's indebted to you somehow. Like you can say I'm absolved or not, like some priest."

"It kind of feels like I might exploit you somehow, or take advantage of you. Am I doing anything that you take to mean that I might misuse this power you think I have, or that might say to you that you are indebted?"

He thought for a moment. "No, I guess not. It's just something I'm sensitive to, I guess."

"You said you would like me to absolve you somehow, like a priest . . . bless your choices?"

"It's not a fucking choice, okay?! I'm bisexual; that's the way it is. Do you think I wouldn't rather be straight and not have all this to deal with?"

"Okay. When I said that you heard it as questioning your sexual orientation, as if you could just choose that, I don't mean that."

"What did you mean?"

"I mean that you still have to respond to your sexuality . . . to make choices in response to the things over which you don't have control. You have said that this is where your struggle is and that you need something new to happen for you."

"Oh." Tim sat sullenly, legs crossed, arms folded, staring at the floor. "I think you're right about that, but that's the tough part isn't it? At this point in my life I'm not confused about my sexuality, just about what to do now that I'm not. I would like to be more open. It's a theme that came up in my dream."

"Would you like to tell me about your dream." His eyebrows raised, and he shook his head, as if he could not make sense of something.

"I almost begin to believe in this stuff. I had a couple of dreams that were so obviously about our conversation. In one you came to the house and rang the bell on the front door. I looked out the window and saw you, and thought 'Hell, Maria's home, I've got to get rid of him.' So I pretended not to be home. But you came around to the back door and wanted to get in, and you were pounding on the door, but I wouldn't answer. Then you went down to the cellar door and were banging on that door. So I went through my workshop for some stuff to put up so you wouldn't be able to look in the basement window and see what I had been making there. I began to panic, so I came outside into the yard and pretended that I had just noticed you. But things switched and it looked like you were nervous about something. You said, 'Don't you tell anyone I was here.' And I said that I had never told anyone anything about you. You said, 'Good, keep it that way.' Then you started walking down the street dressed in this long black coat, like a gunslinger. But you turned, like in the movies, and put your finger up to your lips, and said, 'Shhhhsh.' That was it." He shook his head again.

"So as you reflect on that dream, what comes to mind?"

"Just that sense of you standing in front of all the neighbors, knocking on the door."

"I would compromise your secrets. I was knocking on the door for all to see, and I wanted to get into the house when Maria was at home."

"Yeah, you were very persistent," he chided and wagged his finger at me, as if I were responsible for my character in his dream.

"How do you experience me in here . . . as being very persistent?"

"No, more patient in here. It pisses me off sometimes. You could do more to help me." This seemed overtly confrontational. Like a breath of fresh air!

"What would I do to help you?"

"I don't know. It doesn't make sense as I say it aloud. I guess the persistence is that you want me to talk about everything in here, and I'm not used to that. I want you to do something, but I can't think what that might be. But this dream . . . ," he seemed to become lost in thought.

"What else strikes you about this dream? Anything that comes to mind?"

He shrugged. Tim was aware of the "intrusiveness" of the imagery, he either did not see, or did not want to acknowledge, the pervasive homoerotic imagery in the dream. Was this the pause in his presentation? Was this an erotic transference toward me? I did not yet want to interpret this; our relationship didn't seem developed enough. If Tim referenced it, we could explore it more safely. Then there was the "shift" in the dream in which it was *I* who did not want *him* to disclose some secret. The figure was a gunslinger, commanding him to silence.

As if tuned into my thoughts, he said, "I don't know what to make of that gunslinger. It's kind of the opposite of how I see you in waking life, wanting me to always talk, to not keep my mouth shut and keep secrets. The gunslinger is like the anti-you."

"All right, so what is the first thing that comes to mind when you think of someone—not me, since you have said that doesn't seem to fit—who wants *you* to be silent about *their* secrets. You said in the dream that you *'never told anyone anything about'* that gunslinger person."

Tim shifted nervously in his chair, dug his fingers into the hollow of his knee, and narrowed his eyes again suspiciously. "I can think of something, but I don't think we need to get into it." He was holding out again.

"Okay, whatever you just stumbled across seems a little too anxiety producing to talk about. It's okay if you're not up to it." We sat for a bit.

"What the hell," he resumed, and I noted once again that Tim seemed to want to elicit in me a confrontation, but that he responded positively to my stepping aside. "It reminds me of my first sexual experience," he said tentatively. "It was with an older man, he was a deacon in our church. He took an interest in me, and I really liked him. We had sex a few times. Actually, it was more than a few. I was confused those first couple of times, and he was always worried that I would tell someone."

"How old were you?"

"Fifteen. It went on for a few months. He eventually got really paranoid and started threatening me if I told anyone. I think I was more disappointed that he had turned on me than anything. It was pretty confusing. He's dead now. Bastard."

As Tim further explored these memories, I let the session pass beyond the 50-minute mark, something I rarely do. "It does feel like a relief to talk about this stuff," he admitted. "I think as a kid it was like the boogey man, you know, like he would know somehow if I told anyone about it. It's something that I didn't think bothered me that much until I'm saying it now. I guess in some way my relationship with him was important to me too. I discovered something about my sexuality that was important to me, but it was messed up too, the whole 'secrets' thing."

"*Sexual abuse,*" I said deliberately, "often seems to engender that kind of ambivalence and confusion. I hear that right now you're more aware of the feeling of being exploited and used."

"Yeah."

He didn't seem to want to continue. I switched gears.

"Let me return to your dream for a minute. It seems like in the dream you have me fused with this figure; I turn into him. Can you say something about that?"

"I don't know; you are both like confessor figures I guess."

"Ah . . . yeah, you said that now that you have confessed to me about your double life that I have power over you . . . that I could punish or manipulate you, just like he did."

"Yeah, as if we are *conspirators* in some pact but that something could go wrong."

"He was intrusive sexually, and you sometimes feel that I'm intrusive psychologically. You might agree to this now, but I might turn on you like he did . . . appear at the front door and want to intrude."

"Or around the cellar door, wanting to see what I have in my workshop, that I don't want you to see."

"Your homosexual side?"

"And my deceitful side with my family."

"Yeah, then there's this sense of you wanting absolution about how you have chosen to live your life. Did you look to him for some kind of absolution?"

"Sure. I felt a lot of guilt about it all. He was the one who caused this guilt but also the one who could forgive me for it . . . like he represented God or something because he was this big church figure, like a priest. I guess that's maybe the long black gunslinger coat! His uniform." Tim's face brightened, he seemed pleased that his interpretation seemed to capture a truth for him.

"Ah, I see. And now you feel I have power over you, but you also look to me for absolution. And you said that you are frustrated that I have not done something more to help you in that regard."

"Yeah. Talking like this makes it seem crazy, like I'm all messed up . . . like all this stuff is happening at once. I want to say this is all bullshit, but I guess it also feels really real, you know what I mean?" he said, looking up at me.

"Yeah. You are not accustomed to looking at yourself the way we are doing in here," I offered.

"No, and it makes me *more* nervous rather than less nervous . . . and more depressed. Like there's no hope. I thought this was supposed to help, but it seems to make things worse. Isn't it your job to help me feel better?" How quickly that tone of aggression and cynicism could return to his voice. For more than a few moments I had experienced a sense of mutual participation.

"I hear from the change in your tone that you feel some resentment about me not helping to improve your mood, but don't you think your mood might be related to your life situation? So, to answer your question, no, it's not my job to help you 'feel better' but to know yourself better. How you feel about seeing yourself more fully is up to you. I know that might sound a little harsh. I can say that many clients coming into therapy feel worse, a lot worse, before they feel better. It seems like you have a lot of stuff that has been stomped down for a long time. But I think something has happened here between us today. You seem very available to our conversation right now, and I find myself able to talk with you quite easily. You have let me see you even more fully, and I understand you better. I really get how difficult your struggle is. How have you experienced our session today?"

"Good, I guess. Well, not 'I guess.' It's been good. I think I've been worried that you will use what I've told you against me somehow. I guess I'm a little paranoid that way . . . distrustful." Tim's posture had relaxed, and he seemed alert, but not closed.

"So maybe now that you are beginning to feel some trust toward me you can begin to experiment with what having trust might feel like in other relationships."

"Maybe," he said, smiling . . . not cynically, but skeptically.

"What was the other dream?"

"What?"

"You said that you had 'dreams' about our session last week."

"I dreamt that termites were eating the joists of my house. The floors were kind of spongy, and I was really upset. I called you to tell you, and you said, 'Can you rip up the floors and start over?' I said, 'No, they're in the walls too.' You said, 'Sometimes fumigation works, otherwise you have to start over and build a new house.' I said, 'That's easy for you to say, you're not the one who has to pay for it.' Then you said don't worry about the money, things always work out, and that we could work on it together."

"I guess that one doesn't need much interpretation," I smiled.

"No, I think I can do that one myself," and there was the hint on his face of what a smile might look like if it were clear and unmarred by self-loathing.

———

I was feeling good about our work together. In the next two sessions, Tim continued to speak openly, though a little less immediately. He seemed to need a break from the intensity of the "big" session, as he called it, but these sessions felt relevant and meaningful. He talked about his early family life, his feelings of disappointment in himself that he had never become what he was "meant to be," and that now it was too late and that life was passing him by. He mused on his failings as a parent and a spouse. He compared himself to his own parents who he described as "good people," though not warm or supportive in the ways that he would have liked. His father's criticism, he said, was always under the surface, never overt, but somehow expressed in myriad ways. His mother was strict and conservatively religious, but at least, unlike his father, you knew where you stood with her. She ruled the household. He was proud of his own children, despite his failings, and felt that though he was no longer as emotionally close to them as when they were very little and dependent, that they respected and liked him. Maria, he said, was a good mother. Maria and he seldom shared pleasurable activities and moved in their own circles, but their lives intersected around domestic life and occasionally in the bedroom.

Tim had turned a corner in therapy; he seemed more willing to participate and was using his sessions well given his capacity for limited engagement. We missed a week when he went away on business, and he returned wanting to talk more directly about his sexual activities. He explained that he had experienced his usual ambivalence but found himself in an adult bookstore backroom that connected to another room by means of a "glory hole," an opening through which one could engage in anonymous sex without even seeing the face of one's "partner." Much to his dismay, he found that he could not perform sexually, and he left the scene in shame and embarrassment, fortunately, he said, having never seen the face of the other participant.

"Sounds like progress to me," I said, risking a reframe of his "failure."

"You think my failure to perform sexually is progress?"

"Yeah, I do. I'm happy for you." I hoped this would confuse him, and it did.

"On the one hand, I think you don't know what the hell you are talking about, and it pisses me off to hear you say that. Thanks for the sympathy," he said sarcastically, but this sarcasm didn't have the same edge.

"But on the other hand?" I inquired.

"On the other hand, as you say that I wonder is this something that has to do with all the stuff I've been dealing with? I mean it makes a strange kind of sense."

"Help me understand what kind of sense it makes to you when I said that."

"Well, I mean, what the hell is that anyway . . . having sex through a plywood partition. I guess in some way I was relieved to get out of there. I always feel kind of sleazy when I leave after those sorts of sexual encounters."

"That sounds new. There's another part of you that says 'What the hell is that? I don't feel good about myself when I do that. I want something else here.' What would the something else look like?"

"Yeah, it is kind of new. I didn't used to notice it because . . . I don't know. I'm not sure how I feel about it. As we talk about it, it reminds me of this guy I know from seeing him in a bar. I tried to pick him up one time, and he said, 'Sorry, I don't even know you.' I said, 'I'm sorry, I thought you were gay,' he was, after all in a gay bar. He said, 'I am, I'm just not a slut.' That really struck me. I apologized to him, and we talked a little, and he said, 'You'll eventually come to the end of that kind of sex and want a *person* on the other end of that dick.' That kind of struck me, you know?"

"Yeah. So maybe your inability to perform sexually in that situation in the bookstore expresses the ambivalence you've been feeling about these encounters being impersonal: objectified and not part of some kind of deeper relationship."

"I don't know about *that.*"

I thought, "Yeah, that did sound more like what *I* want for you to feel."

"I think it's a matter of degree. I at least should see the face of the person I'm with. I should at least know his name, or have a drink or something. But I'm not looking for a deeper relationship, maybe just a friendly relationship. I also think it has something to do with acknowledging the secrecy about the abuse," he continued, "which, I guess I never really thought about it as 'abuse,' but I find myself being really pissed off about it the more I remember what happened."

"Somehow the secrecy and anonymity go together."

"Yeah . . . and if it's anonymous, it's like, did it really even happen?"

"It vanishes, it's hardly even there, like having sex through a partition."

"Yeah, you're kind of protected from the repercussions."

"Oh, really?" I thought. This seemed like a perfect opportunity to broach the subject that had been troubling me ever since Tim revealed his other life. "Let me ask you something I've been wondering about that has to do with being protected and repercussions. Do you practice safe sex during these encounters?"

"Of course I do. I'm not stupid."

I nodded. I wanted to believe him, but somehow, with all those anonymous encounters, I doubted that he had always been so deliberate.

In our next session, however, the issue of safe sex came up again in our discussion.

"And you don't know what's out there, you know, and it's not something you like to think about," he said.

"Do you mean in terms of sexually transmitted diseases? You said last week that you always have practiced 'safer' sex, I won't say 'safe,' because when you have that many partners I don't think it can be safe."

"Yeah, I mean, you know, there have been slip ups. I mean, when I first was going out. I guess I lied about that."

"More recently you have been more diligent about it."

"More . . . yeah, I guess. But you know, sometimes stuff happens pretty quickly, and sometimes things go wrong. So, there have been many times when I can't say that it was safe. It's not something that I'm real proud about."

But as I looked at Tim, he did not seem abashed. He looked angry that I had brought up the question again. "'Many times,' you said. Have you ever been tested for STDs?" I asked.

"No." His face looked set in an attitude of defiance.

A long silence hovered in the room between us. "You look angry right now that I am focusing on this, that I'm saying that maybe that's something you should think about."

"It's not really your concern. Can't anything be private here?" Another long silence. "What?" he said.

"I guess we're also talking about the rights of others as well." I said it as gently as I could.

"Now you're out of line."

"You feel like I'm meddling now."

"Damn straight."

"But Tim, come on," I said impatiently, matching his energy level, "you've told me that you and Maria are having sex. Are you using a condom with her? I guess I wonder; what if your choices are also affecting the lives of others without them having the opportunity to participate in those choices. Aren't you potentially victimizing her in the way that you have been victimized in the past? How can she make choices about her own life unless she has all the information?"

This was pretty strong, and I found myself being more emphatic than I would have liked, but Tim didn't walk out of the room. He did cross his arms again, and his voice assumed that intellectual tone that communicated to me that he was withdrawing.

"If I thought I had something, I would do something about it. I told you, the unsafe encounters haven't really been flagrant . . . well, most of them, and it was a while ago. I've been much more careful in recent years. I would know if something were wrong." He looked like a petulant little boy, arms crossed, a set look on his face.

"Okay. I can see that you feel I've overstepped here."

"Why is it so important to you?"

"Do you really want me to say?" I asked, surprised that he was continuing to pursue the issue.

"Why not?"

"Tim, I don't think you're being honest with yourself or me. You are rationalizing the risks and talking yourself into a desired reality. I can't see it. If you believe I can usually hear you pretty well, and yet my perception is very different from yours, maybe that should give you pause. We're talking science here, not how you would like things to be. You say there's very little chance that you have a sexually transmitted disease. But you also say you've had a number of 'slip-ups.' I think the risks are high and that Maria is sharing those risks with you without her consent. Explain to me why putting her at risk is any different from her being a victim here." I was very aware that I was imposing my "categories of experience" on him in this moment, but this clash between our subjective worlds still felt important, even if there was little agreement. At least it gave him something to "push off of," which he had said was important to him.

"I would know if there was something wrong," he maintained doggedly.

"In that case, there's no reason not to be tested, since you are certain to get the result you want." I felt like Galileo saying "Look into the damn telescope!" persisting in making sense to an irrational and superstitious mind.

"I would have to consult my doctor, and those records might go to my insurance company," he rationalized.

"You can get tested anonymously. I can give you a card. Will you take it?" I persisted.

"I'll take it, but I doubt I'll use it," he said heatedly.

As we argued, I felt like I was articulating a competing impulse in *him*. Why else would he have kept the discussion going? "You know what?" I said, suddenly doing an about-face, "You're right! This is really my agenda. You're your own man, you can make your own decisions."

Silence. He looked confused. "What do you mean?"

Ha! I knew it! I thought I would really "pee in the soup" by combining an acceptance of his choice with an endorsement of his irrationality. "Just what I said. It's clear that you might find out something you don't want to know, and I'm not respecting your desire to remain uninformed, though it *is* at odds with what we're about here. My assumptions are getting in the way. My assumption is that you share this idea that it's better to know than not know on all levels. But you seem to be saying you are *making a choice* not to know. You are defending your right to remain in the dark about this. I guess there is a culture in some parts of the gay community that believes you may as well 'fiddle while Rome burns' and go down in fine style. You know, the whole 'And the band played on,' thing. We all deny some things we don't want to see, and it's your right to deny the parts you don't want to see. Garrison Keillor is right I guess, 'Sometimes you just have to stand up to reality and deny it.' I would ask you to say, 'I choose not to know,' knowing that your choice affects others, to say that to honor the work we're doing in here."

A long silence. I thought, "He's confused now. Good!"

"I choose not to know," he said finally.

"Okay."

"You respect my choice?"

"No, I don't. But it's your choice, not mine."

"That's right, it is."

———

Tim missed our next appointment. And the next. I made my usual phone call when any client fails to appear: "Hi Tim, I missed you for our appointment. Hope everything is okay. Please call me to reschedule." After that, I don't pursue. A few weeks later Tim called and arranged to meet. He made flimsy excuses for not keeping the previous appointments and spent the first half of the session with trivia. I was about to interpret this when he inquired, "Well, aren't you going to ask?"

"You want me to ask you something?"

He snorted, "You mean you don't remember . . . about the test."

"Of course I remember, I didn't know if that's what you meant. Did you get tested?"

"Yeah . . . it was positive."

"Positive for HIV?" I asked softly.

"What else?"

"Tim, I'm so sorry."

He looked at me curiously. I suppose I was the only one who knew, and the first to express sympathy.

"Thanks. As you can imagine, I was quite surprised." His face was flat and emotionless. His gangly limbs seemed collapsed in the chair like a dead spider. I thought, "He is still in shock. The long denied implications have suddenly slammed him in the face."

"Yes, you thought it was unlikely." He looked forlorn, and I wanted to somehow comfort him, to say words that would give some meaning, hope, or solace to him. But I knew no words that could do this.

"I was stupid. During the days when I was waiting for the results, I remembered lots more times of being unprotected. The more I thought about it, the more I remembered. It's a nightmare," he said flatly.

"I'm so sorry, Tim."

I sat with him, gently reflecting back to him the little he was able to express of his emotions. I reminded him that new drugs greatly improved treatment and quality of life, but he said that he felt his life was over. The meaning he assigned to contracting the virus was that this was a final proof of his unworthiness; even that God had caught up with him at last. I gently helped him pick apart the barrage of self-deprecating generalizations and interpretations that followed. Toward the end of our interview I asked, "Have you thought about how you will handle this information with Maria?"

"There's nothing to think about. I'll keep my mouth shut like I always have. It's not going to help her any to have to deal with this too."

I sat in disbelieving silence. Could he be serious? "What about your sexual relations with her?" I inquired.

"What about them?" he shrugged. "I guess I'll have to make up some excuse for wearing a condom," he said, as if this was an afterthought. "I'll tell her it helps me delay my orgasm."

"You feel okay not telling her even after all this? What if you start to need medical treatment; what about all the drugs you will have to take?"

"I don't know . . . I haven't really thought about it. I'll figure it out."

"What if she is already HIV-positive . . . shouldn't she know?"

This seemed to give him pause, but he only said, "heterosexual transmission is much less likely. We have sex infrequently these days, so it would be a long shot."

"Like you said it was a long shot for you to be positive."

"I could use a little more support here," he said.

Support! Despite my sympathy for his plight, I had to monitor my rising indignation at Tim's disregard for those he claimed to care for. Suddenly, the regard I had felt for Tim evaporated. But I also had the impression that this reaction would be exactly what Tim would expect from someone whom he had let really "see" him. Was he intentionally trying to elicit rejection to confirm feelings he already felt for himself in his crisis? Was he trying to get me to reenact with him old traumas, to endorse his belief that he must be punished? Did he think that I, like his parents, like God, should revile him? As we sat in silence together, these thoughts gave me hope . . . hope that there was, latent within him, an opposing impulse waiting to be confirmed, an impulse toward respect for the rights of his wife, a need for affiliation and acceptance. He had, after all, followed through on getting tested and had brought this information back to our conversation. He was setting me up to condemn him. I would not reenact this with him.

"Tim, I feel almost like you want me to punish you, but I'm not going to do that. I do have real concerns about your not wanting to disclose you HIV status to Maria. I do believe you when you say that you care for your family. I think that kind of caring means that Maria has the right not to be exposed to the kind of danger that is possible with STDs. Only someone who is incredibly angry and hurtful would deliberately expose another person. I don't believe you are that angry at Maria to further put her in harm's way."

"You don't know how angry I am. But my being angry is not why I'm going to keep it from her. You're right. I'm not going to deliberately expose Maria. I want my family together . . . that's what's best for the kids especially. I'm not going to hurt anyone."

"Tim, I believe you. You will find your way with this."

"It's not going to be your way."

"I understand that. It's going to be your way, but you have some hard choices ahead of you. I don't believe you will continue to live as you have in the past. It was hard then, it will be harder now. You'll figure it out."

Between sessions I ruminated on Tim's case and my ethical dilemma. I contemplated breaking confidentiality, reasoning that I could make a case for "intent to do harm to another." What if Maria were HIV-positive? She would need immediate treatment. And if she were not infected, intervention might prevent her from becoming so. I found that there was little legal support for such an action. "A penis is not considered to be a weapon in a court of law," one colleague reminded me. In addition, Tim had said that he would "protect" his family from harm, which made my position, legally, less tenable. Ethically, however, it was another matter. I possessed information that directly and significantly affected the well-being of someone's life. I decided that all I could do was work with Tim to get him to be more honest with Maria. If he did not, and revealed to me that he was putting her at high risk, well, then I might have to make another choice.

"I wonder if you've thought any more about what we talked about last week," I inquired, "about sharing your situation with Maria?"

"I thought about it a lot." This was encouraging. "I think I'm doing the right thing not telling her." This was not encouraging. "We had sex the other night, and I didn't have a condom, but I made it so we just stuck to other stuff, you know. I think she thought that's just what I was in the mood for. I mean, there was very brief oral but I redirected her."

"You surely know that a person can become infected from oral sex."

"Well, it was brief, and anyway, she doesn't like me to, you know, come in her mouth," he said, a grin spreading over his face, "a lot of women don't you know." I felt a sense of anger rising from my chest, seeking words. Don't take the bait, I reminded myself.

"Tim, I'm not sure how to respond to that. On one hand I feel angry that you seem cavalier about describing this encounter. But I also sense that maybe you are trying to shock me so I will chastise you."

"Whatever you say, Doctor."

We sat silently for a moment. "Tim, tell me about your relationship with your wife. How did you meet? How did you fall in love? What drew you together and made you want to have kids together?"

Tim told the story of how he met Maria on Martha's Vineyard. How they courted and fell in love. She liked that he was intense, quiet, and serious. He liked that she was outgoing enough for both of them. As the story unfolded, Tim seemed to recall details that made their union make sense . . . as if he had lost that part in the years that followed.

"I know what you are trying to do," he said.

"What am I trying to do?"

"You're trying to get me to remember how I love Maria so I won't put her at risk. But you don't get that I don't need to be convinced that I care for her."

"And, as you consider our differing views on this, how is it for you to have that tension between our positions . . . it seems like a significant thing between us."

"I guess I like that you're straightforward about how you see it, no beating around the bush, but you're not demanding that I do it your way. Even though I can see you are pissed. It makes me want to at least consider what you are saying." This was more than I had hoped for. "I thought you might pull some power thing on me and tell Maria. The truth is, there's a part of me that even hopes that you would. Maybe you're right about me wanting you to say stuff to me that I want to say to myself, but somehow can't."

"Oh! There's some part of you that wants her to know, but you don't want to be the one to tell her, to take responsibility for that? So that's why I sometimes feel pulled to respond in a way that I feel reflects a part of your own experience?"

"I don't know. Maybe so. The picture I have as we're talking about it is that you would tell her, and then I guess *everybody* would be against me . . . and that would probably be about right. That's probably what *should* happen. At least she would have some support. She's going to hate my guts; I won't be able to do anything for her."

"But you would like to do something for her. And perhaps you would like me to do something for her."

"Yeah, I would. It still doesn't make sense to you that I care for her does it?"

"No, it does make sense, though I admit I have struggled to reconcile the choices you make with your expressions of care for her."

"You don't know how hard it is being in my situation. Don't you think," he said suddenly angry, "that if I could have suddenly become straight that I would have? Don't you think I want my life to be easier? Do you think I want my life to be this way? And now it's too late, even if I could somehow make it right."

"You keep assigning to me feelings I don't have toward you. I think maybe it's you who feels punitive toward yourself about your sexual orientation."

"That's true," he said with resignation. "All along I have been thinking that there are no choices left to me. That was beginning to change as we talked. But now, with the HIV part, I feel that sense of hopeless-ness. You used a word once that shook me up, stuck in my mind, and it's been bothering me because I never saw myself like that. You said I looked 'furtive,' and that was very different than my view of myself as somehow, I don't know, just keeping a part of my life from other's view. But when I talked about how I would like things to be if there was some kind of miracle, I knew that could never happen, but I at least knew what I would *like* to have happen. I had never thought of that, that there might be a whole different life. Well, that's not true. Maybe that's why I have to push things to the limit."

"What do you mean?"

"Maybe that's why I've gotten myself into this situation, where the old way can't continue."

"In other words, maybe your denial about the consequences of your actions is pushing you toward a resolution that you couldn't choose with full awareness, but that you have been gravitating toward for a long time, a choosing without choosing."

"Yeah. I think that's the part you don't fully get; you don't get how I need to just have it happen."

"I get it loud and clear right now."

"I guess your way would have been better; it's a pretty high price for not just doing it intentionally."

"But you couldn't accept it in yourself. It would be fully owning what you have wanted to deny but also feared giving up."

"Well said."

"Say more about 'it.' What is it you would like to happen now?"

"Living the life I need to. I haven't been able to keep this going; I think I knew it somehow. I just never thought it would be like this. So I guess you have no intention of telling Maria what's happening?" I sud-denly wondered if that was the primary reason for Tim seeking therapy, telling someone of his secret life so that they would take action or at least enable him to do so.

"No, sorry, that's your job. I'll tell you what I can do. If you want to have some joint sessions with Maria, talk to her in a more controlled setting, we could meet together. I could be there to support both of you, perhaps even bringing in a female co-therapist who could be avail-able to work with her if she wants. What do you think?"

"That would probably be best," he said. He looked tired and resigned, and his expression was suddenly childlike, sad and reflective, as if many years of struggle had resolved into a singular moment of acceptance.

After another preparatory meeting, Tim did bring Maria to the session where he intended to disclose to her both his bisexuality and his HIV status. I picked them up in the waiting room, and she politely and nervously greeted me holding out her small hand. She was as diminutive as Tim was tall. Her plain round face wore no makeup, and though it was now lined with worry, seemed younger than her years. Her sandy blond hair cascaded down the back of her blouse to the waist of her jeans like a horse's mane. Tim's demeanor betrayed nothing of what he was about to tell her. They followed me down the hall and entered the room. She looked around quickly, then took a seat next to Tim on the couch. Tim had said that he wanted no prelude to talking to Maria, but as they sat on the couch they *both* looked at *me* expectantly.

"Tim, you have invited Maria to be with us today in our session. How would you like to begin?"

"I don't know. Maybe you could give us a start." Damn! This was not what we had discussed. Was he going to try to get me to tell her after all?

"Maria, I'm wondering if Tim has mentioned anything about the purpose of our meeting today?"

"He just mentioned that you both thought it would be a good idea for me to come to the session and talk about the things you have been discussing. He didn't say much about it." She turned and looked at him nervously. He was supposed to have let her know that he wanted to talk to her about something very important in the safety of the therapy setting.

"Tim, would you like to begin?"

"Maybe it would be best if you gave Maria a brief overview of some of the other issues we've been discussing in therapy to prepare the stage," he offered.

What issues? It was all about what he wanted to disclose to her at this meeting!

"What is going on?" Maria said anxiously.

"Tim, I think it's best if you just talk to Maria about the issues you have invited her here to discuss. I don't feel it's my place to do that for you, but to help you both. Please begin."

"Well, I wanted to talk to her about . . . ," he began, looking at me.

"Tim, please talk directly to Maria, not to me."

"I wanted to talk to you about something I've been dealing with for a long time. I haven't been able to tell you about it because I was afraid you'd be so unhappy about it that you'd leave me. I don't want that to happen."

"Oh, God," Maria moaned. She put her forehead in her hand.

"What?" Tim inquired. Maria shook her head silently. "So, I've been wanting to tell you about a side of me that's difficult to talk about. But I think it's important to talk about. I don't know how you'll feel about it, well, I guess I do know. But I want you to know that our family means so much to me and . . ."

"You're gay," Maria said under her breath, without looking up or moving her head from her hand. Tim seemed shocked that she had anticipated his revelation. "Do you think I don't know that you're attracted to men?" she said, suddenly animated. "Do you think I could live with you all these years and not know that? How many times have I found your stupid magazines hidden in the garage? I knew soon after we were married, maybe even before, that you had something going on in that direction. I was stupid. I thought that once you married me it would go away. Yes, it broke my heart for a while, but I thought, 'he can't help it,' and I learned to live with it. But I hope you haven't been in here 'exploring your gay side,'" she made quotation marks in the air with her fingers. "I hope you're not encouraging him to 'come out,'" she said, looking at me. "Because you have a family! You've dealt with it up until now; you can continue to deal with it. Just stick to your magazines. Did you really have to make this an issue?" she said in my direction. "For all this time we've managed. Then he comes here and we have to . . ."

"It's a little more complicated than that," interjected Tim.

"What do you mean?" She looked at Tim, then at me. "Oh, God." Her head dropped back into her hand. "What?" she said, not looking up, "You have a boyfriend?"

"No, I don't have a boyfriend." Maria looked up hopefully. "I'm afraid it's a little worse than that," he said. Maria's shoulders slumped, and her face went slack. "I've been having some sexual encounters . . . with men."

"What? Where . . . when did this happen?" she said.

Tim offered a highly edited version of his out of town encounters. Maria asked the questions that all betrayed partners seem to ask: how many times, who with, how it compared with what they shared sexually. Tim, while sticking to the main truth, offered her an account that was heavy on "spin." I mediated the discussion as best I could, mainly supporting Maria in her struggle to accommodate what she was hearing and helping her express her reactions, which were naturally shock, anger, and sadness. Tim began to share a little too much detail and I intervened.

Maria had put her face in her hands and began to cry silently.

We sat quietly for a while. "Maria," I said softly, "I can see that this is very difficult for you to take in, and that you're very upset. From what you have said, it seems like you knew Tim has this other part to his sexuality and, though it was disappointing to you, that you found a way to live with it. It seems like neither one of you wanted to talk about it openly." She nodded her head slowly.

"It would have been better if he had never come in here," she said.

I looked at Tim, and nodded. We weren't finished.

"I wish I had talked to you about it," said Tim. "I didn't know you would understand." Maria snorted dismissively.

"I didn't have a choice, did I?" she said. My God, this attitude seemed to run in the family.

"There's something else I have to tell you," Tim said. His voice was meek and wavering. She looked up at him suspiciously. "Apparently, I've had some bad luck despite my efforts to practice safe sex. I have been diagnosed with a sexually transmitted disease." Maria's face seemed to instantly drain of color.

"What disease?" she asked quietly.

"HIV," Tim said.

"Oh God," she said in a whisper. "Oh God, Oh God." She sat silently. She looked numb. She didn't cry. Tim reached over to her and put his arms around her. She didn't move except for shaking her head slowly back and forth.

"Maria, I know this comes as an incredible shock," I said. After a while I said, "Maria, can you say a little about what you're feeling right now?"

She looked up at me. "If I could, I wouldn't say it to you!"

"You feel that if Tim had not come here that maybe this wouldn't have happened?"

"We were doing fine until he came in here!" I looked at Tim to prompt him to explain to her that his extracurricular activities had been going on before he came to therapy.

He averted his gaze and tried to comfort his wife. All he said was, "No, it's not his fault. This needed to come out eventually." Oh man! He was going to let her assumption stand!

"Maria, it's important that you get tested as soon as possible," I said.

"Don't you think I know that?" she said. "I have to go," she said suddenly. We were about two-thirds of the way through the session.

"Maria, I'd like to encourage you to stay and talk a little longer," I offered. "This has been a big shock to you, and it's best if you talk about your reaction."

"My reaction! What do you think my reaction is?" Then turning to Tim she said, "I can't believe you would do this to our family!"

She stood up and walked toward the door. Tim stood, but seemed not to know what to do. Maria paused at the door and said, "Are you coming or not?"

"I think we should stay," he said.

"I'm leaving. Come if you want."

He looked at me. "You'd better go," I suggested. "Call me and let me know how it's going."

After days of anxious waiting, Tim called to say that Maria's tests indicated that she was HIV-negative. They decided two weeks after this news to come in together for a session. Maria had regained her composure and seemed eager to talk.

She said she thought of Tim and she as "good friends" but not good companions for a marriage. She admitted that she had not been happy for a long time, she said, and only stayed in the marriage because Tim was a good father and that she too wanted to keep their family together. But she also revealed that she had been fantasizing for a long time about getting out and getting her own life back and finding a more suitable mate.

Maria said she had been thinking it over, and she did not want to immediately dissolve the family (a big surprise for Tim). Rather, she wanted to plan for an eventual separation and divorce to take place within a year or two. This would give them time to work out living arrangements, prepare the children, and experiment with living apart. She was for full disclosure to the children about Tim's sexual orientation and HIV status. After long deliberation, they negotiated to reveal Tim's sexual orientation closer to the time they separated and to not reveal his HIV status until he became symptomatic, potentially many years down the road.

She seemed, Tim observed, to be suddenly energized. It was as if she had been preparing to meet this crisis for a long time. She was like a general with a battle plan for living arrangements, kids' needs, visitation, and property settlement. She seemed to need the efficacy of meeting the crisis proactively. She followed through on a referral I gave her for a female therapist with whom she could do individual work. I gave them the name of a couples' counselor. Tim trailed along, agreeable to what she wanted and seemingly relieved that it wasn't worse.

I had intended to continue working with Tim, but after one more joint meeting, they both decided that further sessions with me were unnecessary. They seemed suddenly a team, and they had made a joint decision. It was as if everything we had discussed had led to this single resolution . . . as if the only self-exploration required was that which made this conversation between them possible. One part of me felt relieved. But I also felt let down and disappointed. I had the feeling that I had been central in upsetting the apple cart, and no matter how much each of them privately wanted and needed this to happen, they both, on some level, resented me for it. Sometimes the relationship is not mutually gratifying.

I saw Tim one more time about seven years later. I was walking downtown on a cold fall day. As I paused at the crosswalk, shivering, I heard someone call my name. I turned to see Tim sitting alone at a bus stop, wrapped in a long coat. It took me a moment to recognize him. He, too, was hunched against the cold. He said his car was in the shop, and he was going to visit the doctor. I sat down next to him, and we talked and shivered together. He and Maria were divorced now, he said, and it had been less traumatic than he had feared. They were still friends, and he saw the kids all the time. He had discovered a support group that had helped him "come out." He didn't need to keep his sexual orientation a secret anymore. It was all good, he said. Well, almost all. His T-cell count was pretty high despite his regimen of drugs, and I could see that his face was much thinner. He had recently discovered the first lesions. That was pretty depressing, he said. The bus rolled up and we stood and exchanged parting remarks. The doors opened and he stepped out of the bright day and disappeared into the shadow of the entry as the doors closed behind him. The bus rolled away. Brown fall leaves were blowing and rattling down the sidewalk on a coming winter wind. I walked on. As I turned the corner of a building, a melody was drifting into awareness . . . what was the name of that song?*

---

*In the American/Texas folk song, the man wrapped in white linen is dying of a gunshot wound to the chest. In the original Irish/Appalachian ballad, he is dying of mercury poisoning associated with the 19th-century treatment of venereal disease.

CASE SEVEN DISCUSSION
Psychotherapy and Change: Some Principles

LIKE MANY CLIENTS seeking therapy, Tim felt that his problems emerged from circumstances beyond his control. He was helpless to respond to or change his life because he framed his difficulties in such a way as to prevent any alternatives from becoming apparent to him. He felt trapped in a no-win situation, and his attempts to solve the problem became even more troublesome to him than the problems themselves. In other words, because Tim viewed himself as a victim of his circumstances, he avoided directly meeting the conflicts he felt in his relational and sexual life, and the various forms of this avoidance became a primary source of his unhappiness and dissatisfaction. Tim led a fractured and untruthful existence, and he knew it. Unable to be direct and intentional, he nonetheless unconsciously made choices that moved him inexorably toward a crisis, a crisis in which change would be forced upon him. His last ditch decision to come to therapy represented one of the first intentional choices he had made in response to his intolerable situation.

Why are people who come to therapy not able to change on their own? Why, when they do come, can they not embrace what seems to the therapist to be an obvious solution to the problems they present? Why, even more mystifyingly, would an empathic and understanding therapist demeanor activate the client's resistance, while falling asleep in a session (I don't recommend this as an intervention) provoke a change in the course of the therapy? Often the therapist does not know what particular experiences will help create change for the client. However, the therapist can use some principles of change to guide the process.

The Repetitive Nature of the Client's Problems

Like most persons who are stuck in a cycle of self-defeating behavior, Tim's particular symptoms and behavior stood in for a constellation of needs and unrealized potentialities he was not addressing directly and honestly. This pattern is familiar to observant therapists. The person substitutes an action that stands in for a primary and critical human experience that has been frustrated or unrealized in its original form. Most often these inner wounds derive from a history of disruptions in connections with important others. These problematic interpersonal traumas and frustrations play out repetitively across many new situations and relationships. But the behavior or symptom that substitutes for the primary longings and needs fails to be truly sustaining, and the self-defeating behavior repeats with ever-greater intensity.

These "repetition compulsions" become apparent to the therapist as he or she notices a pattern of ever-increasing intensity where the client is essentially saying, "That didn't work, I think I'll try it again." Clients often have a kind of blind spot for the repetitive nature of these efforts, and depression and anxiety often follow close behind whatever initial gratification derives from these compensatory efforts. The depression seems to stand in for a challenge that has yet to be truly undertaken, as if to mark its location within the being of the person. It is as if some wiser part of the person is saying, "You cannot be content until you pay attention 'here.' I will not allow you to escape the imperative of growth." In other words, at some level, a person potentially preserves a clear idea of what he or she needs. The degree of anxiety or depression can mark how far away that person is from his or her own center.

One obvious example of this repetition compulsion is that Tim seemed to be reenacting the wounds pertaining to his sexual molestation as a teen. This traumatic event seemed to crystallize what must have been a host of additional interpersonal disruptions and ambivalent feelings. Not the least of these were his conflicts over his sexual identity, his failed attempt to deny his disturbing impulses through marriage, and his belief that he had failed to live up to his parents' wishes and values. The secret life he constructed in response to these disowned aspects of himself preserved something important to him, but it also set him on a path that only increased his conflicts.

These conflicts played out in his secretiveness about huge parts of his sexual identity, his concern over "power" issues in relationships, his evasive and passive-aggressive style, and his fear (and desire) that I might betray him. All these seemed to express another important feature of his inner world, the underlying and pervasive shame and self-loathing his cynicism tried to mask. His transference dream that substituted me as the molester, his reenactment of his molestation with anonymous others, and the driven quality of his compulsive sexual exploits pointed out that these wounds and conflicts continually sought expression in a host of indirectly related behaviors.

While Tim's self-development certainly unfolded in the context of many other developmental influences, it is a well-recognized phenomenon that sexual abuse almost always significantly disrupts a person's identity consolidation. One feature of this disruption often manifests as a defensive style of *hypersexuality*. Tim's compulsive and anonymous sexual behavior seemed particularly driven.

It seems paradoxical that a person might choose the area of behavior in which he or she is wounded to enact some attempt at resolving the wound. I first encountered this paradox when I worked with a client who made her living as a stripper. She described early sexual molestations and later pervasive hypersexuality in her erotic life. She had obviously chosen a line of work that placed her in a situation that was resonant with symbolic reenactments of her most loaded traumas, conflicts, and emotions. This client described, tellingly, that each time a man tucked a $20 bill into her stocking, it was as if she had prevailed over her molester. Her trauma and her power over it were contained within the same enactment.

This paradox has important implications for how relationships unfold in therapy where, because of the intense nature of the encounter, these enactments can become even more energized. The client will unconsciously attempt to create the same interpersonal dynamics that indirectly contain *and* address the conflict in an unproductive and repetitive enactment. This combination of motivations for stasis and change can be very confusing to the therapist.

The Motivation to Change

Tim marshaled a host of effective psychological defenses to protect himself from the anxiety associated with the conflicts that plagued him. He rationalized his behavior to himself and to me, reframing his actions to always justify the choices that were merely compromise solutions to facing his dilemmas. His expectation of rejection and abuse made him suspicious and cagey. Tim's use of the defense of denial screened from his view many unpleasant realities, especially the reality of just how "unsafe" he had been in his sexual encounters. The lack of emotional integration that he felt became greater as he dissociated the many domains of his life from one another. As he said, "It's like I live in two worlds, and neither contacts the other. I kind of switch between them." All of these fairly "deep structure" personality features impaired his ability to have sustaining and close interpersonal connections and to relate with immediacy, directness, and sincerity.

When Tim first sought therapy, he would have liked for me to somehow ease his suffering. I believe that at first he resented me for not providing him with some easy solution to his difficulties. But every client eventually comes face to face with the existential issue that is at the center of the potential for change: one cannot change the circumstances of life (one's parentage, sexual identity, ethnicity, traumas, and so forth). Over these things one has no control, and blame, regret, and rage merely end in exhaustion. Søren Kierkegaard (as cited in Friedman, 1992) called these existential givens of life one's "throwness," as in each person is thrown into a set of conditions in life over which he or she has no choice. But each person has the ability to *respond* to these surrounding influences and conditions, and this idea is at the heart of therapy. Clients have often forgotten that no matter how much of a "raw deal" they feel they were handed, they still have the capacity to *relate* to their conditions on terms that they create. As Victor Frankl (1959) illustrated in describing his experiences in a Nazi concentration camp, even in such extreme circumstances a person can choose to respond to suffering in ways that increase rather than diminish one's essential humanity, value, and meaning.

Therapeutic change is hard, though. As Leslie Farber (1966) has observed, therapeutic change is not passive. It does not merely *happen to* the client. Rather, it demands a commitment of participation and *will* on the part of the client. The client must discover some impulse toward growth and change for any productive movement to happen, because no matter how much trouble is caused by the client's particular way of constructing reality, psychological organization provides a sense of stability. Like all organized complex systems that achieve some sort of balance, the system resists whatever might disrupt its homeostatic equilibrium (Becvar & Becvar, 1988). The process of therapy is inherently destabilizing (even if only temporarily) to the existing self-system. Knowing this, the client sometimes chooses the known misery over the anxiety that accompanies the unknown, whatever prospect of fulfillment change may hold. However, in the balance between the client's will to change and the desire for stability, the client's misery may, paradoxically, prove to be a prime motivator.

Fortunately, as Carl Rogers (1980) observed, the impulse toward stasis is not only disrupted by misery and unhappiness but is also countered by the human tendency toward positive growth and change. Perhaps that is the corrective function of boredom. Somewhere between the need for predictability and the subjective sense of psychological fragmentation attending too profound a change lies a potentially transformative medium—an optimal tension therapists must discover with their clients. When I stumbled across this with Tim, it came as a surprise to me. Because nothing seemed to happen in our work despite my best attempts, I had been ready to give up as we approached the end of our first course of sessions.

When I nodded off in the session, and then (feeling I had nothing to lose) explicated to Tim my perceptions of him, this sparked a new process between us. I did not realize at the time that it also tapped into a complex group of associations for him. On one hand, he felt affirmed that I asserted that there was more to him than he was willing to reveal. On the other hand, because it felt insulting to him, I also appeared more "real" to him than a person who would not show what he perceived as any "negative" reaction to him. The event evoked both sides of one of his generic conflicts. It was interesting to me that he could not trust my former attentiveness because "nobody is that nice." My attentiveness and empathy had more greatly activated his suspicion that I might then exploit, punish, or reject him than had my nodding off! An optimal and safe distance had been created between us by my confrontation. Worried about trust and judgment, he paradoxically felt safer when I essentially said, "Your worry is legitimate . . . here is how I see you." It suddenly felt safer to him to be confronted, even criticized (that he understood!), but to feel that he had accurate information.

I had been working hard to create a greater sense of interpersonal connectedness without realizing that for some clients this can be highly intimidating. My assumption that a high level of interpersonal "presence" in the session was a good thing was, in this case, wrong. I realized later that some clients cannot tolerate too much immediacy and possibility for affiliation, and that Tim was certainly one of those clients.

The ability to engage with another, I realized, exists on a continuum for any person. In Martin Buber's (1958) paradigm, Tim was much more comfortable in the "I–it" than in the "I–Thou" mode. Most of the people in his life were functional, like tables and chairs, except that their legs and arms actually moved. He was much more comfortable objectifying most of the people around him and being objectified by them. Occasionally, however, Tim's deeper longings for affiliation allowed him to reach past his fear and cynicism and to participate in an unguarded moment. I realized that finding an optimal distance was not something I had been striving to do.

Clients are rarely aware that they are attempting to re-create their primary conflicts in the relationship with the therapist. Sullivan (as cited in Greenberg & Mitchell, 1983) equates the client's reenactment of interpersonal processes as remnants of early "security operations," behaviors designed to manage anxiety and gain control in problematic relational exchanges with caregivers. These enactments are usually far below the client's self-observation. But the client's unawareness does not mean that when the therapist responds differently the resulting corrective effect of new relational experiences is any less powerful.

Evoking the Client's Potential for Change

Of course, it is often helpful for the client to gain insight into *how* the same problematic relational dynamics that frustrate him with others are playing out in the current encounter with the therapist. But the *experience* of the event is almost always a more powerful agent of change than an interpretation about it. I teetered on the edge of failure with Tim in this regard, because the part of Tim that wanted me to chastise him as he chastised himself intentionally evoked in me a sense of anger and rejection. He did this by pretending that he could completely objectify, and be indifferent to, others for whom he claimed to care. But I trusted (barely) that there was another opposing impulse in him that longed for confirmation, an impulse that endorsed what he was also telling me all along—that he cared for and loved his wife and family.

I chose to try to elicit this other part of his conflict and self-experience rather than condemn the "ugly" or "repulsive" parts that he made immediately visible to me. As Jung (1952) observed, every psychological extreme contains its own opposite. Fortunately, Tim's hidden and sequestered feelings toward greater care and affiliation appeared. In his own way, the evocation in our sessions of Tim's greater humanity became a more visible reference for his future choices with regard to others in his life. I had to continually remind myself that sustained empathy and unconditional positive regard must be directed toward the essential humanity of the person, and that this did not mean that I had to also endorse the choices of that person.

In the beginning of our work together, Tim resented that I did not have any magic solutions for him. He came into therapy expecting that I might have some ability to make him "feel better" without him having to do the hard work of self-examination. I think he felt that if he just "confessed" he would find absolution. Clinicians-in-training are especially susceptible to wanting to respond to a client's appeal for relief. But as Freud observed, the therapist's goal is not to remove suffering but to turn neurotic suffering into normal suffering (as cited in Brenner, 1973). Though the client may indeed experience relief and hope at the commencement of therapy, as the real work of therapy is engaged, things often get worse before they get better. Sometimes

I even share this possibility with a client in the beginning of our work together.

The therapist's task is not to make the client feel better directly but to help the client know himself better. The therapist uses the relationship to disrupt the client's old patterns but also to facilitate the client's ability to flexibly participate in a new encounter, and to be self-reflective and aware in its process. The sustained empathic inquiry of the therapist reactivates the frustrated developmental impulses in the client and serves to reintegrate aspects of the client's potentialities and emotions that have been ignored, repressed, and sectioned off (Kohut, 1984). Becoming more whole and integrated enables the client to become more able to create the life he or she wants. An important point is that "happiness" and "pleasure" emerge as secondary states from an integrated and relationally engaged self that is not debilitated by neuroses. Happiness, like pleasure, cannot be aimed at directly, and if it is, it proves highly elusive.

How is it, then, that therapy makes it possible for the client to change? As mentioned previously, one important aspect is that the therapist must not reenact with the client old problematic patterns but supply a new relational experience. The client will attempt to re-create in his relationship with the therapist the same problematic dynamics that trouble other parts of his life and interpersonal relations. The therapist, however, recognizes the gambit, refuses to play the expected part, and resolves to maintain a sustained empathic attitude of inquiry. When client and therapist explore the resulting relational dynamic in the here-and-now, the client not only gains an experience of something unexpected and new but expands his awareness about how he creates his interpersonal world. When I refused to play my role in punishing or reviling Tim despite behaviors designed to elicit these reactions in me, it evoked the other side of his conflict: the desire for some level of affiliation and affirmation.

Of course, the process of therapy also evokes change by helping to restore to clients *their own capacity* for greater self-understanding, choice, and action. Aiming to directly attack and solve clients' problems rarely proves effective. Understanding and illuminating the principles by which clients create their own reality, however, often leads to the resolution of clients' difficulties. With Tim I gained a lot of practice at not making a "frontal assault" on clients' problems. Perhaps no other client evoked in me as strong a desire to cajole, to direct, to hammer away at his irrational and self-defeating thinking and to control the outcome, especially after he revealed his HIV status.

The judo metaphor applies to many forms of "stepping aside," using the client's own energies to foster discovery and change. One such therapist stance is the "I'm not from around here" attitude (Presbury, Echterling, & McKee, 2002). Essentially, the therapist communicates that it is as if he or she is a newcomer to town, is lost, and needs the client's guidance, illumination, and help in grasping the layout and terrain of the client's inner world. This posture seeks to elicit the client's own resources in uncovering and explicating important self-experiences. It keeps the therapist from hogging the expert role and subverting the client's own growing abilities.

One thing is certain, the therapist cannot *merely explain* clients' problems to them, provide rational and practical solutions to those problems, and expect clients to change. Common sense and logic almost always fail in addressing clients' repetitive problems.

First and Second Order Change

To avoid the pitfall of trying to talk clients out of their difficulties by logic, it is helpful for the therapist to distinguish between first and second order change (Watzlawick, Weakland, & Fisch, 1974). These ideas, first formulated at the Brief Therapy Center of the Mental Institute of Palo Alto, deal with action-oriented approaches to change in complex systems and are an important complement to the therapist's repertoire. The authors observed in their therapy work that common sense and logical approaches to problem resolution often failed and even compounded existing problems. Paradoxically, seemingly illogical and unreasonable actions succeeded in producing the desired change.

First order change happens when change occurs within a system that itself stays invariant. It is change from one behavior to another *within* a given way (or class) of behaving. First order change attempts mostly occur at the level of rationality and logical thought and look like common sense. Different behaviors out of a limited repertoire of possible behaviors may be combined into different sequences, *but these different behaviors always lead to identical outcomes.* First order change is like rearranging the deck chairs on the *Titanic.* With Tim, I found myself wanting to use rational arguments to convince him to change in certain ways that seemed obvious to me. These attempts were mostly unproductive, but they were hard for me to resist because I perceived that some form of problem resolution was urgent.

Part of why first order change is ineffective is that all stable systems (including clients' self-systems and relational systems with others, such as family systems) tend to achieve a homeostatic balance that helps to preserve the existence of the system. In first order change, the problematic homeostatic balance or stability of the client's self-system has not really altered. First order change might represent the client trying on some new behaviors to directly solve a problem. For instance, what could be more sensible to relatives and friends than to try to cheer up a depressed person, to remind him of all the good things he enjoys, and to take him out to a ball game? Such problem solving often appeals to the client's desire for things to fit into existing schemas of thought and self-organization. First order change may add something to the client's repertoire if the client welcomes the addition. But most clients have a pretty good grasp of how the thoughts or behaviors that motivate them to seek therapy are problematic. If his difficulties could be addressed merely by pointing out how they are self-defeating or illogical, or by revealing a better method for living, the client would have discovered it and acted on his own a long time before needing the therapist's help.

First order interventions are easy for the client to fend off or resist because they are so obvious and aim at the client's rational capacities. They essentially say, "Yes, I can see that's a problem, why don't you stop doing that." They rarely shake up the client's world. Clients are motivated to only provisionally accept first order interventions because they are often privately *ambivalent* about changing or giving up repetitive patterns of thought and behavior that, on some level, serve them well. Interventions that aim to merely make logical sense are easy for the client to refute at the logical level. The therapist can't talk the client out of his thoughts, feelings, and problems, no matter how sensible the solution the therapist provides.

Second order change is change that alters the system itself. It is a change in the rules that govern the system, and, therefore, it interrupts the homeostatic balance and repetitive circularity of the system. The Palo Alto authors offer the example that one can do many things in a nightmare: run, scream, hide, or fight, but these first order change behaviors do not alter the fact that they occur within the nightmare. Only by a second order change in state (waking up) can the nightmare end. Second order change often involves a logical jump or discontinuity that is paradoxical, abrupt, and unpredictable. Sometimes second order change relies less on clients' intentionality or insight and more on the effect of systemic disruption and reorganization. I found that my sudden change-ups with Tim sometimes produced second order change. One example was when I abruptly switched from trying to reason with him that it's "better to know" to defending his "right to remain uninformed."

One example from the Palo Alto group involved a married couple and their in-laws. The couple complained that during the husband's parents' visits (which lasted up to three weeks a few times a year) the parents virtually took control of the young couple's lives. The couple made frantic efforts preceding the visits to take care of anything the parents might notice and correct. However, the parents insisted on "helping" in every aspect of running the house (which they had chosen and bought for the couple). The father serviced the cars, maintained the lawn, painted rooms, power washed the deck, and insisted on getting the check at every restaurant outing, and so forth. No matter how much the young couple explained, argued, insisted, and confronted, these sensible first order change interventions produced only greater insistence from the parents. The couple had come to dread the visits.

The therapist listened carefully to the couple's efforts, which had by now become as problematic and misery producing as the parents' behavior, and which were causing significant marital tension. The therapist reasoned that any intervention would have to be in a "language" the parents would interpret as affirming their role as "good parents." The therapist then instructed the young couple that preceding and during the parent's visit, they were to stop cleaning the house, let the lawn and garden go, not clean out the cars, and let the kitchen get dirty with unwashed dishes piling up in the sink. They were not to stock the house with groceries, and any defects in the house, such as burned out light bulbs and dripping faucets, were to be left unattended. When the parents invited the couple to help remedy these situations, the couple was instructed to cheerfully invent excuses for being unable to do so, such as "I'm watching the game . . . I'll be along later," but to praise the parents' efforts. The couple was to encourage the parents to pick up all checks and bills and to generally revert to an intentionally dependent state in relation to the parents. Above all, they were discouraged from making any attempt to get the parents to acknowledge that they had a right to their independence. They were to accept everything the parents did for them as expected and to thank them very perfunctorily.

When the couple returned they explained that the parents had cut their visit short. Before leaving, the father had taken his son aside and told him in friendly but firm terms that the son and his wife were far too pampered and that they had gotten much too accustomed to being waited on and supported by the parents. They felt a little taken for granted, he said. It was high time, the father explained, to behave in a more adult fashion and to become less dependent on them! In other words, instead of overindulging the young couple, the parents now dedicated themselves to the gratifying parental task of weaning them.

The therapist effectively helped the couple to stop repetitively behaving *within* a limited class of behaviors (which had contributed to the perpetuation of the problem) and to change the class of behaviors itself. It is important to realize that these second order changes deal with *what* is happening, not *why* it is happening. The action is here-and-now and not concerned with causality. In other words, there can be change without insight. This is not to say that these second order "nonsensical" and disrupting interventions don't serve as an important component of a parallel process of fostering self-reflective awareness.

It is useful for the therapist to wonder, "What is being done in the here-and-now that perpetuates the client's problem, and what can be done to disrupt the client's repetitive 'solutions'?" The client's solution is often reflective of the "Be spontaneous" paradox. For instance, a man who has trouble falling asleep tries even harder to fall asleep. He says, "I must make myself go to sleep." What is, by its very nature, a nondirected and spontaneous act is addressed by a solution that itself becomes problematic. The obvious second order change intervention would be to instruct the man to attempt, by all means, to stay awake . . . to lift him out of the paradox by a counterparadox that changes the rules of the game. Rational solutions point out the obvious, but the way out of the maze is often through the least obvious opening.

Second order change interventions are difficult for the client to refute because they fly in under the logical radar. They are most often experiences with the therapist that nudge the client off center while at the same time maintaining an empathic connection. Second order change interventions are often events of which the client cannot make any sense, and which are therefore all the more intriguing. The old Zen koan "What is the sound of one hand clapping?" captures something of the disorienting but useful uncertainty that precedes change. A second order change intervention is the pond pebble that falls in any spot but ripples through the whole of the person's consciousness.

Tim had repetitively tried to "get rid of" his depression by a variety of solutions. These solutions had themselves become a problem such as demanding of himself that he "overcome" the depression and "pull himself up by his bootstraps." But these efforts only left him feeling guilty and ineffective. He then resorted to trying to "distract" himself with activities that he later regretted. When I reframed the problem by offering that maybe he needed to become more depressed because his depression stood in for something to which he was not attending, this altered the class of behavior being applied and in a small way helped him out of the paradox of trying to overcome his depression by intentionally "feeling good."

Similarly, when Tim rejected the notion that he had the ability to change or to make a choice, I could sense that he wanted me to take the opposing view. This would have locked us into a power struggle regarding how much change was possible given his "impossible" situation. When I agreed with him, rejecting the notion that there was an acceptable solution and that he had to choose, this evoked in him the other side of his ambivalence—the side that desired efficacy, control, and change.

De Shazer (1984) argues that the counselor's interventions must take into account the client's natural impulse toward homeostasis as well as the client's capacity and motivation for something to change. The counselor's interventions aim to perturb the former and facilitate the latter. The idea is that when one part of a complex system is perturbed, this perturbation has the capacity to affect every other part of the system. De Shazer quotes Maruyama (1963), who contends that a "second cybernetics" operates on principles that later became known as *chaos*, the *butterfly effect,* and *complexity.* The idea is that when a system is given sufficient push or kick in the "right direction," it will enter into a deviation amplifying process resulting in change that is disproportionately large compared to the initial perturbation (Cowan & Presbury, 2000). The metaphor is that a butterfly moves its wings in China, and later there is a hurricane in Florida. There is interconnectedness at all levels of the system, and a therapist-induced change at one level, however small, may resonate at other levels of the system not specifically targeted. Although this may feel disorienting to both therapist and client, the desire for something concrete after inducing confusion often serves to set up a climate of acceptance for new opportunities and interventions.

The therapist may, however, have to do something a little more perturbing than flap the butterfly wings of his empathic listening to offer optimal influence on the client's self-system. If we assume, as in Tim's case, that clients want change but no change is happening, then the therapist has not introduced sufficient perturbation to the system. The therapist has not offered a "difference that makes a difference." Strangely, when I nodded off on Tim, this initiated a series of interventions, discussions, and changes in our relationship that I could not have predicted. This initial disruption led to further opportunities to participate and intervene at different levels (cognitive, dream, and relational) of Tim's experiential world. This deviation amplifying process is a feature of second order change.

I found myself wanting to argue with Tim, to refute his decisions and to explain to him his rationalizations and denial. These were first order interventions that he could easily ignore. Second order interventions were aimed at eliciting Tim's ambivalence, subverting his denial processes, and allying with disowned parts of his inner world. Second order interventions also involved confronting the discrepancies and rationalizations of which he was only half aware, or stepping aside and forcing him to work to show me both sides of his conflicts. Sometimes a single word can provoke a second order change: Tim ruminated on my description of his demeanor as "furtive" (which was incongruous with his self-image). What he discovered in his willingness to engage with the "miracle question" surprised him as he created a new picture laden with possibilities. Surprise is a feature only of second order interventions.

Tim reminded me that often the therapist must let go of the idea of "removing" clients' problems and difficulties. Sometimes the best the therapist can do is to help the client discover other alternatives that are more expressive of the client's greater capacity for self-determination. As with many clients where ingrained personality traits contribute to problematic life circumstances, Tim's deep structure personality issues were largely intact at the end or our relatively brief work together. Yet there was second order change as well; his life would not have looked so profoundly different if there had not been.

✂ ✃

The Dance of Nayana

I resemble everyone
but myself, and sometimes see
in shop windows,
    despite the well-known laws
    of optics,
the portrait of a stranger,
date unknown,
often signed in a corner
by my father.

    — "Self-Portrait," A. K. Ramanujan

B reathe, Nayana, breathe!" I said earnestly.
    She reached out the hand that was not clasped to her heaving chest. I took her hand and sat next to her on the couch holding it. I put my other arm around her hunched shoulders. "You're all right," I said confidently, "don't worry . . . take long, deep breaths."

"I . . . I . . . can't," she managed to say between gasps.

"Yes, you can. I'm right here, and you're okay. This will pass in a few moments. Your heart's slowing down as we speak, and you are going to breathe like this. Watch me." She fixed her terrified eyes on me as I took a long, deep breath. I exhaled loudly. "Do as I do. Okay, in . . ." she took a breath, "good! Out . . ."

"I'm . . . going . . . to . . . die!" she gasped.

"No . . . eventually, but not today," I smiled reassuringly. Nayana tried to smile back at the joke out of courtesy but couldn't. "Okay. In . . . out, excellent! Again, together, in . . . out, good! Now you're breathing. You're doing fine, keep going."

She started saying something in Hindi.

"No, English, Nayana."

"My heart!"

"I know. Don't worry. It's slowing down right now. Can you feel it slowing down?" She shook her head, no. "Yes you can. Feel my hand squeeze yours, that's how slow your heart is going to get in just a little while. Feel that?" She nodded quickly, her eyes still fixed on me. I waited a while, keeping a steady rhythm on her hand. "It's slowing down now, isn't it?"

She nodded, "A little. Yes, a little."

"Good, don't forget to breathe." She obediently took another deep breath.

Ten minutes later I was saying, "Now you're doing fine. See. You're all right," I said soothingly.

We sat on the couch together, and slowly Nayana's panic attack passed and resolved into tears. She sobbed as I sat with her for a while trying to offer whatever reassurance I could.

"That's pretty scary isn't it?"

She nodded. "I'm sorry to surprise you," she said remorsefully when she could speak again. "It is so awful. I was in the car, and I didn't know what to do. I was only a few kilometers away when I felt it coming, so I rushed here. I didn't know what else to do. You must have a patient waiting for you."

"No, don't worry. I don't have anyone waiting."

This was Nayana's third panic attack in as many weeks. During these attacks, her heart would race, she would become short of breath, and she would be overcome by a horrible sense of dread, a foreboding feeling that she would die. Although I'm sure she would not agree as she sat there slowly regaining her composure, it looked to me like Nayana was making progress in therapy. At least her anxiety was now closer to the surface, even if it was overwhelming her at times.

Nayana's medical doctor had referred the 27-year-old Indian graduate student to me four months earlier. She complained of stomach and chest pains, headaches, muscle tension, and a variety of gastrointestinal maladies. She seemed to be "falling apart," she said. She reported to her doctor that she had always had minor medical problems, but it seemed as if all of them were happening at once and much more intensely than in the past. Stumped by her symptoms and unable to make a diagnosis (all her tests came back negative), her doctor made a series of referrals to specialists who, likewise, could find nothing wrong with her. Since she had recently returned from a visit to India she even consulted a specialist in exotic parasitic infections but he, too, could find nothing medically wrong with her. There was little question that Nayana was suffering from *something,* so her doctor referred her to a psychiatric resident who took a complete history, noting that Nayana met almost all of the symptom requirements for somatization disorder. He referred her for outpatient therapy and sent her file to me.

When I met Nayana in the waiting room for our first meeting, Ben, her American boyfriend, sat next to her holding her hand protectively. She asked if he could join us for our first meeting, and I agreed. Because of her cultural background, I wondered if Nayana might feel uncomfortable being in a room alone with a strange man.

"I'm not sure we need to be here," Ben explained, taking the lead as we sat down. "Nayana's got something wrong with her that the doctors can't find, and I think they just don't know what to do. It's not like she's crazy or anything. I mean her pain is real."

I nodded in acknowledgment, "Yes," I said to Nayana, "I understand from Dr. Meyers that you have been suffering from a lot of physical problems, and I don't doubt, like Ben said, that your pain is real."

"Oh, it's real all right. I can tell you it's real." She spoke in a lovely resonant voice, made even more interesting by the melodic inflections characteristic of English spoken with an Indian accent. "I have to suffer with it all of the time, and nobody can tell me why I have to do that," she said, holding an upturned palm under her heart, as if to refer to it. "I am not making it up at all." Her round light-brown face was earnest, and her large dark eyes seemed to appeal to me to believe her. Ben reached over and stroked her long, straight jet-black hair.

"I believe you, Nayana. I don't doubt that your pain is real," I said.

"Her *physical* pain," interjected Ben.

"Yes, her physical pain. I have no doubt that you are suffering real physical complaints. I believe you when you say that you have headaches, dizziness, nausea, cramps, stomach problems, and back pain," I recited her symptoms so that they would know I had the specifics. "I don't think for a moment that you are faking."

"Do you think that she's a hypochondriac?" Ben said, persistently. Something about his protectiveness was both amusing and endearing. I could see that he felt she was out of her range of experience with Western health care and was running interference for her.

"Yes, do you think that?" echoed Nayana. "Ben says that's the only reason Dr. Meyers would send me here, because I'm making it all up in my head."

"Nayana, do you often believe that your physical symptoms mean that you have something terribly wrong with you like cancer or a tumor or some disease?" Her eyes got wide.

"No, I don't. Do you think that?" she asked, alarmed.

I shook my head. "I'm not a medical doctor, but, no. So, I don't think you are a hypochondriac."

"What then? Why do I need to come here to meet with you?"

"I'm not sure that you do, but sometimes when a person is really stressed-out or emotionally upset or is troubled at a deep level about important issues in life, those problems can get translated into real physical problems that cause real physical pain. It's not a matter of it being all in your head. You can't separate the body from the heart and mind. Body, mind, and spirit are all just different aspects of the whole person. Often, when a person is out of whack, the trouble can show up anywhere in the system. It's not like the person can intentionally control just how this *imbalance* shows up. I don't know if you feel this might fit with what's happening for you, but it might be something for us to consider."

I wanted to frame what I suspected were her troubles in language that addressed their fears that I might think Nayana was "crazy." This was an explanation for which they were unprepared. Even Ben seemed to pause.

"It's a Western idea," I continued, "that you can split a person up into all these separate parts, separating the mind and body." She began nodding. "In your culture I think there is more attention to keeping them all together, yes?"

"Yes, that's right," she turned to Ben, confirming this.

"So, my question to you would be, and you don't have to talk about this right now" (I was thinking it might be better to wait until Ben was not in the room), "what might be happening in your life or in your private thoughts and feelings that might be troubling you, knocking you off center? Sometimes these troubles are not so discrete and go pretty deeply and the person can only describe a little part at any given time. Also, sometimes it helps to wonder, 'Why is this happening now?'"

They turned and looked at one another significantly but said nothing.

"I gather from your faces that you are thinking of something."

"I can think of many things," Nayana said in her musical voice, clearly articulating every word. "One thing is that we are having many troubles together right now because soon I am supposed to return to India, and Ben would not be able to go with me. My family says I cannot stay here in the U.S. It is very upsetting to us. We would like to marry, but my family is strict Hindu, and they say I cannot marry anyone but a Hindu person." She looked over at Ben. He was frowning. "I always thought that I would obey my family, but I have been in the U.S. for four years now and I would like to be able to make my own decision. But this is very hard." Her eyes suddenly brimmed with tears. "My family does not understand this. I live with my uncle, and he tells my family *everything* that I am doing here. It is this way in Indian families. They are very close, you know."

"Naturally, I want her to make her own decision," Ben said, taking her hand, "to do what she wants so that we can marry. I'm Jewish, so I know what it's like when parents want their kid to marry someone with the same faith and culture, but my family loves Nayana. They're crazy about her. They would love it if we married. We're hoping her family can adjust, and if not, well, I know it would be hard for her, but you can't let your family control your life forever."

"Ben's family is very good to me," Nayana confirmed. "I think they were a little suspicious at first, you know, but I am very close to Mrs. Zimmerman."

"No, they weren't suspicious of you," Ben said with a wide grin, "they loved you from the instant they met you. And Dad loves you too, he thinks your nose ring is exotic." Nayana laughed and smiled back warmly. These two were clearly very attached to one another. I enjoyed the feeling of bright, fresh romantic love in the room.

"So, it's very hard for you both. You both know what you want, but there are pretty serious obstacles to overcome before you can be together." It seemed clear to Ben, and at the time to me, that the plan for therapy would entail encouraging Nayana to voice her feelings and her new independence to her family. It was clear to the American men in the room what was supposed to happen.

"I don't know if we can overcome the obstacles," Nayana said.

"Don't worry," Ben reassured her, "we will."

"So, you think that my body is sick because my mind is troubled? They are talking to one another but not with my voice?" Nayana said, turning back to me. I liked her perceptive explanation.

"I don't know. Maybe it would be better to say that maybe your body is expressing some feelings and conflicts that are hard for you to experience directly or to put into words."

"What do I do?"

"Well, one thing is that you could come here each week, two times a week to start, and we could talk together and see if that's true. After a month or so you can tell me if you think our talks help you."

She looked at Ben. He smiled and tilted his head, as if to say, "You might as well give it a try." So Nayana entered therapy with both of us wondering how she might be somatisizing whatever distress was not finding a more direct and conscious expression.

———

"I don't know what to say. How do I begin?" Nayana asked at our next meeting. She must have felt safe with me, as she had come to the appointment alone.

"Why don't you begin by telling me all about yourself so I can get to know you better as a person."

Nayana paused for a moment and then offered a very articulate account of what she thought was most relevant. She explained that she came from an upper-middle-class family in Bombay. Her father is a businessman, and her mother raised the children. She has two older brothers who are also college educated in Indian universities. One works in computer software, the other as a civil servant. Her family is not wealthy, but they are comfortable. They are all very committed to their Hindu faith, she explained. Her parents are very committed to the idea of immediate and extended family staying in close proximity.

Nayana came to the United States to attend graduate school in both civil engineering and architecture. She excelled in her studies and was about to graduate with her master's degrees in each of these fields. Her parents recognized that Nayana, at a very early age, demonstrated an extraordinary talent for mathematics, science, and anything that involved solving technical problems. (She had recently taken an IQ test and scored in the top 1 percent for these sorts of technical abilities. This contrasted with her verbal reasoning skills, which were "only" above average.) Her parents invested significant time and energy cultivating her special abilities and nurturing her talents. Their expectations were very high, and Nayana always met those expectations, often pushing aside her own desires in order to achieve and excel.

"I felt like I was different from the other girls," she said. "I rarely played or had free time because I was always working and studying."

"It seems like there was a lot of pressure on you to make the family proud, carry the family banner, even more than your brothers."

"Yes, because I had this special talent. That is normal for us. If you are a middle-class Indian family, education is everything. It is your way to get ahead, especially in the technical fields. And yet I always knew that I was supposed to get married and have children too. I think even my parents did not know, still do not know, which is more important to them. It is as if they want me to do it all, but I am only one person, you know."

"So that's a lot to carry. That must have been hard for you to reconcile, those two conflicting expectations. How do you feel about it now? Which is more important to you, career or marriage and children?"

She moved her head in that uniquely Indian side-to-side wobble that indicates that one is faced with insoluble mysteries. She seemed to have few words for expressing her feelings about it.

Nayana's parents were reluctant to allow her to attend graduate school in the United States for fear of her becoming "Americanized." She gently persisted, and they relented when it became apparent that scholarships would pay her tuition and she could live with her uncle who promised to keep a close eye on her. The prestige of graduating from an American graduate program and the status this would confer on her and the family tipped the scales in favor of allowing her to leave India. She was sent abroad, she said, with a clear understanding that she would return to India to be near the family, accept an appropriate husband, have children, and eventually serve the family and her homeland with her new credentials.

All had gone according to plan at first. Although Nayana disliked much of what she experienced in American culture, she quickly discovered that she reveled in the extraordinary freedom she had as a woman on a college campus. Though Nayana lived with her uncle's traditional and strict family, she was free during the day to structure her time, activities, and social life as she chose.

Two years into her studies, she met Ben. He was intelligent, warm, and respectful of her newfound autonomy. He introduced her to his warm and caring family. Soon, secretly, because she could not reveal the relationship to her uncle, she began dating Ben. A few months into the courtship she had her first sexual experiences when she and Ben became lovers. She bashfully explained that she experienced some guilt over this compromise of her religious and family values. She was, she explained, expected to be a virgin on her wedding day. But she felt fulfilled in her emotional and sexual connection with Ben, and in her new culture it all seemed acceptable and normal. Ben was a sensitive and affectionate partner. Her feelings of guilt about being sexually involved and that she was deceiving her family gradually subsided as her connection with Ben became even closer. She began to fantasize about marrying Ben and staying in the United States, and she even convinced herself that her family might accept this arrangement.

"Then came the letter," she said.

"The letter?"

"The letter saying that since I would be coming home soon my father has arranged for me to be introduced to a number of eligible men. These, of course, are possible marriage partners who are from good families my father knows. He said they are waiting to meet me and that everyone is happy that soon I would return. It also said that I should listen to my uncle because they were unhappy to hear that I was spending time unsupervised with a Jewish boy. They said they hoped I was behaving like a true Hindu girl should do. They do not like that I would spend time with a man, especially a non-Hindu. My father, he is very stubborn. My cousin told my uncle about Ben, and he told my parents. Now they want me to come home to marry. They are waiting."

"So, even though you come from an upper-middle-class and educated family, your parents still expect that you will have an arranged marriage?" I had a hard time imagining that this bright articulate woman who in many ways seemed thoroughly modern had so little say in her own life choices.

"Oh, yes." From how I framed my observation she picked up its underlying values and went on to explain, "But it's not like it used to be, where you don't even know the groom. Now they introduce you to different men, you know, and you are expected to eventually find one who is acceptable."

I thought that these improvements to the system still left a long way to go. "But the parents of both groom and bride are still involved, proposing the mate?" I had a skeptical expression on my face.

She was amused by my expression. "Oh, yes, very much so. It is a marriage, in some ways, between families and not to be undertaken lightly. Perhaps it is a little more traditional in my family than in many Indian families. Some women in India have remarkable freedom. It all depends on the class and the family. But my family is very conservative."

"So how do you deal with that? It must be very hard for you after you have experienced the freedom you have as a woman here to contemplate going back into a more constricted role."

"Yes and no. My culture is very rich, and the closeness of the family and between families is a great blessing. In America, I meet many people who feel isolated like they have no family. It is remarkable how people live *alone*. In my culture, you are hardly ever alone," she laughed a wonderful throaty laugh, "everyone is always into your business! It is impossible to get away and be by yourself like you can do here. But you feel safe too, and a part of a community. I never thought that I could marry an American boy until I met Ben. He is wonderful, and he comes from a family like an Indian family . . . very close. I suppose I never expected to fall in love! It was not in my plan, you know?"

"Yeah, sometimes it is unexpected."

"But where I come from it is only unexpected in the movies. It's fine if it is just a story and everyone says, 'Oh, isn't it a wonderful thing.' But don't try to make it happen in real life!"

"So now you have a real dilemma. You either go back to India soon . . ."

"Within the next five months."

"Okay. Or you stay here where you have more independence and the freedom to be with Ben and try to convince your family to accept this very different picture of their daughter's life." I thought as I said this that my own biases were leaking out everywhere in our conversation. Independence, autonomy, freedom, self-determination, these were all assumptions and ideals that I took for granted as psychological achievements. But in Nayana's culture I had to remind myself, these were not the ideals that served the values of service, family, community, and obligation.

"Exactly. That is my dilemma. Stay here with Ben, or go back to India and meet those men my father has waiting and eventually marry one of them."

"And how are you leaning?" I began trying to keep my "values" questions as neutral as possible.

"I have been thinking that I must stay with Ben. I don't know how I can go back. I don't know how I could leave Ben. He would eventually find another, and I cannot think how I would feel about it."

"Well, let's talk about that. How do you feel when you think of staying with Ben here in the U.S."

"Very good and very bad. Good because I would be with him and his family. But my family will be very, very mad. Very mad," she said again, shaking her head. "They will think I have betrayed them. They will not accept that I marry a Jewish man who is not even an Indian. They might try to come here and force me to go back with them. If I did not come, they would say very bad things." She shifted in her seat nervously.

"What might they say?"

"They might say that . . ." She stopped. She seemed stuck. It was like her mouth suddenly went into "pause" mode. The defense of "isolation of thought" was so obvious that I was startled. I waited. She seemed blank. I prompted her.

"You were saying that what your parents might say about you is hard for you to put into words." I realized as I said it that I probably should have respected her effort to defend against whatever was too anxiety producing for her to say. Too late.

She began wringing her hands, her face became worried, and suddenly she grew *very* agitated. She looked like she wanted to jump out of her skin. "Doctor Cowan, I have to go now. I should not have come here. I should not have talked badly about my family to you. That was wrong." She got up and grabbed her coat, and walked toward the door.

"Nayana, please stay. You're upset. We don't have to talk about it."

She paused considering, "Thank you, I must go, I must go."

I could see that I wasn't going to be able to stop her without physically restraining her. "Nayana, I will see you the day after tomorrow at our time," I said definitively. She did not respond to my statement but was too educated in courtesy to simply walk out.

"Thank you very much," she nodded, and then walked briskly through the door.

"What the hell was that?!" I wondered, standing alone in the middle of the room, shaking my head, trying to figure out the exact trigger. It was like a switch had been thrown. Was it what her family would say to her if she asserted her independence and married the man she wanted to? Or was it the tenor of the whole discussion of freedom, autonomy, defiance of her parent's wishes? She had said that it was wrong of her to talk badly of her family. How had she talked badly about them? Clearly whatever was going on in one part of her thoughts and feelings was forbidden by another part. I could see that I was dealing with a whole different set of internalized cultural reference points that I would have to understand more fully.

I had always had a fascination for India and its cultural and religious traditions, had read the *Bhagavad-Gita* three times, planned to eventually travel there. But what did I *really* know about what it was like to live inside the culture and to have that culture as part of the very structure of my psyche? Her culture was the metanarrative that permitted what was possible in her personal story; I had some idea of it but would need to better understand how it shaped Nayana's perception of herself.

One thing I did know. There was a rift in the continuity of Nayana's self-experience that mirrored the gulf between the two cultures she sought to bridge in her love with Ben. "East is East, and West is West, and never the twain shall meet," seemed to describe not only the vast differences in worldview between two cultures but between the areas of her own identity as she participated in these two entirely different worlds.

I was relieved and pleased when Nayana appeared in the waiting room for our next session. When I met her, she was wearing a beautiful and flowing crimson sari. She wore sandals and ankle bracelets, and there were rings on her toes. Little bells tinkled from her wrist bracelets as she moved. I smiled as we walked down the hall, and I heard the delicate tinkling behind me. We entered the office, and she smiled and shook her wrists a little as I stepped back to admire her costume. Her black hair was pulled back and tied with a decorative band of silk, and her clear complexion was subtly made up with traditional Indian cosmetics that heightened the effect of her already large dark eyes. She smelled of sandalwood perfume. No wonder Ben was smitten! She had appeared rather plain in her T-shirt, blue jeans, and tennis shoes at our first meeting. She explained that she was dressed for an Indian traditional dance, which she was going to perform with some other students at a cross-cultural fair on campus. She was going there after our meeting. We settled into our chairs and talked of her costume and her upcoming dance for a while.

"Perhaps you would like to come to a dance sometime. You will learn a lot about Indian culture," she offered.

"I'd like that," I said.

I knew that after these easy subjects she would look to me to set the agenda, and for this session I was happy to do so. "Nayana, last session we talked about your feeling torn between two worlds that make very different demands on you. Actually, it helps me to see you dressed like this today, to see aspects of those two worlds represented in your clothes between last week and this. But last week you became very anxious and needed to leave our session early." She nodded bashfully.

"I'm sorry. I didn't mean to be rude." She made a deprecating gesture with her arm.

"I didn't think you were rude; I thought you were very distressed about thoughts and feelings that seemed to come to you as we talked."

"Yes, there are many things that I should not think about because they are not good; they upset me."

"And what do you do when troubling things upset you like that?"

"I try to not think bad things. I try to think of something good and positive to avoid getting a negative attitude. A negative attitude is very bad. I concentrate on my studies so I can get something done."

Good, bad, positive, negative, upset. I realized that these impoverished and sterile words stood in for Nayana's masked feelings. I had not heard Nayana use any emotionally descriptive words like sad, angry, bewildered, pensive, hopeful. She may be a technical genius, I thought, but what had happened to her emotional world?

"Nayana, let's reflect on your experience of needing to leave last week." She shifted in her seat nervously. The bells tinkled. She nodded her assent. "Describe to me when you first felt very uncomfortable and anxious."

"I don't know, it happened so fast. That happens to me sometimes. I know that I felt bad that I had said bad things about my family. And right after that I said how I wanted to stay here with Ben against their wishes."

"Okay, so it seemed that you could talk about your life and family in India very affectionately. And it also seemed that you could talk about Ben, your love together, and about liking your freedom here, but when . . ."

"But when I talk about them together, at the same time," she interjected, suddenly animated, "it upsets me very much. I never do that! When I am with Ben, I try not to think about all those other things. I don't think about my parents and what will happen. I don't think bad things about them. It is like I am in a pretend world, you know, and Ben and I can be there together. But it is over here," she reached with her arm as far as she could to one side and touch the arm of the couch, "and this other life is over here," she did the same thing on the other side.

"You keep them apart."

"Oh, yes. Very separated. They must be. Otherwise I would not be able to be with Ben."

"Now I'm going to ask you something a little harder. You say that last week that sense of needing to get away came on you suddenly," she nodded. "Let's explore some of the feelings you were having right before that. What can you recall?"

She nodded, and paused. "I felt a little nauseous, and that always worries me. I am sometimes afraid when that happens that I will vomit."

"That would be very embarrassing, wouldn't it?"

"Oh, yes. I would be very ashamed. I felt a little dizzy too."

"Okay. So you were having those physical sensations. What emotions were you having?"

She paused and reflected. This appeared to be more difficult for her. "I don't know, maybe I was afraid about what will happen if I stay here with Ben."

"Afraid. Okay, that's one that's right there that you can get to easily. Keep reflecting, you're doing well," I encouraged.

She paused. She shook her head.

"Okay, let's do a little experiment." I thought she might resonate to framing our interaction like this. She nodded. "When your cousin broke your secret and told your uncle about Ben, and your uncle immediately told your parents, how did you feel?"

"Ashamed," she said instantly. Okay, another experience that was close to the surface and, I noted, one that was safe because it was a "negative" feeling directed toward herself, not disruptive to others or directed outward. It obviously endorsed her sense that she was doing forbidden things.

"Okay, and what about your feelings toward each of them."

She paused. "I didn't like that my cousin did that. I was upset. It was a secret. You should not break a secret." Now she was concentrating on the technical issue of breaking a promise.

"So when she *betrayed* that secret," I continued prompting, "did you feel something *toward* her?"

She paused. She looked hesitant, and she averted her eyes. "I suppose I was very *angry* with her. And I was angry with my uncle for telling my parents."

"What did you do when you felt that anger?"

"I went to my room and *wanted* to cry, but I share that room with Gita, so I just worked on my studies. Then I felt bad at being so mad at little Gita, so I took her to the movies." She said this without the least bit of irony.

"Did you say to either of them your feeling of being angry or sad?"

"Oh, no!"

"That's not allowed?"

"Maybe to my cousin, but not to my uncle. I am a guest, so I don't say anything to anyone that would be bad."

"So you had angry feelings that you couldn't express because it would be ungrateful to your host," she nodded, "and you had sad feelings that you dealt with by studying," she continued nodding, "and you feel that you must keep your love for Ben a secret for fear of discovery. Nayana, I'm wondering where in your life it had been safe to express your emotions?"

She pondered this, a confused look on her face. "Do you think this is why I am sick all of the time?"

"I'm noticing that before you describe your emotions you name what is happening in your body. Nausea, dizziness." She reflected on this silently. "How about with Ben, do you share your inner thoughts and feelings with him?"

"Oh, yes." Then, "To a point," she corrected. "He does not want to hear too much about my family's desire for me to come home. He wants me to make my own decisions and do what I want to do. He sees more of the American me. He does not understand what that means to have my family's expectations, what I would have to give up if I tell them I will do what I please."

"So you don't push that. It becomes invisible."

"Yes, that is very, very true. With my family, my real life here in the U.S. becomes invisible. With Ben, my life in India becomes invisible."

"And as you try to satisfy all of them, you become invisible to yourself, your feelings and thoughts become lost to you as you seek to please them all. How do you do it? It sounds exhausting," I said softly.

Her large dark eyes became very wide as I was saying this. Suddenly they brimmed with tears, and she began crying. "I don't know how I do it. I can't do it anymore."

"Okay, Nayana, let's work on this a little," I said, gently. "What are you feeling right now?"

"I'm crying."

"Yes, but what are you feeling."

"Upset."

"That's not a feeling. It's safe to say *whatever* you want in here. It's like no other place in the world for saying things, because no one else can know what you say." I had the sense that her emotional life had become dammed up because different parts of it were either compatible or not in her different relationships. Each valued relationship variously required that some aspects of her experience be elaborated and other aspects hidden. Her physical symptoms seemed to contain these conflicts and to express the squelched and forbidden emotions that disrupted her different relationships. The appearance of her tears was a very good sign.

"I suppose I am sad. Very, very sad," She whispered. Ah, that was a good start.

"Okay, tell me about that sadness, say *everything* that comes to mind about it, no matter how silly, scary, or ugly it seems."

Nayana did. In fact, she surprised me with her ability to give voice to her inner world. She was not nearly as unskilled as I has supposed. Rather, she seemed only to lack the complete interpersonal receptivity she required to risk such disclosure.

She cried as she described the hopelessness she felt about resolving others' competing expectations and the sense that no matter how much she achieved it was not enough. She cried because she missed her family and because they had made her the family standard bearer when she just wanted to belong. She cried because no one understood how she could not do it all: have a career, a marriage, children. She did not know how to balance her desire for freedom with her desire for duty and filial obligation. She wanted to marry the man she loved, and she wanted to go home. There was no way out.

Just before she met Ben, she revealed, she had been bulimic for a short while and then had stopped eating almost entirely. She lost 20 pounds. After she met Ben, she felt happy and content. But as her final year in the United States progressed, the reality of her predicament asserted itself into her secret and insulated life with him. Time was running out. She suddenly felt like a stranger in a very strange land. It was as if her "Indian self" became larger and larger and competed with the Nayana she had become through her new experiences with Ben in America. She was sobbing now.

"Then I just started getting more and more ill. The sicker I got, the less I could do my work. I'm not even sure I can graduate unless I catch up, and I don't know why I'm getting sicker."

"Nayana, as I listen to you there are a number of good reasons for you to get sick. Let me ask you something. What physical complaints are you feeling at this moment . . . nausea, dizziness?"

"No. Nothing. Just very sad and unhappy."

"Exactly. That's good." She looked up at me confused. Her makeup had run down her cheeks in long lines, as if the stream of color had drained from the reservoir of her dark iris.

"It's good that I'm unhappy and sad?"

"Yes, it's good that you're unhappy and sad, not ill. Unhappy is honest and direct and expresses what you really feel."

"I don't want to be unhappy."

"Of course not, but you are unhappy sometimes, and when you express it like this in this safe place, speaking to all the parts of your feelings, you don't need to trade your tears for being sick."

She nodded. "I think you are right. It is hard to do that though. I don't like to be unhappy and sad. You don't know, because I am caught between in too many expectations."

"You're right. I can't fully understand, but I see that you are trying to stand in your own ground and reconcile your Indian self and your American self. At the same time you are trying to honor all the people you love. You want to be able to please them all and have that be okay."

"That's exactly right," she said. "But nobody understands that. Even Ben cannot fully understand that. He loves me too much to see the other side." She took a tissue and began to wipe her face. "I have ruined my makeup, how will I dance?"

I liked the metaphor. "Perhaps it would be okay to see you, the dancer in the dance."

She got it. "I will stand out too much. You must fit in with the others."

"Is there any part where you are free to make up your own dance?"

"At some part, each dancer takes turns and comes forward to the center while the others move back. Then you can do something that you have made up while the others do the steps together."

"Ah!"

"But that is just a dance," she smiled, "but maybe someday in life too."

I tried, unsuccessfully, to mimic her Indian head gesture in response, and she laughed at me, then put her hand to her mouth for fear she might offend me. But she was still smiling.

"Nayana," I said at our next meeting, "you mentioned that unless you feel better soon you might not be able to graduate." It was our sixth session. Nayana's physical symptoms had already started to moderate significantly as she gave voice to her inner world in our talks. But I felt some resistance emerging around her giving up more of her symptoms.

"Yes, I'm behind for the first time with some projects," she said, "I have been feeling good a lot more, but then I sometimes feel too tired and ill to work all the time."

"And what happens if you do not graduate right now?"

She shrugged. "It just means that I have to stay until it's finished, maybe another semester at the most."

I decided to risk an interpretation that I had been pondering. "So if you are sick enough and you can't work, the whole issue of what happens next is put on hold. You don't go back to India, and you have a legitimate reason to stay with Ben for a little while longer. That sounds to me like a powerful incentive to stay ill. What do you think about that? Do you think that what I have just said could describe a part of what's happening for you?"

"You mean that on the one hand I don't want to be ill because I feel bad, but I do want to be ill because it keeps me with Ben?"

I shrugged. "What do you think?"

"I love Ben very much. It's true that I would rather be with him sick than not at all."

"But at this time I hear that you don't want outright to say that you are not going back to India. You are not sure enough to go that far."

"I cannot say that right now, even though that is what I want to say to my family. I only want to say it if they will accept it. I don't want to say it if they tell me . . . if they tell me I can no longer be their daughter." She put her hand to her mouth, as if she would have preferred that those words not have been said.

"Ah . . . those are very high stakes indeed." I said, softly.

She nodded, keeping her hand to her lips.

In the following sessions Nayana and I continued to organize our efforts around a central theme: we went hunting for squelched and forbidden affects. We searched for those feelings that were hiding, cut off, reclusive, and shy. This process between us seemed revolutionary to her as we wondered aloud together, and I helped her to uncover and give words to parts of her emotional life that were merely waiting for a unconditionally supportive climate to become revealed. She reported that after our sessions she felt relieved and even happy for the rest of the day. Sometimes she felt better for the day or two after the sessions. She wanted more of that. But soon the sense of dread would creep up on her again, and she felt the foreboding oppression.

As the sessions progressed, I realized that Nayana's translation of emotion into symptoms was more accessible to scrutiny and analysis, less "deep structure," than most clients who tended to somatize their conflicts. Her feelings were not buried so deeply or inaccessibly as I had supposed. Nayana's complaints coincided with the impending crisis looming in her life, the time when she would be forced to choose between her life of freedom in the United States with Ben and her constrained but emotionally connected family life in the homeland where she felt more grounded in her culture and religion.

Nayana remarked that my interpretation about the "secondary gain" as one part contributing to her physical symptoms made a lot of sense the more she thought of it. "I would do almost anything to stay with him," she said, "even make myself sick."

As we talked and she was able to address many of the emotions that had been waiting for a receptive and fertile relational soil, these emerging feelings increasingly took root in her own consciousness. She began to journal as well as to record her dreams. She brought both to the sessions, and they became richer as time passed. She was able to speak to her feelings of longing for her family while simultaneously expressing her resentment that her desired connection with them came at the price of the freedom she had learned to cherish. She spoke of her grief at the losses that were soon to come regardless of which way she chose, the path of self-determination, and choices in love, or the way of cooperation and affiliation and duty in family and marriage. As her inner world became more elaborated, so did our relationship. It felt more and more like we were partners. And always we could feel the looming crisis as the time for her expected return to India approached, the time by which she must make a decision that would change her life forever.

I must admit that I had to constantly monitor my own impulses to sway her to assert her independence. I sympathized with her desire to be free to create her own life, and I had to be careful to be empathic about the losses she would incur if she chose this route. I had to be careful to not see her father as overbearing and despotic and accept that, though Nayana experienced her father as stubborn, she also saw him as a model of devotion and caring. In her eyes he was doing what any good father would do from within his own cultural frame of reference.

One session Ben joined us. He was clearly getting nervous about what might happen as he began to understand just how deeply Nayana would be affected even if she did stay with him in the United States. I felt for him as he began to understand the dimensions of her predicament, began to admit to himself that there was a danger of losing her. Nayana's parents had written to say that they intended to come to her graduation and to help her get ready for the move back to India. They also wanted to visit her uncle and his family.

But Ben had a plan. He wanted to introduce Nayana's parents to his own so that their families could meet in the hope of easing the news that he and Nayana hoped to wed. We all discussed the possibilities, and the lovers looked to me for suggestions about how they might manipulate the situation. Together we schemed. I felt a little like Friar Lawrence in *Romeo and Juliet,* trying to circumvent impossible barriers or distill some potion that would get around the obstacles and free the young lovers to be together. But I had no potions, and Nayana and Ben had to reconcile themselves to the fact that the best they could do was to invite her parents to meet Ben and his family in the hope that this person-to-person contact might soften the strong resistance they expected to encounter. Nayana said she did not know if her parents would even agree to such a meeting. She pointed out that inviting them to meet Ben's family also meant revealing to her parents that she had defied their wishes and had pursued a relationship without anyone's knowledge or consent. She was ready to do this, but she was worried because such a disclosure indicted her uncle. His stewardship of his niece should have been such as to prevent her from such a deep connection. This could create some upset in the family and cause her uncle to become embarrassed and ashamed that he had not fulfilled his promise to appropriately watch over his niece. This was complicated!

One session, a few weeks later, Nayana reported this dream. "I was walking down my street at home in India. But on this street there was a wonderful temple, and my house was next to it, which is not true in real life. As I approached the end of the road, I saw a huge tornado coming down the center of the street from the other end. I watched in terror as it destroyed one house after another in a row. Then it would go to the other side of the street and destroy the buildings there. I thought, 'There is no way it will destroy my house; my house is too strong and God will protect it.' All the people were fleeing into the temple for safety. Then the tornado crossed the street and came to my house, and I was terrified because it started ripping my house to pieces. I was so afraid. Then it stopped. Then I saw with amazement that the temple was the only structure on the street left standing. I ran to where my house had been but all that remained was the foundation. I walked around inside where the rooms used to be. I was looking for my room, but I fell down a hole where the stairs had gone to the cellar. The dark cellar was now filled with water and debris, and it was swirling around and around. I cried out for help. I was being sucked down, and just as I thought 'I am going to drown!' the dream switched. I was suddenly riding in a car along a dirt road. I never looked to see who was the driver of the car. The car turned off the main road and went up and up a long hill. It seemed like it went up forever, but it finally stopped just before the final crest of the hill. I got out of the car, and there was an old man with a shovel. I asked him, 'What are you doing with that shovel?' and he smiled and nodded toward the crest of the hill. I walked up to the top, and I saw that I was on the highest mountain in a whole long range of mountains as far as I could see. I could see forever from that spot. I looked down at the ground, and I saw that a new ditch had been dug to put a new foundation for a house. I thought, 'This house is meant for me!' It had been prepared for me."

What a rich and multilayered dream! And how relevant to the circumstances of her life and therapy. I asked Nayana for her associations with the images and events. We didn't need to look far for the tornado; she was clear that all of the emotions that we had been evoking and exploring were like a huge storm. Her physical symptoms had lessened significantly, but she alternated between feeling relieved and being even more anxious and fragmented.

"And this storm, in coming down the center of the street, it's like it's tearing apart the two different sides of my life. Going from one side to the other."

Yes, the tornado had destroyed her personal house, a metaphor for the familiar structures of her inner life that were changing and being dismantled as her emotions became more accessible. But the temple, that larger and stronger structure of culture, faith, and belonging was left intact. The powerful metanarrative could not be buffeted by these storms. Did this mean that there was safety within for the dislodged aspects of her self-experience—all the people running to take shelter? When she stumbled into the cellar of her old house, the forces that still threatened to suck her under were waiting.

"I thought, even though my house is destroyed, I will die in it. I was always afraid to go down into that basement as a little girl."

The vortex of water swirled with the debris of her anxieties, her fears, her conflicting emotions and loyalties, and threatened to drown her. But she managed to transform her crisis of being "sucked under" into a journey. In this journey she was not being sucked downward but was ascending higher and higher.

"The man standing there with the shovel, he seems to know that you are coming," I observed.

"Yes, he had prepared the site even before I got there, even before I knew I might build a house up there, you know."

"So what comes to mind when you think of that old man?" I was thinking, "This is a part of you that anticipates what you need as you seek to build new houses in your inner life."

"You do," she said without hesitation in her distinctive Indian inflection. "You are always digging around," she chided, wagging her finger at me. "You are always preparing the site!"

Nayana had fully engaged in her therapy and was making huge strides. She had come to understand my role and what I could offer her as she looked for a new foundation for her life. I had my trusty shovel ready. But then something happened.

Two sessions later Nayana reported that she had been driving and had become lost in what should have been familiar terrain.

"I know the city. I don't understand it. It was as if everything looked like it should, but I did not know where I was or where to go. It was terrifying. I didn't know which way to turn. I asked someone how to get to a certain place, but they had never heard of that place so they didn't know either. I began to get panicky. I have never been this lost. I had to stop and call Ben, and he came and got me, and he couldn't understand why I would get lost in that place. I went to his house and cried and cried. You see what this therapy is doing to me! I cannot even remember where I am."

Her sense of dislocation made sense to me. Nayana's relief in our work not only evoked the sad, painful, and anxious aspects of her struggle but also left her feeling lost and disoriented.

As the time approached for her to either leave for India or announce to her parents her intention to marry Ben, she became more and more fragile. Then she had her first panic attack. It happened when she was shopping in a big department store.

"I was going to buy a gift for my mother, and a feeling came over me, and I knew I was in trouble." She had to sit on a bench and wait until her breathing and heart rate became normal again. But this event combined with her previous experience of becoming lost made her reluctant to leave the house.

The second attack happened a week later. I gave her a referral to a psychiatrist to consult about a medication to help control the attacks during this delicate phase of our work together. I didn't want her shutting down her involvement with therapy under the assumption that "putting the lid back on" would prevent future attacks. Apparently the medication was not enough.

"So what was happening right before you had the attack?"

"I was just driving, and I was reminding myself not to miss that exit or I couldn't turn around for a long time, and as I looked for it I thought, 'Did I already miss it?' and I began to get shaky and nervous, and then it happened, and I couldn't breathe. I pulled over, but it didn't get any better. I felt as if I would die. I just lay down on the seat and I thought, 'They will find me here dead!' Now I don't want to go anywhere without Ben."

"Does Ben take you everywhere now?"

"No, because he can't really come to my uncle's house. I have to drive myself. But now I'm afraid to leave the house."

"But you find yourself relying on him more when you are together?"

"Yes, I do. That morning I received another letter from my father. He is making the arrangements for their trip and to prepare for me to come home. I think I want to be with Ben all of the time because it seems like . . . I don't know."

"It's happening, isn't it? The two paths are coming to a single intersection." She nodded. "What are you telling Ben about what you intend?"

"Our hopes are in the meeting of our families. I have not said what will happen if it does not go well. I fear it will not. I think Ben assumes that even if it does not go well that I will stay here with him, but he knows better now that it is very hard, very hard, and he is uncertain what will happen. I don't know what I will do."

The following week, 10 days before her family was due to arrive from India, she was stricken with yet another panic attack.

"Breathe, Nayana, breathe!" She clasped my hand.

Nayana was, as she said, "in the jaws of the tiger." Though she was now better able to articulate in our sessions what was happening in her inner world of thoughts and feelings, and though her physical symptoms had drastically reduced, her crisis was upon her.

Nayana brought Ben to her session two days before her parents were to arrive. They described how Ben's family was prepared to have Nayana's family to dinner. Nayana discussed how she would wait until halfway through their visit to broach the subject of her relationship with Ben and her desire to marry him. For his part, Ben was prepared to move to India if that should be the only impediment to their being together.

Nayana invited me to attend a multicultural fair the following week where she would be dancing. Many of her family and friends in the Indian community of San Diego would be there. She said she would like to introduce me to her parents. Apparently they had been informed that Nayana was seeing me to, as she had described it to them, "help her cope with her medical complaints."

On the Saturday afternoon of the fair, Balboa Park was alive with activity, music, and people from all over the world. I wandered through the stalls and exhibits and past the demonstrations and performances. Mingling smells of spices floated on the air from tables filled with food from various countries. I sampled as many as I could before I went to the stage where Nayana was scheduled to begin. Most of the women, young and old, wore saris, the men wore plain white shirts and baggy trousers and sandals. All of them spoke with Nayana's voice and intonation. I was delighted to hear that the music would be live as a tabla drum began playing, a sitar began singing a melody, and the other instruments whose names I didn't know joined in. The dancers emerged from the tent and onto the low stage. Nayana was there. How graceful they were as they danced to the exotic sounds and rhythms. How beautiful the women's garments and movements were as their limbs undulated fluidly in unison. The audience applauded gratefully.

In the middle of the final dance, first one, then another, of the dancers moved from the group into the center and danced alone. Each improvised her own unique dance, apart from the others. Nayana moved forward, and as her head came up and her arms unfolded, she saw me sitting near the front of the stage. She smiled happily. She seemed perfectly at ease. I had the impression that she seemed so in context, so "fit" with all of her surroundings in her beautiful garments with these people. I remembered our conversation about the metaphor of the dance, how it is both individual and collectively expressive, and I knew as we caught each other's eye that she remembered it too. She was in the center now, and she danced beautifully, improvising expressively, her arms, like reeds, bending gracefully, perfectly in tune with the half note scales and rhythms of the players. Then she moved back and merged with the other dancers once again. I knew then what her decision would be if her parents did not approve of her marriage to Ben.

After the dance Nayana came over to me with her father and mother on each arm. She introduced us, and they were aglow with pride after their daughter's performance.

"Thank you very much," her father said sincerely, with his daughter's same crisp enunciation and intonation. He continued to hold my hand after our handshake, "Thank you very much for what you have done for our daughter. She has been having many troubles coping with her sickness." Nayana's mother nodded, "Yes, yes," she said, "you are good to her."

"You're very welcome," I said, taken with how sincere and gracious they were.

"Thank you, very much," he repeated. "In our country, we don't have so many like you . . . what do you say?" he asked his daughter.

"Counselors."

"Yes, not so many counselors; we have teachers . . . gurus who help the soul," he said, placing his hand gently on his heart while still holding my hand. "You are a good guru to our daughter."

"Your daughter is a wonderful person, and if I have helped her soul then I am very glad."

"Oh, yes," her mother nodded.

Nayana smiled, "Come on, Papa, let's get you something to eat or you will not be so pleasant soon. Thank you for coming, Dr. Cowan. It really means a lot to me."

"I wouldn't have missed it. Good luck," I said as they walked away. Nayana looked over her shoulder at me and nodded.

"How did it go?" I asked her as soon as we sat down. But looking at her, I knew how it went. Her eyes were puffy, and she looked exhausted.

She sighed loudly, "It did not go too well."

"Tell me, tell me what happened," I said, not even bothering to constrain my own impatience to get the story.

"I told my father and mother three days ago. I brought them to the park, away from my uncle's house. We had a picnic, and I told them that I was in love with the man that my uncle had told them about and that I wanted to marry him. My father was very angry. He couldn't yell because we were in a public place. He demanded to know everything, and I told him all about Ben and how I wanted to stay in the U.S. with him, but that Ben was willing to move to India if he forbade me to stay. My mother was crying all of the time we were talking. He said that they should have never allowed me to come here, that it was all a big mistake. He demanded to know if I was a virgin." She paused.

"What did you tell him?" I sat utterly attentive.

"I told him not to ask me such questions. I told him it was unseemly for him to pry into such things. It was not something I wanted to discuss with him. I was suddenly very angry at his reaction! It surprised me so much that I could speak to my father in such a way as that. My heart was pounding and pounding so much. I thought, 'Oh no, I am going to have a panic attack!' "

"But you didn't have one, did you? The sword had finally fallen, and your own reaction surprised you. How did they react to your assertiveness?"

"My mother just cried. But my father said, 'You have been in this country for too long. You are becoming like an American girl.' I said, 'You have sent me here to become an American student, you have allowed me to come here and learn new things. I cannot help it if I have to change. If you lived here, you would change too.' I don't know how I said this to him."

"You really took him off guard! How did he react to your proposal for meeting Ben?"

"I did not tell him right away. We went back the house, and there he was yelling and yelling. Somehow, seeing him after all this time, he looks a little older . . . I don't know. I have gotten a little older too. Somehow, with all that yelling going on, I was not as frightened as I thought I would be. It was very unpleasant, and I cried and cried. My mother came to my room, and she was very kind. She brushed my hair and talked to me. She said that soon my father would calm down. The next day we were sitting at breakfast and I said, 'Ben's family has invited us all over for dinner, and I have accepted because to not accept would be rude.' My father became mad all over again. He yelled and yelled. He refused to go. He said we were going back home that day, but of course we could not. He got very mad at my uncle, but my uncle argued with him that it was not his fault, that it was his own willful daughter who had disobeyed."

"So the whole house was in an uproar!"

"Yes, even my little cousin came to me crying. She said, 'I'm sorry I told your secret.' She thought it was all her fault, you know. I told her no, that it was good that she told, that I didn't like that secret anyway. My mother said to my father, 'We must go to this dinner, otherwise they will think we have no manners. Nayana has already committed us. She should not have, but she has, and there's an end to it.'"

"How were you through all of this?"

"I was so sad and angry. I felt like I would do what I want to do, and I don't care what happens. Then I would think of missing my family and my home, and I would just want to say to Papa, 'Don't be mad, I'm coming home.' Then I would cry again for Ben."

"You know, Nayana, what I'm *not* hearing you say is that you felt ashamed or guilty. You seem to be feeling grounded in yourself in a new way in relation to your family."

Nayana slowly nodded as I made this observation, and a little bit of a smile livened up her tired and exhausted face. "Yes, I hadn't thought of that. That's very true. I did not feel ashamed, even about telling my father to stay away from my sex life."

"So did you all go to the dinner?"

"Yes, we went."

"My God, and that was the first time they met Ben?"

"Yes, the first time. Ben's parents were very, very nice. My father does not know any other way than to be polite in return. Ben was very good and polite to my parents. We all talked of many things, and nobody talked about Ben and me being together. But at the end, when we were getting ready to leave, Mr. Zimmerman said to my father how he knew it must be very difficult to have found out that his daughter was attached to a boyfriend. He said that if he were my father he would feel the same way. He just wanted to say that they thought I was very special and that they should be very proud. Ben's father runs a company, and their house is very nice. It overlooks the ocean in Solana Beach. We were standing in the foyer, the door open and the ocean below, and Ben's father said how much they think of me and that they hoped my parents wouldn't be too upset because Ben was very devoted to me."

"Wow! So that got to your father?"

"Well, no. I think it got more to my mother. And she and Mrs. Zimmerman seemed to like each other. On the ride home, I asked Papa, 'Does meeting Ben's family change your mind?' He said, 'Of course not, but they are very good people. Ben is a good boy.' He was less mad, and there was no more yelling in the house."

"Ah." So, she was still forced to choose. "So what now?" I asked gently.

She paused, and managed a weak smile. All her tears were used up. "Now I will go back to India with my family on the 8:30 flight the day after tomorrow."

"Ah." There was a long silence. "You don't feel that you can make your own decision?"

She looked up at me. "No, I *can* make my own decision. I *am* making my own decision," she said. "It sounds strange to you, I'm sure, but my family is too important. I want to marry Ben. I love him. But where I come from this is not everything. I could tell them that I will not go. But, in many ways, I want to go. I have been wanting to get back to my country where I belong."

I remembered how gracefully she danced across the stage in the park with the group of saried women, how relaxed and at home she seemed. The brief move to the center for her individual improvisation, then back to the choreographed dance with the others.

"You know, I think if my father had said, 'You are no longer my daughter,' that I would have stayed here. I would have defied him. But between all the yelling he said, 'You are my daughter, and you belong in India with your family that loves you and is proud of you.' And do you know what I said to him?"

"What?"

"I said, 'Papa, you are being a stubborn papa. But I have decided to come back home with you because I love you and my family too much to stay here. But you must do something for me. You must allow Ben to come to India to visit me. You must give him a chance too.' As I said this, I saw my mother, standing behind him, smile."

"Did he say yes?"

She shook her head sadly, and then she looked up at me. A smile played on her lips. "He didn't say yes, but he didn't say no either. He didn't answer at all; he just took my face in his hands and kissed me on the forehead."

CASE EIGHT DISCUSSION

Intersubjectivity and Culture

THE THERAPIST SEEKS to enter the personal world of the client and to understand and make explicit how that world is structured and expressed. When the therapist and client come from similar ethnic and cultural backgrounds, they often possess a kind of "shorthand" of communication because their individual consciousness is shaped by shared larger developmental influences and forces that surround them. They have in common recognizable cultural reference points. This similarity is not often the focus of awareness because it is latent and contextual. Of course, the therapist must be careful not to carelessly assume too much similarity. No culture is homogeneous, and the various influences of family, socioeconomic class, education, and so forth will play a significant role in forming the client's interpretive systems. It is challenge enough to explore the client's differently constructed subjective world when client and therapist share a cultural milieu. In this sense, *all* therapy is cross-cultural. But fundamental assumptions about "how the world is" diverge even further when client and therapist possess differently organized personal *and* cultural subjectivities. Then both participants are forced to examine what would ordinarily tend to be the invisible cultural "container" for their dialogue. The added differences in race and ethnicity, nationality, language, and values all must become available for scrutiny. The differing worlds of client and therapist can then come into contact and become explicit and open to change in the therapeutic conversation.

Locke (1986) argues that therapists must attend to their own multicultural awareness by making sure they have engaged a number of issues in their own development. This begins with self-examination regarding one's own biases and prejudices and a good hard look at how these are shaped in the context of the culture from which they emerge. Often the therapist must make a concerted effort to recognize subtle configurations of racism, sexism, and classism that are latent in one's values and attitudes. The therapist must cultivate sensitivity to individual differences and the diversity that exists within cultural groups. Finally, the therapist–client encounter must reflect appropriate techniques and approaches that will help both participants reach across the gulf between differently organized self- and worldviews.

When Nayana entered therapy, I understood how her anxiety and physical symptoms were interrelated. There is universality in the various ways in which repressed powerful emotions and developmental longings become expressed as symptoms. It seemed clear to me that what Nayana needed was to break free of the constraints imposed on her. She needed to honor her legitimate but squelched feelings and ambitions by differentiating herself to a greater degree than she previously had been able to achieve. It was only later that I came to see how my own cultural biases initially *centralized* this liberation and set the agenda for its achievement.

At first I resonated mostly to the part of her self-experience that fit with my values and cultural reference points. Partly this was because she and Ben were also focused on the new possibilities available to them as a couple. And what seductive possibilities they were: Her longing for romantic love, and her desire to realize her individual ambitions apart from others' expectations. When I saw Ben and Nayana together, these were impulses I was glad to endorse and support. My enthusiasm for these ambitions, however, made me somewhat less sensitive to her equally important and no less apparent desire to preserve her cultural identifications and safeguard her family unity. My bias was for independence before the costly sacrifices of affiliation, assertion of individual rights over compromise with family demands. But Nayana and I both quickly came to realize that she did not seek to reject one way of being in favor of another. Rather, she struggled to reconcile these conflicting forces, to balance them all within her so as not to entirely lose what was most valuable to her. Hers was the art of compromise, to find a new integration that would allow her to preserve not only the important aspects of herself that were becoming lost but as much as she could of what she most loved.

Interestingly, it was when Nayana appeared for her session dressed in her traditional Indian clothing that I became more alert to watch my own frames of reference. When she wore blue jeans, a T-shirt, and tennis shoes, I tended to see her through the lens of what she described as her "American self." When I saw her in traditional dress, especially when I saw her dance, it seemed to evoke something very different from us both. Whereas before I identified with the part of Nayana that most represented her and Ben's ideas and objectives for their relationship, her flowing sari and tinkling bells invited me to see her in the context of her "Indian self," the self that connected to her family and faith. It was then easier for me to set aside my skepticism that she, or anyone, could be fulfilled while under such obligations as her family and cultural values demanded.

Significantly, it was this creative tension between our worldviews, I believe, that helped Nayana get the most from her therapy and arrive at a kind of resolution and integration of conflicting forces. As she struggled to accommodate her new and developing "American" identity, I tentatively represented one pole of that experience. At the same time I attempted to understand and be sensitive to the other pole of her Indian identity, one which she helped me value as it became revealed in our relationship. My initial bias that psychological health was represented by complete autonomy and independence gave way to honoring other cherished realms of her experience. Nayana did not seek a resolution by choosing one pole over the other. Rather, she used our dialogue to illuminate the conflict itself. She was able to explore dimensions of her opposing emotions and conflicting impulses that had, until then, no legitimizing and clarifying interpersonal process in which to take shape. Once the sectioned-off and denied thoughts, fantasies, and feelings became more available to her, she was able to forge a new reconciliation of them with her deeply ingrained cultural and family imperatives. Nayana was able to find a way to *choose* her way of responding to their differing claims even though this involved sacrifice.

It is an important idea that differences in background ethnicity and culture can significantly contribute to the potentialities of the therapeutic dialogue rather than impede those opportunities. The naive notion that a therapist must share with the client the same race, ethnicity, gender, or nationality entirely ignores the basic premise of all therapy, which emphasizes the relationship. This premise is that elaborated empathy, that deep engagement with the client's inner world, reveals the various dimensions of that person's reality. We are always learning the culture of another person's life when we strive for this level of participation. The trick, when the client is from a different culture than the therapist, is to *centralize this part of the dialogue,* to explore how and where each person's subjective frames of reference intersect, or not, with the other's. Illumination is the goal, not uniformity, agreement, or even confirmation of existing internal structures. If I were in Nayana's shoes, I would not choose in the way that she did, and she knew this. But I value, respect, and honor the choice that she made. Through our work together, she was able to make that choice with deliberation and awareness, not unconsciously and because of anxiety-reducing capitulation. For those therapists whose worldview was formed in the milieu of the dominant or privileged culture, this means a deconstruction of attitudes and values in the service of self-awareness. Just as therapy challenges the client to try on new ways of perceiving, the therapist must also develop the ability to see the world through other lenses. Therapists not from the mainstream of the culture, who may, in fact, come from marginalized groups, are taxed with the same imperative, just in a different direction. They must also make a leap of imagination and empathy to read the blueprints, as it were, of another's culture and the self-architecture that it shapes and supports.

Therapists who have practiced with diverse populations have repeated experiences in their work of these cross-cultural illuminations. An incident that humorously highlights one such incident involved my

work with an expressive Hispanic lesbian. In the second month of therapy she observed that she could never talk to a "straight" therapist, man
or woman, because the therapist wouldn't know "anything about where
I was coming from." When I asked her why she presumed that I was
gay, she advised me not to be elusive. She was certain I was because her
friend, who had seen a gay therapist, had referred her to me. She also felt
that I was able to understand her in a way that would be impossible for
a straight man. After exploring her feelings about how my sexual orientation might influence my ability to help her, I revealed that I was, in fact,
heterosexual, married, and had children. "Oh, my God," she exclaimed,
"you're a *breeder* too!" Despite having a good laugh together, it took a
few sessions for my client to get her "mind around" this "mix up." It
later became apparent that her friend, in referring her to me, had not
meant to imply that I was the same gay therapist he had been seeing.
My client admitted that she felt our therapy, thus far, had gone well. At
the end of therapy she disclosed that our therapeutic relationship had
been the vehicle for her examining her own prejudices and fears. It provoked her to forge friendships with a number of persons who were not
only "straight" but some of whom were straight men, a population that
formerly she had completely avoided. Through our work, her own categories and biases, she said, had been shaken to the core.

Each culture and each family within that culture shapes rules for the
expression of internal states and behavior. Nayana had learned early on
in her life to censure any expression of emotion that might lead to discord. This censure was one significant contributing factor to her translation of emotional conflict (and that conflict's attendant anxiety) into
symptoms. Her learned constraint of affect was one aspect of Nayana's
familial and cultural inheritance that I felt clashed with her personal
disposition. It bordered on a kind of psychological oppression, and I felt
comfortable challenging her to examine how it undermined her psychological cohesion.

This raises an interesting question with regard to cross-cultural therapy: In the therapist's efforts to respect the client's cultural background,
must the therapist ipso facto *endorse* the client's internalized cultural
mores? Does challenging cultural imperatives that also seem to cause
the client distress reflect insensitivity on the part of the therapist? If so,
does this not place the therapist in the role of an enforcer of the prevailing culture's standards, morality, and values? Is this the role the therapist wants to play?

My work with Nayana illustrates that while the therapist must honor
the client's values, those values and attitudes must also be fair game for

examination and revision. When internalized cultural precepts and mores are subverting rather than promoting the legitimate growth of the person, then these, too, must be called into question. Being sensitive to cross-cultural issues is not a politically correct, namby-pamby assumption that all values, ideas, and cultural mores are good, that they are all equal and deserving of unthinking affirmation. To be multiculturally sensitive is not to affect a sham respect for superficial differences under the guise of appreciating diversity. Rather, being cross-culturally aware means to have attuned oneself to the social and developmental origins of another person's existence. It means to understand the interpretive frames of reference, emotions, thoughts, and conflicts that existence contains. Only then can the therapist help the client to place his or her personal story within the larger metanarrative of the culture. Only then can the therapy process illuminate and examine that personal story and discover what promotes or subverts the client's potentialities. A therapist who is merely the representative of the prevailing cultural ethos would have, perhaps, counseled Rosa Parks to deal with her unresolved anger and sit at the back of the bus.

I prefer to think of my role of therapist as similar to that of the artist or poet. The artist, poet, and therapist must necessarily stand both within and outside of the culture so as to understand and reveal its dimensions. Perhaps this role contains something of that slightly disaffected observer, the odd fellow or witchdoctor who lives on the edge of the village, the one who is able to see the culture from a distance and not merely be its servant but to probe and question it. I feel queasy thinking that the therapist's job is to help a person who might be a casualty of the culture to "adapt" to that culture's demands so as to achieve the "normal." Instead, the reference points must emerge from within the client as to what will be preserved and what must be challenged or even discarded. In this sense therapy, like art, has the capacity to become a freedom creating, perhaps even subversive, activity in relation to the client's culture. The fundamental premise of therapy is to explore the possibility of new modes of being, and the therapist cannot ultimately predict where this will lead for the client. Nor can the therapist predict the implications of change for the people and institutions to which the client will return after leaving the consulting room.

Nayana's explorations led back to embracing her culture but with a different perspective as well as the self-efficacy to articulate that emerging creative power. Perhaps there is nothing more productively subversive than that. I challenged Nayana to question herself, to express previously forbidden affects and ideas, and through this she changed her way of relating to others and to her cultural heritage. Nayana was no longer merely compliant with demands that she herself did not endorse. She no longer repressed her anger in the way that her previous "acculturation" demanded. She was able to both respect and confront her family and to protect the boundaries of her sexuality and feelings. Choosing to return to India and continue to negotiate for her relationship with Ben did not feel to her like subjugation but like a chosen compromise that aimed at preserving what she valued most, including her own feelings and wishes. She no longer needed to get sick to express herself but could use ideas and the courage of words.

As Nayana learned to accept and express her thoughts and feelings more freely and to censure herself less, she ultimately did not need to bind her anxiety by translating it into physical complaints. However, during the middle phase of therapy, when she had learned to better use language to identify and express her conflicts, her anxiety was much closer to the surface of her conscious life. During this phase she did not yet possess enough of a new "system" of meanings, a new consolidated self-image strong enough to contain this anxiety. Her panic attacks in this transitional period revealed that she was overwhelmed and fragmented. I must admit that during this period I questioned whether I had been a good steward of her growth and progress by allowing her upcoming "deadline" to rush the process. Ideally, new self-structures emerge gradually as the client internalizes aspects of the therapeutic relationship that provide strength and support and a container for emerging configurations of experience. Nayana, however, seemed to have her own schedule for growth. She had been poised and waiting for the right interpersonal environment, the right stage on which she could dance both parts of that graceful unfolding. One part of the dance was fixed, guided by the choreography of culture, history, and conformity. But that other part, that dance within the dance, broke free of established forms and came from her heart alone.

Conclusion

I began this book by likening the therapeutic process to the partnership of Ariadne and Theseus as he sought to find his way in the corridors and chambers of the labyrinth. It is the therapist's stance of sustained empathic inquiry that is Ariadne's silver thread, spun so that the client can go to the heart of self-experience, encounter the forces that dwell there, and discover a new understanding and way of being. Through these tales of therapy I hope it is apparent that the therapist's empathy involves much more than emotional resonance with the client and support for the client's objectives. Rather, therapeutic empathy implies deep engagement with the client's inner world, which is evoked in the encounter, made explicit in its dimensions, and therefore becomes open to change. This inner world includes the client's emotions and also his or her thoughts, fantasies, conflicts, relationships, and ways of organizing and interpreting experience.

The underlying value assumption in therapy is that this holistic self-knowledge is a good thing, affirming, as Ralph W. Emerson said of the Socratic ideal, that the unexamined life is not worth living. That self-knowledge should best be found through participation with another is the wonderful paradox of the therapy process. I know this participation is central to understanding because my own life has taught me that I become revealed to myself (for better or worse) in the various facets of my relations with those whom I love. But this is true in the therapy relationship as well. The process of remembering all of the encounters with the clients described in this book evoked in me many of the feelings and impressions I experienced during the time I shared with them. They are not lost to me, or I to them. Each of us carries within ourselves the experiences that took shape between us. In each case the client changed through our encounter. But I know that I, too, changed through my meetings with these clients, though I might not always have realized it at the time.

The therapist's empathic participation as a type of intervention with the client points to another paradox in the practice of counseling and psychotherapy. On the surface, the therapeutic endeavor appears to be

governed by techniques, principles, and procedures that, when applied
by a skilled practitioner, should lead to amelioration of the client's suffering. But unlike the surgeon with his scalpel or the priest with his
doctrine, the therapist's only real instrument in therapy is him- or herself. As is clear from these cases, I sometimes struggled with how best
to use this instrument effectively in service to the client's growth. No
amount of "technical" proficiency can guarantee an effective therapist
unless the therapist is also capable of a person-to-person relationship
that is dimensional enough to include another person's existence. That's
a tall order, and it is not something easily learned in a classroom. It is
life's curriculum that is the therapist's other classroom.

The prospective therapist must be something of a risk taker in his or
her life and relationships. He or she must be willing to sustain a few
bruises, to turn personal suffering into areas of expertise about life. The
therapist must be willing to live deeply and sincerely to acquire the req-
uisite abilities, or perhaps, "sensibilities," required to spin the thread.
Becoming a therapist is not just a vocation, it is a high and difficult
calling. When Arpena's father referred to me as a counterpart of the
"guru" in India, I was amused. As I thought about it later, however, I
wondered if he were not far from the mark. If being a guru means
addressing the potentialities of a person's existence and helping that
person to actualize these in life, then, perhaps, in Western culture the
therapist as a helper is potentially a guide for another's soul.

Self-Awareness of the Therapist

It is daunting to a student laboring to get through graduate school to
realize how much of a project must be made of his or her own life; to
cultivate both the specialized knowledge *and* the self-awareness
required to be an effective clinician. However, if the student finds such
an endeavor not merely daunting but onerous, it would probably be
wise to find another profession. It is labor enough, as Henry Thoreau
said, to subdue and cultivate a few cubic feet of flesh. In this sense, the
therapist's education is never finished.

Though the development of both a high level of self-awareness and
obtaining a graduate school education are corollary processes in becoming an effective helper, the latter is much more easily achieved. A bright
and intellectually curious person can comprehend the pedagogical
aspects of counseling and psychotherapy. To comprehend the human
condition as it is inflected through a unique person, however, is another
matter and a never-ending project. To work effectively, the therapist

must also have taken a journey, entered and explored the labyrinth, and mostly integrated the forces within his or her own personality. Many graduate training programs require that the student participate in his or her own therapy as a condition of graduation. I have personally found it essential to have occupied both the client's and the therapist's chair during the course of my development as a helper. There is no better reminder of Carl Rogers's poetic assertion that each of us is a "being in the process of becoming" than to be a student of one's own life.

The imperative of maximum self-awareness is most relevant as the therapist-in-training encounters the infinite variety of transference and countertransference possibilities that emerge in the person-to-person encounter. As can be seen from the cases presented here, the client will necessarily reenact old and problematic relational patterns as well as project a host of affectively charged attributions and perceptions, which can be confusing to the therapist. It is a very complex interpersonal environment in which to maintain one's balance! The effective clinician responds to this complexity by cultivating a kind of multidimensional perception. The clinician registers and experiences the client's expressions in the here-and-now while simultaneously experiencing his or her own immediate responses and feelings. At the same time, however, the therapist must "bracket" his or her own perceptions and reactions to the client to be able to track the "data" emerging from this shared event. The therapist who participates fully with the client in the here-and-now but who fails to simultaneously cultivate an "observing" function will miss the big picture. Conversely, the therapist who observes well and analyzes the client's issues brilliantly but who fails to cultivate the emotional energy and power inherent in the here-and-now, person-to-person engagement, will make elegant and perhaps even accurate interpretations that have little effect in the client's life. Clearly, the ability to fully participate with the client but also to reference and bracket self-experience demands that the therapist know a lot about his or her own emotional makeup, interpretive processes, and relational patterns.

The Therapist's Shadow

Carl Jung (1983) mythologically described the unexplored regions of a person's psyche containing powerful forces as the person's "shadow." The shadow is simply those forces and aspects of a person he or she would prefer not to integrate and acknowledge. But it is precisely these unacknowledged forces that can undermine a person in his or her life and relationships. This is especially true for therapists in their work with clients.

Robert Bly (1988) described the shadow as the long bag we drag behind us that contains the sectioned-off aspects of the self and the energies that go with those dissociated parts. As therapists-in-training with clients, they are sometimes startled by (and forced to make the acquaintance of) their shadow. This happens as the therapist's counter-transference reactions appear in response to the client's expressions and potentially begin to subvert the relationship. It is certain that the study and practice of therapy will uncover and prod the helper's own unresolved issues. The therapist's shadow may involve disowned and forbidden parts that were never confirmed in relationships and that are evoked in the current encounter. Often, the shadow involves those largely unconscious motivations to which the person may attribute a "negative" affective valence. Sex, anger, envy, desire for control, or dominance, any of these forces, if unacknowledged, can be a part of a person's shadow. Even self-deprecation, low self-esteem, and a too strong desire to please others may compose these aspects of self-experience and trace the outlines of the shadow. The therapist's shadow is only a problem if he or she ignores or denies these forces and begins to unconsciously enact them in relationships with clients. The idea is not to somehow become completely purged of these qualities; they often contain elements essential to the therapist's vitality and powers. The therapist must be reconciled to casting a shadow and self-aware enough to channel its energies: it is the monsters that you don't see and acknowledge, the ones that you run from, that get you from behind.

Preserving the Client From Pain

Just as therapists must be courageous enough to face their own distress and life wounds, they must also be willing to stand with the client in his or her struggle and not flinch from the client's necessary pain, pain that is a part of growth and transformation. This sounds easy, but it is often difficult in practice because it sometimes *appears* to lack compassion. Therapists at the beginning of their training often become activated by the client's distress and try to find a quick fix to ease the client's suffering. They often want to "love the client out of" misery. This is especially true if the therapist believes his or her interventions are provoking additional distress in the client as conflicts and anxieties become more accessible through the therapy work. The therapist may tend to view any intervention that disrupts the client further as problematic. The result is that the client stays stuck, merely feeds off the therapist's support, hides the parts that seem to threaten the therapist, and does not do the difficult and sometimes agonizing work of transformation.

There are many reasons for therapists to become seduced by the illusion of being able to relieve suffering in this manner. Therapists have often entered the field to be of service to others, to be helpers and to ease suffering. In Karen Horney's paradigm, therapists often possess a "moving toward" style of relating to others and do not realize that they are tending to their own feelings of security *before* responding to the client's situation (Teyber, 2000). It is imperative that therapists examine the origins of their own "altruistic" motives. Usually therapists' aversions to elevated levels of client distress have to do with their own countertransference anxieties, unresolved life wounds, and need for soothing—not the client's potential to engage in productive struggle. Therapists-in-training sometimes imagine that they will be merciful helpers to others, dispensing comfort and relief. They may not realize that they are seeking something highly gratifying to their own legitimate but (in the context of therapy) narcissistic need to be appreciated, valued, loved, and soothed themselves.

Therapists Feel Responsible for the Client's Progress

Unfortunately, therapists' efforts to soothe the client's pain communicates that it is the suffering alone, not the existential situation from which that suffering emerges, that needs attention. Therapists-in-training often assume that if the client's suffering is not quickly reduced they are not "doing their job" and are failing in their duty to the client. But suffering is a part of life, growth, and change. Often clients will only be as brave as their therapists and will attenuate their expression to honor the capacities of therapists to receive their distress. It is not uncommon for clients to irrationally believe that the aspects of themselves that are "forbidden" and "repulsive" have the power to drive away, or even to somehow damage, the therapist. The therapist's attempts to solve the problem and get the client to quickly feel better, without a parallel process of exploration, seem to the client to confirm these feelings.

Therapists' Fear of Confrontation or Challenge

Therapists-in-training often fear interventions designed to confront or challenge the client for the purpose of destabilizing old and unproductive patterns. They equate confrontation with unproductive *conflict* in the relationship and fear the negative reactions of the client. Every therapist would like for the client to like and appreciate him or her all of the time, but this, of course, is impossible. It is the client's job to work through, in the relationship with the therapist, all the problems and difficulties that arise in other relationships and that have become structuralized as part of the client's self-organization. Therapists must make themselves and the relationship available for the client to experiment in this way and not predicate the dialogue on mutual gratification. Clinicians who tend to be "conflict reducers" to bind their own anxiety can often trace this tendency to their role of peacemaker in their families of origin. In their subsequent therapeutic relationships, they fear confronting the client with important interventions because they imagine that something terrible will happen. The concern is that the client will leave therapy, feel misunderstood, disappointed, or even condemn the therapist. In addition, therapists fear further upsetting the client who may already be in distress. If these fears are present, would-be helpers tend to avoid any elevation of energy in the relationship of any kind, but they especially avoid energy that feels remotely like conflict or disagreement.

But, of course, in the process of therapy the client will sometimes become disoriented or confused, upset, angry, or frightened. If the therapy is *always* comfortable and soothing for the client, then probably not much is happening therapeutically. The therapist who always hopes for smooth sailing fails to recognize the value of the client's transference enactments, wishes, and fantasies, which can energize the therapy and lead to important and relevant issues. Another dimension of this dynamic is that the therapist who fears the emergence of the differences in the subjective worlds of therapist and client tends to overly personalize the "negative" reactions of the client. The therapist may not realize that he or she stands not only in the ground of the current existential encounter but *stands in for* a host of others who must be addressed in the client's psychological world and process of healing. Learning how to cultivate an always-ready curiosity regarding the *phenomenon* emerging in the relationship allows the therapist to permit new and unexpected things to happen in the immediate and then to step back curiously and say, "Huh, I wonder what that was?"

A Unique Interpersonal Culture

I hope these cases have conveyed that the therapeutic dialogue is not subject to the same ingrained conventions as social intercourse outside of the therapy setting. Our interpersonal habits of discourse are often deeply embedded, but there is no quicker way to sap the power of the therapeutic relationship than to import conventional social behaviors into the therapeutic dialogue. Just as the therapist invites the client to "say anything," and assures the client that the safety of the therapeutic relationship is unlike any other, so the therapist must struggle to break the habits and confinement of conventional restraints in participation. One former student observed that she hesitated to point out some contradictions in her client's motivations because "it would be rude." Another stated that he was reluctant to process with his client her flirtations, and his own response of feeling flattered, because it would be "embarrassing" and "unprofessional." Another clinician couldn't help but respond to her client's endless small talk with her own chitchat, even though she was frustrated and bored. When these sorts of rules govern the discourse, then the clinician becomes disempowered and hesitates to exercise his or her capacity for real participation. It is ironic that therapists sometimes fear taking the risks of participation, hiding behind a pseudo-professional mask, even as they ask clients to unveil their deepest fears and conflicts. Falling back on social habits masks a desire to be protected, to play it safe, and to hide behind a function and role. Clinicians-in-training must learn to relish standing with their clients in front of the clear image of truth and find language that speaks directly and immediately to describe it.

Creating "Presence" Through Encounter

Therapists-in-training seek another kind of safety net. They would like to trade the imperative to create a real "encounter" with the client for appearing to be highly skilled and expert in their knowledge and interventions. Naturally, we each have a desire to be seen as competent and capable, and clients do need to be reassured that they are in good hands. However, clinicians-in-training sometimes assume that their teachers and other experienced clinicians know what they are doing in the session at all times, and they would like to emulate that expertise. The real truth is that to be an expert clinician partly means to be willing to be uncertain, confused, and to not have the answers. It also means allowing this uncertainty to show, even to the client! Discovery and creativity are inherently fluid and lack familiar reference points. To be an expert clinician really means to be able to find out what is needed as the need arises in the encounter with the client, not to doggedly apply a single method or technique.

The clinician can best imbue the sessions with this sense of expectancy and potentiality by cultivating a sense of "presence" and immediacy in the person-to-person encounter. The therapist's demeanor embodies a sense of "happening" in the here-and-now relationship that is vitalizing and charges the therapeutic encounter with energy. Cultivating this sense of presence is perhaps the most essential skill in determining whether the sessions feel significant and meaningful or lifeless and tedious.

Listening Empathically

Therapists-in-training, especially those who hold an oversimplified view of the client-centered approach, assume that if they track their clients well and are emotionally resonant and understanding, this alone is sufficient to create transformative change. Alas, this is not often true. Although emotional resonance is an essential component of therapy, most clients benefit from the therapist being able to understand underlying patterns of client self-organization and to make these patterns overt in the therapeutic dialogue. There is a give and take between therapist and client that makes visible and illuminates the outlines of the soul. The ability to listen for clinical themes and underlying configurations of experience, and to include these observations in the conversation with the client, is a powerful component of therapy. It often demands that the therapist give up his or her latent desire for the client to make logical "sense." As is clear from these cases, the client's issues and symptoms often do not make rational and logical sense when viewed out of the context of the client's referential world. The client's behavior and expression does have meaning and value, however, in the larger context of the client's perceptions of self and others. It is the combination of emotional resonance and a willingness to meet clients on their own turf that reveals the dimensions of the client's inner life and existential situation and makes those dimensions available to the relationship. The way through the labyrinth is to track and understand the client's expression in the present, to enter the client's world, to understand how it makes sense in its own context, to grasp the underlying themes, to listen for conflicts, and then to help the client articulate it all in the current relationship, making it overt with language.

A Sense of Accomplishment

As I wrote about these cases and contemplated my own path through the pitfalls just described, I was reminded that the difficulties in clinical training are in proportion to what the therapist can expect to enjoy from becoming a skilled helper. There is an abiding sense of accomplishment and gratification in working with clients. It is a privilege to be admitted into a client's inner life and to participate with a person who is seeking to meet the challenges of life more honestly and fruitfully.

It is my intention that each case in this book conveys the spirit of the therapy with that person. However, I have intentionally left parts of the picture unfinished. I have not fully explicated important dimensions of each case nor explored every issue to which I have alluded. In some instances I have offered provocative material or countertransference reactions without elaborated comment. My intention is to give clinicians-in-training and their teachers and supervisors room for discussion, debate, and conjecture. What I do hope comes through fully is the sense of reward and gratification that even the most difficult cases can sometimes offer the therapist. Often the reward is more than what the therapist and client think is possible. Though graduate training and licensure in the helping professions is long and rigorous, the prospect of real fulfillment that comes with so meaningful a professional life must be sustaining to the student. I have the sense in working with clients that my labors do not end even when our therapeutic work is done. The important and meaningful conversations emerging in therapy don't just cease; they resonate through time and through other present and future relationships. The work lives on after our parting.

It was this sense of accomplishment and inherent value to the work that drew me to the helping professions. I became a clinician relatively late in my professional life and did not follow a conventional course. As a young man I found college disappointing. I was after big game philosophically and spiritually and, in those early years, was unable to find the right mentors. I pursued my own "great books" approach to education. I dropped out of college to be a folk musician, which in the mid-70s was still a cool, if not entirely original, thing to do. In my late teens and early 20s I kicked around in Africa and Europe, sailed across the Atlantic and across the bay in sailboats. I married, had kids, fled the city for the country with my little family, and landed in the picture framing and art gallery business. This was lucrative enough for material comfort and satisfying for a while. But in my late 20s I was still restless, longing for a profession that mirrored my interest in self-discovery, in meaning and value, in spirituality and art. I wanted a profession that was important to me and allowed me to have a deeper level of engagement with others around significant human concerns. I decided to become a therapist.

With a family in tow it was a long haul through a master's degree counseling program and then through a doctoral program in clinical psychology. All along the way, however, I was sustained by the idea that this profession was my calling and that I was happiest when attentive to the process of my own self-exploration and engaged with others around theirs. I thrived in the parts of my training I loved and held my nose and endured during the parts I didn't. And I have not been disappointed. I have a sense in doing therapy with clients and also in training therapists that I am involved with something larger than myself. My professional concerns are never irrelevant to the most important things in life, and there are few fields of work where this is so completely true. Especially given the difficulties in the current managed care climate and the shrinking incomes of mental health professionals, the primary gratification in being a therapist will always be the sense of intellectual and spiritual accomplishment, the reward of participating with and serving others at the deepest levels of human engagement.

As I was writing these final words, I received a confirmation of this—a letter in the mail from Chloe. She writes to say that she is doing well and has graduated with a master's degree in fine arts. It has taken her longer than she wanted because she had to work at the same time she was taking classes. As I read her letter, I feel as if she is reaching out and sharing this victory with me, wanting me to be pleased in her accomplishment on many levels. She includes photos of all the works in her master's portfolio. One is a self-portrait in oil. Her dark hair frames her serious and composed face, her arms are draped across her torso. She appears languid and composed at once. Her eyes are looking directly out from the canvas across the time since we last met. They are not averted, but clear and confident. The painting is too good to not have been rendered honestly, and there is neither a lack nor a surfeit of pain. I can see from her expression, from her pose, from her eyes as she looks out, that she can now embody her life. She writes on the back, "I wanted you to have this so that you could see me as I am now, and to tell you that I still remember our talks." A simple line like that sometimes stands in for months or even years of struggle, tears, and discovery. A simple line like that can make it all worthwhile.

References

Anderson, H. & Goolishian, H. (1990). Beyond cybernetics: Comment on Atkinson and Heath's "Future thought on second-order family therapy." *Family Process, 29,* 157–163.

Alexander, F., & French, T. (1946). *Psychoanalytic therapy.* New York: Ronald.

American Psychiatric Association. (2000). *Diagnostic and statistical manual of mental disorders* (4th ed., text revision). Washington DC: Author.

Bateson, G. (1972). *Steps to an ecology of mind.* New York: Ballantine Books.

Bateson, G. (1979). *Mind and nature.* New York: E. P. Dutton.

Becvar, D. (1997). *Soul healing: A spiritual orientation in counseling and therapy.* New York: Basic Books.

Becvar, D., & Becvar, R. (1988). *Family therapy: A systemic integration.* Boston: Allyn & Bacon.

Bly, R. (1988). *A little book on the human shadow.* (W. Booth, Ed.). San Francisco: HarperCollins.

Brenner, C. (1973). *An elementary textbook of psychoanalysis.* New York: Doubleday.

Bruner, J. (1990). *Acts of meaning.* Cambridge, MA: Harvard University Press.

Brunner, J. B. (1986). *Actual minds, possible worlds.* Cambridge, MA: Harvard University Press.

Buber, M. (1958). *I and Thou.* New York: Charles Scribner.

Buber, M. (1988). *The knowledge of man: Selected essays edited with an introduction by Maurice Friedman.* New Jersey: Humanities Press International.

Bugental, J. F. T., & McBeath, B. (1995). Depth existential therapy: Evolution since World War II. In B. Bonger & L. E. Beutler (Eds.), *Comprehensive textbook of psychotherapy: Theory and practice* (pp. 111–122). New York: Oxford University Press.

Combs, G., & Freedman, J. (1994). Milton Erickson: Early postmodernist. In Jeffrey K. Zeig (Ed.), *Ericksonian methods.* New York: Brunner/Mazel.

Cowan, E. W., & Presbury, J. H. (2000). Meeting client resistance and reactance with reverence. *Journal of Counseling and Development, 78,* 411–419.

de Shazer, S. (1984). The death of resistance. *Family Process, 23,* 11–17.

Dolan, Y. M. (1985). *A path with a heart: Ericksonian utilization with resistant and chronic clients.* New York: Brunner/Mazel.

Erickson, M. (1980). The varieties of double bind. In E. L. Rossi (Ed.), *The collected papers of Milton H. Erickson* (Vol. 1). New York: Irvington.

Erickson, M. (1994). *In Ericksonian methods: The essence of the story* (Jeffrey K. Zeig, Ed.). New York: Brunner/Mazel.

Everill, J. T., & Waller, G. (1995). Dissociation and bulimia: Research and theory. *European Eating Disorders Review, 3 (3),* 129–147.

Farber, L. H. (1966). *The ways of the will. Essays towards a psychology and psychopathology of the will.* New York: Basic Books.

Frankl, V. (1959). *From death-camp to existentialism. A psychiatrist's path to a new therapy* (I. Lasch, Trans.). Boston: Beacon Press.

Freud, A. (1966). *The ego and mechanisms of defense. The writings of Anna Freud* (Vol. 2). New York: International Universities Press. (Originally published in 1936)

Freud, S. (1917). Introductory lectures on psycho-analysis. *The standard edition of the complete psychological works of Sigmund Freud* (Vol. 15).

Friedman, M. (1989). *The healing dialogue in psychotherapy.* New Jersey: Jason Aronson.

Friedman, M. (Ed.). (1992). *The worlds of existentialism: A critical reader.* New Jersey: Humanities Press International.

Ginter, E. J., & Bonney, W. (1993). Freud, ESP, and interpersonal relationships: Projective identification and the Mobius interaction. *Journal of Mental Health Counseling, 15,* 150–169.

Grave, R., Rigamonti, R., Todisco, P., & Oliosi, E. (1996). Dissociation and traumatic experiences in eating disorders. *European Eating Disorders Review, 4,* 232–240.

Greenberg, J. R., & Mitchell, S. A. (1983). *Object relations in psychoanalytic theory.* Cambridge, MA: Harvard University Press.

Hycner, R. H. (1991). *Between person and person.* New York: The Gestalt Journal.

Jones, E. (1953). *The life and work of Sigmund Freud* (Vol. 1). New York: Basic Books.

Jung, C. (1952). *Symbols of transformation.* New York: Bolinger Foundation.

Jung, C. (1983). *The essential Jung. Selected essays with an introduction by Anthony Storr* (A. Storr, Ed.). New Jersey: Princeton University Press.

Keeney, B. P. (1983). *Aesthetics of change.* New York: Guilford Press.

Kershaw, C. (1992). *The couple's hypnotic dance: Creating Ericksonian strategies in marital therapy.* New York: Brunner/Mazel.

Kohut, H. (1977). *The restoration of self.* New York: International University Press.

Kohut, H. (1984). *How does analysis cure?* Chicago: University of Chicago Press.

Liotti, G. (1989). Resistance to change in cognitive psychotherapy. Theoretical remarks from a constructivist point of view. In W. Dryden & P. Trower (Eds.), *Cognitive psychotherapy: Stasis and change* (pp. 28–56). New York: Springer.

Locke, D. C. (1986). Cross-cultural counseling issues. In A. J. Palmo & W. J. Weikel (Eds.), *Foundations of mental health counseling,* (pp. 119–137). Springfield, IL: Charles C Thomas.

Mahoney, M. J. (1988). Constructive metatheory: Implications for psychotherapy. *International Journal of Personal Construct Psychology, 1,* 299–316.

Mair, M. (1988). Psychology as storytelling. *Journal of Personal Construct Psychology, 1,* 125–137.

Maruyama, M. (1963). The second cybernetics: Deviation-amplifying mutual causal processes. *American Scientist, 5,* 164–179.

May, M., Angel, E., & Ellenberger, H. F. (1958). *Existence: A new dimension in psychiatry and psychology.* New York: Basic Books.

May, R. (1979). *Psychology and the human dilemma.* New York: W. W. Norton.

May, R. (1983). *The discovery of being.* New York: W. W. Norton.

McManus, F. (1995). Dissociation and the severity of bulimic psychopathology among eating disordered and non-eating disordered women. *European Eating Disorders Review, 3(3),* 185–195.

Natterson, J. M., & Friedman, R. J. (1995). *A primer of clinical inter-subjectivity.* New Jersey: Jason Aronson.

Piaget, J., & Inholder, B. (1969). *The psychology of the child.* New York: Basic Books.

Presbury, J., Echterling, L., & McKee, J. (2002). *Ideas and tools for brief counseling.* New Jersey: Merrill/Prentice-Hall.

Rogers, C. (1951). *Client-centered therapy.* Boston: Houghton Mifflin.

Rogers, C. (1969). *Freedom to learn.* Columbus, OH: Merrill.

Rogers, C. (1980). *A way of being.* Boston: Houghton Mifflin.

Sands, S. (1989). Female development and eating disorders: A self psychological perspective. In A. Goldberg (Ed.), *Progress in self psychology* (Vol. V). New York: Analytical Press.

Shultz, D. P., & Shultz, J. E. (1996). *A history of modern psychology* (6th ed.). Fort Worth, TX: Harcourt Brace.

Stern, D. N. (1988). The dialectic between the "interpersonal" and the "intrapsychic": With particular emphasis on the role of memory and representation. *Psychoanalytic Inquiries, 8,* 241–250.

Stolorow, R., & Atwood, G. (1992). *Contexts of being: The intersubjective foundations of psychological life.* Hillsdale, NJ: Analytic Press.

Stolorow, R., Brandchaft, B., & Atwood, G. (1987). *Psychoanalytic treatment: An intersubjective approach.* Hillsdale, NJ: Analytic Press.

Swirsky, D., & Mitchell, V. (1996). The binge-purge cycle as a means of dissociation: Somatic trauma and somatic defense in sexual abuse and bulimia. *Dissociation, 9,* 18–27.

Teyber, E. (2000). *Interpersonal process in psychotherapy: A relational approach.* Connecticut: Brooks & Cole.

Trüb, H. (1964a). *Individuation, guilt, and decision. The words of existentialism* (M. S. Friedman, Ed. & Trans.). Chicago: University of Chicago Press.

Trüb, H. (1964b). Healing through meeting. In M. S. Friedman (Ed.), *The worlds of existentialism: A critical reader* (W. Hallo, Trans.). Chicago: University of Chicago Press.

Watzlawick, P. (1984). *The invented reality.* New York: W. W. Norton.

Watzlawick, P. Weakland, J., & Fisch, R. (1974). *Change: Principles of problem formation and problem resolution.* New York: W.W. Norton.

Winnicott, D. W. (1945). *Through pediatrics to psycho-analysis.* London: Hogarth Press.

Name Index

Subject Index

350